Global Health Communication for Immigrants and Refugees

This book analyzes important international cases of immigrant and refugee health from diverse health communication perspectives, providing theoretical frames and effective recommendations for designing future health communication campaigns and interventions for global health promotion.

Internationally renowned scholars elucidate the reality of health communication situations that immigrants and refugees experience in host countries around the globe and examine how national and global health risk situations, including the COVID-19 pandemic, affect immigrant and refugee health during difficult health circumstances. Offering effective health communication strategies for promoting immigrant and refugee health, the book also provides lessons learned from past and present health communication campaigns, responses of diverse communities, and governmental policies.

This book with many case studies from major host countries on different continents will be of interest to anyone researching or studying in the areas of health communication, public health, international relations, public administration, nursing, and social work.

Do Kyun David Kim is Richard D'Aquin/BORSF Endowed Professor of Communication at the University of Louisiana at Lafayette.

Gary L. Kreps is a Distinguished Professor of Communication at George Mason University.

Routledge Research in Health Communication

Global Health Communication for Immigrants and Refugees

Cases, Theories, and Strategies

Edited by
Do Kyun David Kim and Gary L. Kreps

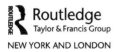

NEW YORK AND LONDON

First published 2022
by Routledge
605 Third Avenue, New York, NY 10158

and by Routledge
4 Park Square, Milton Park, Abingdon, Oxon, OX14 4RN

Routledge is an imprint of the Taylor & Francis Group, an informa business

© 2022 selection and editorial matter, Do Kyun David Kim and
Gary L. Kreps; individual chapters, the contributors

The right of Do Kyun David Kim and Gary L. Kreps to be
identified as the authors of the editorial material, and of the
authors for their individual chapters, has been asserted in
accordance with sections 77 and 78 of the Copyright, Designs
and Patents Act 1988.

All rights reserved. No part of this book may be reprinted
or reproduced or utilised in any form or by any electronic,
mechanical, or other means, now known or hereafter invented,
including photocopying and recording, or in any information
storage or retrieval system, without permission in writing from
the publishers.

Trademark notice: Product or corporate names may be
trademarks or registered trademarks, and are used only for
identification and explanation without intent to infringe.

Library of Congress Cataloging-in-Publication Data
Names: Kim, Do kyun, editor. | Kreps, Gary L., editor.
Title: Global health communication for immigrants and
refugees : cases, theories, and strategies / edited by Do Kyun
David Kim and Gary L Kreps.
Description: New York, NY : Routledge, 2022. | Series: Routledge
research in health communication ; 5 | Includes bibliographical
references and index.
Identifiers: LCCN 2021062122 (print) | LCCN 2021062123 (ebook) |
ISBN 9781032132358 (hardback) | ISBN 9781032136370 (paperback) |
ISBN 9781003230243 (ebook)
Subjects: LCSH: Communication in public health. | Communication
in medicine. | Immigrants—Health and hygiene. |
Immigrants—Medical care. |
Refugees—Health and hygiene. | Refugees—Medical care.
Classification: LCC RA423.2 .G545 2022 (print) | LCC RA423.2 (ebook) |
DDC 362.101/4—dc23/eng/20220121
LC record available at https://lccn.loc.gov/2021062122
LC ebook record available at https://lccn.loc.gov/2021062123

ISBN: 978-1-032-13235-8 (hbk)
ISBN: 978-1-032-13637-0 (pbk)
ISBN: 978-1-003-23024-3 (ebk)

DOI: 10.4324/9781003230243

Typeset in Sabon
by codeMantra

Contents

Contributors

Sameen Ahmed is a second-year undergraduate student at the University of Maryland – College Park, where she is studying public health sciences with a pre-medical focus. She is currently involved in the University's American Medical Student Association and is an active member of the Public Health Without Borders club. Sameen is a research assistant under Dr. Muhiuddin Haider and is involved in other research projects at the University. Sameen hopes to continue gaining clinical and research experience in global health initiatives as her studies continue.

Hedwig Alfred is a journalism lecturer at the Wee Kim Wee School of Communication and Information, Nanyang Technological University, Singapore. She is a former journalist and teaches several journalism classes including the school's signature Go-Far (Going Overseas for Advanced Reporting) course, for which she selects a country every year for a team of students to visit and report on current issues. The team's work has been published on media platforms locally and in the region, and won three prizes in the Majurity Trust's Stories of a Pandemic (SOAP) Awards for best stories, best photographs, and best commentary.

Kyungeh An, Ph.D., is a Professor in the Graduate School of Biomedical Sciences & School of Nursing at the University of Texas Health Science Center at San Antonio. Her research focuses on the relationships between psycho-socio-behavioral factors and cardiovascular disease outcomes. As a fellow of the American Heart Association, she has contributed to advance our understanding of the biological mechanisms underpinning the impact of the psychological factors such as stress and anxiety on acute coronary events, such as acute myocardial infection (AMI) and acute ischemic stroke (AIS). Her studies addressed gender differences and ethnic disparities in etiology of the CVD, health seeking behaviors, and health outcomes, then in adherence to rehabilitation after acute coronary events.

Ambar Basu, Ph.D., is Department Chair and Professor in the Department of Communication at the University of South Florida. His research explores how individuals and communities living at the margins of society communicate about health, illness, and wellbeing. With particular emphasis on theorizing culture as a site of social change, his scholarship documents and analyzes narratives about health that emerge from dialogue between his self (as the researcher) and research participants. His interest is to locate health inequities in the context of cultural, political, economic, geopolitical, and development agendas in marginalized spaces. His scholarship embraces a mix of methods such as critical ethnography and autoethnography, and highlights the implications of knowledge production in collaboration with marginalized communities. Self-reflexivity is an integral lens/method that shapes his work.

Xiaomei Cai, Ph.D., is an Associate Professor in the Department of Communication at George Mason University. She got her M.A. and Ph.D. in Mass Communication from Indiana University, Bloomington. Her research areas include children and online privacy issues, mass media effects, media message analysis, and youth and health messages. She was involved in a series of studies on smoking cessation intervention among Chinese and Korean immigrant populations.

Hilda Patricia Garcia Cosavalente, Ph.D., has worked as a Communication Specialist for the Pan American Health Organization in Washington, D.C., and in the Ministry of Health of Peru. She has taught communication courses at the University of Lima, Peru, and George Mason University and recently collaborated with the HealthyMe/MiSalud project of the Horowitz Center for Health Literacy at the University of Maryland. Her research interests are health information seeking behavior, women's health in the developing world, and health information needs of immigrants and underserved populations.

Leanne Chang, Ph.D., is Associate Professor in the Department of Communication Studies and Co-Director of the Centre for Media and Communication Research at the School of Communication at Hong Kong Baptist University. Her research concentrates on three areas of inquiry: technology and health, culture and health, and public deliberation on public health measures. She has taken a social psychological approach to examining health information behaviors, impacts of m-health interventions on personal health management, and the link between social media use and psychological wellbeing. She has also taken a cultural approach to exploring the importance of cultural values in shaping individuals' health beliefs and health practices.

Xuewei Chen, Ph.D., is an Assistant Professor of Health Education and Promotion at Oklahoma State University. Previously she obtained her

Ph.D. in Health Education from Texas A&M University as a Distinguished Honor Graduate, which was followed by a postdoctoral fellowship within the School of Public Health and Health Professions at University at Buffalo. She has 22 peer-reviewed publications and over 40 national/international conference presentations. Her research focuses on improving health literacy and health communication to reduce health disparities among underrepresented groups including immigrants with limited English proficiency, rural residents, and racial/ethnic minorities such as African Americans, Latinos, and Native Americans.

Tamara Giles-Vernick is the Project Coordinator of the SONAR-Global project (Horizon 2020) and Leader of the Anthropology & Ecology of Disease Emergence Unit at the Institut Pasteur (Paris, France), France and conducts research at the interstices of ethnohistory and medical anthropology, investigating zoonotic disease emergence transmission and global health interventions in Africa. Her other health-related research has included hepatitis B and vaccination; childhood malnutrition; infantile diarrhea in the Central African Republic; an historical epidemiology of malaria in West Africa; hepatitis C transmission in hospital and dental settings in Egypt; a comparative history of pandemic influenza; and a history of global health in Africa.

Maria Gruber is a doctoral candidate at the Institute for Communication at the University of Vienna. Her research focuses on the interplay between media and migration. As a member of the H2020 project MIRROR, dealing with the role of ICT, new media, and new perceptions in the migration process, she published on qualitative interview methodology during a global pandemic and is engaged in qualitative analysis of migrants' media use *en route* as well as their perceptions regarding Europe.

Muhiuddin Haider, Ph.D., is a Clinical Professor in Global Health at the University of Maryland School of Public Health's Institute for Applied Environmental Health. Since 2009, he has been teaching undergraduate courses under the Public Health Science and Global Health Scholars Programs, while also teaching graduate courses in the Global Health Certificate Program offered through the University. In addition to teaching, Dr. Haider is a highly skilled public health professional who has managed/led diverse public health research projects and studies in more than a dozen countries worldwide over the past 30 years, on behalf of several international agencies and universities.

Eun-Jeong Han, Ph.D., is an Associate Professor in the Department of Communication at Salisbury University, MD. The main area of her research and teaching is intercultural communication. Specifically, her research interests include the issues of (1) global migration and diaspora, (2) multiculturalism and diversity, (3) language learning and use among members of a minority group, (4) stereotypes, prejudices, and discrimination against minorities, and (5) Asians/Asian-Americans in the United States. Dr. Han received the *2020 Outstanding Book Award* by the Asian Pacific American Communication Studies Division of the NCA (National Communication Association), with the book she edited with two co-editors, *Korean Diaspora across the World: Homeland in History, Memory, Imagination, Media and Reality.*

Soo Jung Hong, Ph.D., is an Assistant Professor in the Department of Communications and New Media at the National University of Singapore. She earned her Ph.D. in health communication from the Pennsylvania State University in 2016. After completion of her Ph.D. program, she worked as a postdoctoral research fellow at Huntsman Cancer Institute – the University of Utah for two years. Her academic interest centers on health and risk communication, which includes designing effective messages for diverse audiences, and risk information and decision-making.

Elaine Hsieh, Ph.D., J.D., is Professor of Communication at the University of Oklahoma. Dr. Hsieh's work examines the intersections of culture, medicine, and health behaviors. Her latest book, *Rethinking Culture in Health Communication* (Hsieh & Kramer, 2021), extends this line of research by situating culture front and center in conceptualizing health theories and health policies.

David Kaawa-Mafigiri, Ph.D., is a Senior Lecturer at Makerere University, a medical anthropologist with public health training and experience integrating biomedical and socio-behavioral/community perspectives to health sciences research, and clinical trials including vaccines for HIV. Dr. Kaawa-Mafigiri's commitment to child wellbeing is illustrated through his research and publications in child abuse and neglect. He participates in SONAR-Global – a EU funded Social Sciences Network for Infectious Threats and Antimicrobial Resistance (AMR), piloted by 11 collaborating institutions across the globe including Makerere University in Africa.

Francis Kato is a Social Worker and a Trainer of trainers in Migration Health. Over time, Francis has supported child wellbeing focused projects in the area of violence against children (VAC), child health, and institutional care. He has a Master's degree in Social Work and Human Rights from the University of Gothenburg, Sweden, and a Bachelor's degree in Social Work from Makerere University. Francis currently works at Makerere University Department of Social Work as a Project Coordinator. His research interests include gender-based violence and VAC, child trafficking, institutional care, alternative care, refugee health, child trafficking, and community engagement strategies.

Do Kyun David Kim, Ph.D., is the Richard D'Aquin/BORSF Endowed Professor in the Department of Communication at the University of Louisiana at Lafayette. His research and teaching spans dissemination and implementation science based on the theory of diffusion of innovations. His praxis focuses on crisis and risk communication in the context of public health promotion, human-machine communication, environmental communication, and organizational and social change. He has conducted diverse communication projects in several countries in Sub-Saharan Africa, Asia, as well as the United States. Based on his excellence in research and praxis, he has published several books with internationally renowned publishers and many research articles in top-tier, peer-reviewed journals.

Judith Kohlenberger, Ph.D., is a Post-Doctoral Researcher working and teaching on forced migration and displacement. Her work has been widely published in international journals, such as *PLOS One, Refugee Survey Quarterly*, and *Health Policy.* She is affiliated with the Wittgenstein Center for Demography and Global Human Capital and serves on the board of the Integration Council of the City of Vienna and the Schumpeter Society Vienna. Her current research projects focus on the integration pathways of recently arrived refugees in Europe, exploring aspects of gender, health, and education.

Ruth Kutalek, Ph.D., is Associate Professor at the Unit Medical Anthropology and Global Health, Department of Social and Preventive Medicine, Medical University of Vienna and Principal Investigator of the SONAR-Global project in Vienna. She has conducted research in several countries in West and East Africa and has supported the WHO in emergency missions in Nigeria and Liberia. Her main fields of interest are medical anthropology, specifically anthropological perspectives on infectious diseases; migration of health workers; access to health care for migrants; environment and health; medical ethics; and ethnopharmacology.

Agnes Kyamulabi is a Research Fellow at the Department of Social Work and Social Administration. She holds an M.A. in Development Studies with a major in Children and Youth Studies from the ISS, Erasmus University of Rotterdam. Her research focuses on parenting, alternative care for children, child poverty, and violence against children. She participated in the development of a regional training curriculum and manual on Alternative Care for Children (Sponsored by SOS Children Villages International). She is currently coordinating a qualitative component of a research study "Promoting Inclusion in Decent Work for Ugandan Young People: Will Reducing Violence Help?" (2018–2021).

Gary L. Kreps, Ph.D., is University Distinguished Professor and Director of the Center for Health and Risk Communication at George Mason University. His more than 500 frequently-cited published articles and books examine the information needs of vulnerable populations to guide evidence-based policy, technology, and practice interventions. He coordinates the INSIGHTS (International Studies to Investigate Global Health Information Trends) Research Consortium across 20-plus countries. His honors include the Research Laureate Award from the American Academy of Health Behavior, the Outstanding Health Communication Scholar Award from the NCA and ICA, and appointments as an AAHB Fellow, an ICA Fellow, and an NCA Distinguished Scholar.

Moonju Lee, Ph.D., is an Assistant Professor in the School of Nursing at the University of Texas Health Science Center at San Antonio. Her research lies in racial and ethnic health disparities, cancer screening, health literacy, inequality and inequity in healthcare service utilization, community engagement, and capacity building in the linguistically and socially isolated underserved populations, mainly Korean immigrants, Hispanics, and refugees. Her research is based on the Community-based Participatory Research (CBPR) and Patient-Centered Outcome Research (PCOR) models. She has conducted the community engagement and capacity building project in the Korean American community to improve health literacy at the community level.

Ming Li, Ph.D., is an Assistant Professor of the Department of Health Sciences at Towson University. She received her Ph.D. degree in Health Education from Texas A&M University (TAMU). She has published 13 peer-reviewed journal articles and provided 27 national conference presentations. Her research focuses on Public Health Genomics, including genomic communication and education, genomics in disease prevention and control among populations that experience health disparities, as well as the ethical, legal, and social implications of genetic testing. Her honors include the Distinguished Honor Graduate from TAMU and the Public Health Genomics Award from the Genomics Forum of APHA.

May O. Lwin, Ph.D., is President's Chair Professor of Communication Studies at the Wee Kim Wee School of Communication and Information at Nanyang Technological University in Singapore. Her expertise lies in the utilization, design, and assessment of digitally mediated health communication and social media to improve public health in population groups. She is currently in partnership with National

Communicable Infectious Disease Center, leading research programs on COVID-19 infodemic and tracking COVID-19 misinformation. She has authored numerous peer-reviewed papers, books, and book chapters, many of which have received academic awards including the Fulbright ASEAN Scholar Award (2015), Ogilvy Foundation International Award (2014), Outstanding Applied Research Award by the International Communication Association (2019). She received the ICA Fellowship in 2020 and is also a Salzburg Global Fellow.

Elisabeth Mangrio, Ph.D., is an Associate Professor at Care Science, Malmö University as well as a researcher at MIM, Malmö Institute for Studies of Migration, Diversity and Welfare. She has conducted both qualitative and quantitative research regarding newly arrived migrants and their health situation after arrival in Sweden. This research covers aspects of how well Sweden manages to integrate migrants and to what extent they have access to employment after the establishment process in Sweden. She is currently also a researcher within the externally funded project 'Precision Health and Everyday Democracy' (PHED).

Caryn Medved, Ph.D., is Professor and Graduate Program Director, MA Corporate Communication. Medved is a recognized expert on issues of work-life communication. She has published 30+ journal articles and book chapters during on issues such as the discourse and practices of at-home fathering, breadwinning mothers, gender and theorizing work-life, corporate family discourses, single employee experiences, and undocumented immigrant family-life aspirations, among others. Currently, her new research explores the discursive and material tensions of redefining work, corporate political activity, and family in the gig economy.

Kyeung Mi Oh, Ph.D., is research focuses on racial and ethnic disparities in public health, health literacy, cancer screening, and smoking cessation. She has done extensive research on culture-specific influences on health behaviors, tobacco use, cancer information seeking, and cancer screening participation among ethnic minorities, particularly Korean American (KA)s. In her past research, she has worked closely with churches, senior resource centers, and community organizations for KAs and gained valuable skills, knowledge, and experience in conducting community-based health research. She recently conducted a smoking cessation intervention study for Chinese and Korean immigrants.

David Napier is Professor of Medical Anthropology at University College London, and Director of its Science, Medicine, and Society Network. He is the lead for SONAR-Global at UCL, and leads the Global Academic Lead for the Cities Changing Diabetes Programme, a cross-sectoral collaboration aimed at researching and limiting the rise in Type-2 diabetes in cities around the world. Napier's special interests in applied research include assessing vulnerability, primary health-care delivery, human wellbeing, caring for ethnically diverse populations, migration and trafficking, homelessness, new and emerging technologies, immunology, and creativity in scientific practice.

Chitra Panchapakesan, Ph.D., is currently working as Scientist in the Social and Cognitive Computing Department at the Institute of High Performance Computing (IHPC) in A*STAR. Her research interest includes information seeking and sharing, mobile communication, new media communication, and digital health communication. Chitra focuses on understanding public sentiments, information seeking and sharing, and the use of new media. She has also worked on numerous digital communication projects that conceptualize and develop social media applications for bettering public health.

Seulgi Park is a doctoral student in the Department of Communication at the State University of New York at Albany. Her research interests lie at the intersection of health, interpersonal, and intercultural communication. She is interested in health communication and health disparities, patient-doctor communication, and healthcare engagement among immigrant populations, especially focusing on Korean immigrants in the United States.

Emily B. Peterson, Ph.D., is a Health Scientist in the Office of Health Communication and Education at the Food & Drug Administration's Center for Tobacco Products (CTP). At CTP, Dr. Peterson's work focuses on formative and foundational work related to The Real Cost campaign and other tobacco prevention initiatives. Prior to joining CTP, Dr. Peterson worked as a Senior Research Scientist at the University of Southern California after completing a post-doctoral research fellowship at the National Cancer Institute. Dr. Peterson's research interests include nicotine education, perceived message effectiveness, and trust in national sources of health information. She holds a Ph.D. in Communication from George Mason University (2016).

Jaime S. Robb, Ph.D., is an Assistant Professor in the Diederich College of Communication at Marquette University. His focus as a researcher starts by centering language as consequential to the human experience. His research investigates the role of rhetorical communication in shaping the rituals and sense-making necessary for marginalized groups and individuals to maintain their health and wellness. Specifically, he situates culture as a process that deals with how collectives respond to local changes. He documents and theorizes about undocumented immigrants' health by engaging in dialogues between himself and research participants. His interest is to illuminate how rhetorical communication practices situate health disparities for certain cultural bodies due to cultural, economic, political, and social inequities.

Michael Strange, Ph.D., is an Associate Professor at the Department of Global Political Studies, Malmö University, and a researcher at the Malmö Institute for Studies of Migration, Diversity and Welfare (MIM). He directs the externally funded project 'Precision Health and Everyday Democracy' (PHED), which, during 2020 and 2021, has run an international inquiry on the future of healthcare post-Covid-19, with submissions from healthcare practitioners, activists, civil servants, and academics, with a particular focus on health equity. He also leads a Wallenberg Foundation funded project on the multi-level politics of AI in healthcare.

Sachiko Terui is an Assistant Professor in the Department of Communication Studies at the University of Georgia. Her research interests include health disparities and intercultural aspects of communication. She uses both qualitative and quantitative research methods to address communicative challenges pertaining to linguistic and cultural aspects of health and health management, communication interventions, health literacy, and health disparities experienced among marginalized and underserved populations. Her recent projects center in interdisciplinary collaborations, including communities and healthcare organizations.

Jamal Uddin is a Ph.D. student at the Department of Communication, Culture and Media Studies at Howard University. Jamal's research interests include health communication, global health, and health disparities. Some of Mr. Uddin's scholarly works are presented at the National Communication Association, International Communication Association, Association for Education in Journalism and Mass Communication, and the Central States Communication Association. Jamal is also working as a research assistant for "Project, ReFocus," a 1.6 million grant project from the CDC Foundation surrounding the COVID-19 virus, at Howard University.

Eddie J. Walakira is Associate Professor at Makerere University and a child and youth wellbeing expert. His research concerns child protection and empowering the youth as a means for ensuring their wellbeing. He is at the forefront of innovating practice-oriented training targeting in-service workers in Uganda and in the region on child protection/safeguarding and plays a critical role in supporting international and local development organizations in the area of programming, policy development, and implementation. He is a member of several organizational boards, working groups, and high-level university and government committees.

Hua Wang, Ph.D., is an Associate Professor of Communication and Affiliated Faculty of Community Health & Health Behavior at the University at Buffalo, The State University of New York, USA. Her work focuses on leveraging innovative communication strategies, social networks, and emerging technologies for health promotion and social change. Dr. Wang's interdisciplinary research has been published in high impact journals such as the *Journal of Medical Internet Research* and the *Journal of American Public Health* and received prestigious awards from the International Communication Association and the American Public health Association.

Xiaoquan Zhao, Ph.D., is a Professor in the Department of Communication at George Mason University. His research focuses on health message design and effects, evaluation of public communication campaigns, health information seeking, information disparities affecting vulnerable populations, news effects on health and risk perceptions, and the role of the self in health behavior and persuasive communication. Dr. Zhao is a scientific adviser on research and evaluation to FDA's ongoing national tobacco education campaigns. He is also a Senior Editor for the journal *Health Communication.*

Preface

Immigrant and Refugee Health in the Age of Globalization

According to the United Nations' recent report (2020), the number of international migrants worldwide increased to 281 million people, showing an upward trend globally. This is almost the total population (331 million) of the United States, the third largest country (by population) in the world, and more than the population of Indonesia, the fourth largest country. When broken down by continent, European countries hosted 87 million international migrants, followed by North American countries with 59 million migrants, and Africa and Asia accounting for 50 million migrants combined.

The rising number of forced displacements of refugees across international borders is also growing at a remarkable pace, as more than 70 million people worldwide have been forcibly displaced from their home countries (UNHCR, 2020). As a recent example, once the Taliban returned to power in Afghanistan in August 2021, an uncountable number of people rushed to flee from the brutal military governance, seeking places to resettle in other countries that generously accepted and helped them continue their lives. Many refugees confront serious health challenges related to poverty, malnutrition, injuries, and diseases. Nearly 25.9 million refugees are vulnerable youth under the age of 18 (UNHCR, 2020). Communication is a critically important factor to help these vulnerable populations who need to learn about their new homes and seek support and opportunities to promote health and their wellbeing in new countries (Kreps & Neuhauser, 2015).

Since immigrants and refugees resettle to live outside of their home countries, it is not unusual for them to encounter many unfamiliar problems in adjusting to their new countries due to the lack of information, experience, and education about different cultures, policies, traditions, life circumstances, and languages. They must learn about new systems and sociocultural environments to become assimilated into new countries. Especially, if their new countries have different languages, which is a very common situation for immigrants and refugees, their language barrier seriously marginalizes them in the new countries. They would feel like becoming babies who have to learn everything from the very beginning in their lives mainly because they cannot express their needs and emotions and receive information they need. In such dire situations, what if they become sick or get injured? It is certainly expected that their lack of knowledge about everything in the new countries and communication/language problems will inhibit their access to needed health care facilities and services as well as health information.

Immigrant and refugee health is now a major global issue because of the rapid increase of immigrants and refugees worldwide (Mitchell, Weinberg, Posey, & Cetron, 2019). According to the Centers for Disease Control and Prevention (CDC) in the United States, tasks for immigrant and refugee health include, but are not limited to, providing guidelines for disease screening and treatment, disseminating information about disease outbreaks and available healthcare facilities, and educating them to improve their health literacy (2016). In addressing such complex immigrant and refugee health problems, communication is not only a central problem, but also a solution (e.g., Ahmed et al., 2017; Alpern, Davey, & Song, 2016; Antonipillai et al., 2017). Responding to the urgency of improving immigrant and refugee health communication in the age of globalization, this book analyzes important international cases of immigrant and refugee health from diverse health communication perspectives, providing researchers and practitioners with theoretical frames and strategic guidelines/recommendations for designing effective health communication campaigns and interventions for promoting immigrant and refugee health. Cases were collected in many countries from different continents, and prominent scholars participated in this important book project.

Challenges and problems in immigrant and refugee health are complex as they are closely tied to many socioeconomic, educational, cultural, and policy issues. Specifically, immigrant and refugee health communication should deal with many challenges related to lack of language education, cultural conflicts during the assimilation process, insufficient information, systemically embedded prejudice and discrimination against immigrant groups, and ineffective public policies and programs to support health communication among immigrant and refugee populations. Although communication has become more critical than ever to improve immigrant and refugee health, few books address immigrant and refugee health communication from strategic perspectives and provide substantial and implementable recommendations. This book was designed to overcome this shortness in the extant literature by employing comprehensive, strategic, and problem-solving approaches.

This book contains 16 chapters, and each chapter presents three major components: (1) important international cases that focus on successful or failed immigrant and refugee health communication strategies in major host countries. Coupled with describing immigrant and refugee health situations in many host countries, each chapter identifies major health communication problems experienced by immigrants and refugees and diagnoses current health communication strategies that have been implemented to solve the identified health communication problems; (2) theoretical scope to analyze the cases and build a foundation of effective health communication strategies; (3) feasible health communication strategies to improve immigrant and refugee health.

Based on this frame, this book balances theoretical and practical aspects so that researchers, practitioners, and policy decision-makers can apply health communication perspectives to develop, implement, and evaluate their immigrant and refugee health campaigns, interventions, and policies. Moreover, this book has some chapters that examine how nationwide and global health risk situations, such as past, current, and future pandemics (including the COVID-19 pandemic), affect immigrant and refugee health and suggest effective health communication strategies during a pandemic. Scholarly, this book not only contributes to extant theories that have been applied to health communication campaigns, interventions, and policies, but also attempts to build new and evidence-based theories on immigrant and refugee health communication.

This global coverage of immigrant and refugee health from the strategic health communication perspective gives this book a unique position compared to other literature dealing with similar issues. This book will provide readers with a comprehensive understanding of immigrant and refugee health and present substantial health communication strategies that will significantly help improve immigrant and refugee health.

References

Ahmed, S., Lee, S., Shommu, N., Rumana, N., & Turin, T. (2017). Experiences of communication barriers between physicians and immigrant patients: A systematic review and thematic synthesis. *Patient Experience Journal, 4*(1), 122–140.

Alpern, J. D., Davey, C. S., & Song, J. (2016). Perceived barriers to success for resident physicians interested in immigrant and refugee health. *BMC Medical Education, 16*(1), 178.

Antonipillai, V., Baumann, A., Hunter, A., Wahoush, O., & O'Shea, T. (2017). Impacts of the Interim Federal Health Program reforms: A stakeholder analysis of barriers to health care access and provision for refugees. *Canadian Journal of Public Health, 108*(4), 435–441.

CDC. (2016). Immigrant and refugee health. Retrieved from https://www.cdc.gov/immigrantrefugeehealth/index.html

Kreps, G. L., & Neuhauser, L. (2015). Designing health information programs to promote the health and well-being of vulnerable populations: The benefits of evidence-based strategic health communication. In C. A. Smith & A. Keselman (Eds.), *Meeting Health Information Needs Outside of Healthcare* (pp. 3–17). Chandos Publishing.

Mitchell, T., Weinberg, M., Posey, D. L., & Cetron, M. (2019). Immigrant and refugee health: A centers for disease control and prevention perspective on protecting the health and health security of individuals and communities during planned migrations. *Pediatric Clinics, 66*(3), 549–560.

UNHCR. (2020). *Figures at a Glance.* https://www.unhcr.org/en-us/figures-at-a-glance.html

United Nations. (2020). *International Migration 2020 Highlight.* https://www.un.org/en/desa/international-migration-2020-highlights.

1 Health Communication in Mixed Status Latino Immigrant Families in the United States

Caryn Medved

It was a chilly day in November of 2016 when we drove out to Long Island. As we parked, I waved to Cristine on the sidewalk waiting for us; she was ready to interpret and provide support as a community advocate. We walked up the stairs to their modest two-room apartment located just off a small downtown business district. After a warm welcome, Sarah, colleague and project co-PI, went to interview sisters Katherine and Alexa in their bedroom.[1] In the kitchen and with the help of Cristine, I interviewed their Honduran immigrant parents. Claudia and Jose Reyes immigrated to New York almost two decades earlier after the devastation wrecked by Hurricane Mitch in Honduras.

As Katherine explained, "My mom was pregnant so she could not come here. They were giving out TPS (Temporary Protective Status) and my dad was the first to get it and my mom could not get it" because of the timing of her travel to the United States. She adds, "She has been here for 16 years undocumented." During their time in the United States, Claudia and Jose, and most recently Katherine, have experienced significant, life-threatening health conditions; the experiences and meanings of which are entangled with (a) structural constraints and enablements, (b) intersectional cultural narratives, and (c) agency exercised in health and migration family decision making along with intersecting material realities.

Jose spent a decade battling polycystic kidney disease. His TPS status provided access to Medicaid coverage. Claudia described, "He began with dialysis in July 5, 2001." She recalled telling her daughters that

> if we went back, his [health] was in danger because, I could not afford medicine [in Honduras or the cost of] dialysis and he could die. During ten years he was in dialysis. Five years ago, he got the kidney transplant.

Claudia shared that their family "conversations were never about our legal status. It was about the father's health. Our major worry was about if he will live or die because he had a several crisis during the dialysis years." Still Jose's health concerns didn't end with the transplant. Jose

DOI: 10.4324/9781003230243-1

explained that if he went back to Honduras, he would not be able to af-ford his medicine; the "medicine that I take [so] my body does not reject the kidney is around a thousand monthly, plus the other medication. I have to take for life." Then just as Jose was recovering, Claudia was diagnosed with anemia but, unlike her husband, she did not have access to health insurance due to her undocumented status. Katherine recalled,

> she went to the hospital couple years ago. And she does not have any medical insurance. I was really worried that she had to pay for all of that … If she has not have a donor she could die.

Because of the emergency nature of Claudia's treatment and access to information about potential healthcare funding assistance, she was able to apply for and receive financial help to cover her medical expenses.

Katherine's older sister Alexa was born in Honduras; she came to the United States with her mother and was finishing high school when we spoke with her family. Alexa had earned legal status through the Deferred Action for Childhood Arrivals (DACA) program during the Obama Administration. With the Trump administration coming into power at the time of our interview, the family worried that her DACA status as well as the renewal of her fathers' TPS status was uncertain, along with their increased fears of her mother's deportation. Claudia shared that the insecurity of Alexa's DACA status affected her daugh-ter's mental and emotional health; she explained "because we do not know what it is going to happen with the new president in this country. And although she does not express openly, she is stressed, anxious, and worried about it." Claudia's mental health also suffered due to her lack of documentation. She disclosed, "Yes, we are very afraid, insecure. It affects us emotionally and physically. We are afraid because … if I go out immigration will be looking for me." She added that:

> people share in social media or the other time a brother in church send us a text message to let me know and do not go out. So, I try to not go out, but if I do not, it then I cannot work and make money. We need two salaries.

Katherine was the only US citizen by birthright in the family and had dreams of serving in the US military. Yet her ambitions, and health, came into question after she was a victim in a 'hit and run' car accident leaving her with severe and ongoing back pain. Jose explained "every-thing is really hard for her and she's wondering 'why did it happen to me? I did not look for it.'" Jose consoled his daughter by sharing that "as Christians we know God has a plan for her and us." Her mom pro-vided significant daily care. While insurance wasn't an issue given her citizenship status, Katherine worried about what would happen if her mother got deported. She revealed,

> she takes me to physical therapy and all of that. So, it is scary if one day when I come back home, she is not here. That uncertainty kind of scares me. She cannot permanently be here. It is like what I am going to do without my mom?

Katherine also lives with the same kidney disease that necessitated her father's transplant and knows she will struggle with this life-long health condition.

Culture-Centered Approach (CCA)

Often-marginalized experiences of migration, family and health communication are visible in the case study of the Reyes family. This complex and intersectional narrative is constructed through the voices of four family members, all with different legal statuses and varying access to healthcare as well as three critical physical conditions. As of 2018, the Pew Center for Research reported that 44.8 million people living in the United States were foreign born and accounted for 13.7% of the US population. Of the total foreign-born population living in the United States, 77% (35.2 million) are lawful immigrants including 12.3 million lawful permanent and 2.2 million temporary permanent residents and 23% (10.5 million) are unauthorized (Budiman, 2020). And, while the number of mixed status immigrant families is difficult to estimate, more than 8 million US citizens, of which 1.2 million are naturalized citizens, have at least one unauthorized family member living with them (Mathema, 2017). While immigration itself can bring particular physical and mental health stressors (Elder, 2003), health communication in the context of mixed status families is complicated by, at times, stark differences within one family unit to health care access and financing, language abilities, acculturation opportunities, generational health beliefs, as well as perceived safety when seeking healthcare.

Drawing on concepts from the Culture-Centered Approach (CCA) (Dutta, 2008; Dutta & Basu, 2011) as well as empirical research on immigrant and Latino health communication (e.g., Elder et al., 2009; Greder & Reina, 2019; Hubbell, 2006; Katz, 2014), this chapter explores structures, culture(s), and agency in relation to meaning making and negotiation about health and migration in mixed status Latino immigrant families. The Reyes family experiences are connected and contextualized with related research, followed by the provision of recommended strategies for health communication praxis.

Communication-Centered Approach

According to Dutta (2008), the culture-centered approach (CCA) "is value-centered and is built on the notion that the various ways of understanding and negotiating meanings of health care are embedded within cultural contexts and the values deeply connected with them" (p. 2). Different from biomedical models of health communication, CCA begins with culture and challenges dominant ways of viewing health communication in research and practice. Three key concepts provide the framework for CCA: structure, culture, and agency, all of which are deeply embedded in issues of materiality – embodied, economic, and geographic – in the lives of mixed status immigrant families (Bishop & Medved, 2020).

Structure

Structures, from a CCA perspective, are "those aspects of social organization that constrain and enable the capacity of cultural participants to seek out health choices and engage in health-related behavior" (Dutta & Basu, 2011, p. 330). Mixed status immigrant families' experiences and meanings of health and illness are shaped by healthcare, legal/political, economic, and community structures. Although the 2010 Affordable Care Act provided insurance options to previously uninsured individuals, healthcare structures in the United States remain significantly tied legal employment, and, by extension, to citizenship. While basic medical assistance for immigrants of varying legal statuses exists, the extent of assistance and financial coverage of treatment varies by state (National Immigration Law Center, 2021). Jose, as a recipient of federally-granted TPS had access to a life-saving kidney transplant and ongoing prescription coverage through Medicaid. And, as a DACA recipient, Alexa also had access to state funded health insurance. However, health care and insurance for undocumented individuals living in the United States is precarious and, ultimately tied to larger state and federal political structures. Claudia did not have the option to purchase health insurance; yet due to the emergency nature of her health condition, Claudia had access to treatment she could not have afforded without financial assistance. Other barriers that can affect unauthorized persons access to healthcare include discrimination and fear of deportation (Hacker et al., 2015).

The framing of healthcare as a 'human right' vs. 'citizenship right' is a divisive public debate in the United States particularly when connected to issues of immigration (Luhby, 2019). At the same time, professional organizations such as the American Medical Association (AMA) have issued ethics policy statements on undocumented health care. AMA H-440.876 states their opposition to criminalization of medical care provided to undocumented immigrant patients (AMA, 2014). Within individual healthcare interactions, research on Latino immigrant families documents parents often rely on their children to be linguistic, cultural and media brokers or intermediaries when they have limited English language facility in the context of health care and other settings. Immigrant children are able to perform this role due to their advanced language skills and cultural knowledge (Katz, 2014). Katz conceptualizes brokering as not just an individual phenomenon experienced by immigrant children, but also part of family and institutional communication systems.

Health and healthcare structures, and by implication, the families who must navigate within these systems, are deeply intertwined with political/legal structures. Claudia worried about her own and her daughter's mental health with the change in political party at the national level that directly coincided with the timing of our interviews. Artiga and Diaz (2019) reported that changing political messages and policies affect the health seeking behaviors of immigrants, both legal and noncitizen. Research reviewed by these authors for the Kaiser Family Foundation suggested that fears resulting from the former Trump administration policies caused families to turn away from utilizing programs and services for themselves as well as their children, who were primarily US born citizens. And, further, they argue that decreases in coverage for immigrant families "would increase barriers to care and financial instability, negatively affecting the growth and healthy development of their children" (p. 5). Similar to the work of Sun and Dutta (2017), meaning structures, in this case political ones, about the risk of healthcare seeking can intersect with embodied materiality as individuals may choose to delay or forgo necessary health treatments. The ongoing political/legal negotiation of immigration status and related healthcare access can be seen as recently as the June 2021 Supreme Court ruling stating that immigrants living in the United States with temporary protective status – most often granted for humanitarian reasons, including fleeing political violence or natural disasters – are ineligible to apply for permanent residency (Barnes, 2021). Thus, healthcare for these immigrants, such as Jose, is tied to the TPS designation; if the status is revoked, according to the ruling, they are unable to apply for citizenship and will lose health coverage as well as legal status.

Finally, community structures also are critical to understanding immigrant health and health communication. In the context of mental health, for example, research documents the primarily protective value of social support from communities, extended family members, friends and neighborhoods (see Kia-Keating et al., 2016 for a review). Claudia mentions social support provided by community and church members in the form of warnings about sightings of immigration officers in the area. For Claudia, community support also was essential to get information about the existence of health financing in the form of a grant to cover her hospital stay and treatment for anemia. Studies of community health advisor (CHA) interventions in Latino communities demonstrate some success (and shortcomings) in the use of CHAs to disseminate culturally specific health information (Candeleria et al., 1998). In addition, community-based parent support programs for immigrants frequently focus on issues of positive parenting and family communication. In their review of research, Hamari et al. (2021) argued that by improving communication, these programs sought to reduce child health behavioral problems. CCA would suggest the continued development of such approaches by increasing dialogic engagement in communities as a means of more fundamental health transformation (Dutta & Basu, 2011). At the close of this chapter, practices of community participation and dialogue will be drawn upon in recommended health communication strategies.

Culture

CCA research begins with the premise that culture is dynamic and "constituted by the by the day-to-day of its members as they come to develop their interpretations of health and illness" (Dutta & Basu, p. 330). For immigrants, regardless of legal status, culture is inherently and *minimally* bi-cultural – always navigating and negotiating between cultures of origin and the culture of residence (Bishop & Medved, 2019). Culture, in addition to being central and dynamic, also is intersectional (Crenshaw, 1990). National or state/regional geographic cultural identities also are intimately embedded in identities of generation, ethnicity, religion, gender/sexual identity/orientation, class, and race among others (for example, see Gonzalez et al.'s (2018) study of Latinx transgender health communication). Further, living undocumented in the United States also means being a part of a subaltern culture – one literally forced to remain out of view and posing unique challenges (Hacker et al., 2015). Claudia's ongoing mental health challenges, for example, brought on by fears of deportation illuminate one aspect of her experiences in the undocumented subculture. Reviewing research across all potential cultural issues experienced by mixed status families living in the United States is beyond the scope of this chapter. Aligning with our case, select studies on Latinx immigrant health communication are reviewed.

The cultural designation Latino/a or, more recently Latinx encapsulates a wide variety of cultural, socio-economic, and ethnic backgrounds immigrating from Latin American countries including in North, Central and South America (e.g., Mexico, Brazil, Panama, Honduras, Chili, Haiti). Similar to the Reyes family, an estimated 57,000 immigrants from Honduras were expected to reapply for TPS status early in 2021 (Cohen et al., 2019). In 2018, 25% of US immigrants were of Mexican origin. For certain health conditions, Hispanics[2] bear a disproportionate burden of disease (e.g., stroke, chronic liver disease, diabetes), injury, death and disability when compared with non-Hispanic whites (CDC, 2004). Increasing scholarly attention has been paid to health communication in Latino communities in the past two decades (i.e., Davis et al., 2017; Elder et al., 2009; Hubbell, 2006).

Hubbell's (2006) study of the extended parallel processing model (EPPM), for example, of rural Mexican American women's preventative behaviors against breast cancer found that perceptions of susceptibility and severity of breast cancer were more strongly related to protective behaviors and thought processes than perceived self-efficacy. When participants did not enact such behavior, women reported the following reasons: lack of access to care, low educational levels, low socioeconomic status, lack of health insurance, or cultural fatalism and/or low self-efficacy. Digging further into culture, Greder and Reina (2018) found that first-generation rural Mexican American women defined health in two ways that aligned with their cultural backgrounds: (a) health as absence of illness and (b) health as good with family. That is, these women, often in charge of their family's health and healthcare, explained that "good health" meant not having disease or addiction along with having "harmony and peace among family members, not having conflict" (p. 1337). Greder and Reina also reported health challenges for the Mexican American women in their study who often lacked easily accessible and culturally responsive health care (e.g., transportation to clinics and trustworthy translators). Follow cultural beliefs these women also perceived that their family's health came before their own and may cause these mothers to delay or forgo their own care. Finally, the lack of healthy physical housing environments also was perceived to negatively affect family health outcomes.

Citing a lack of research about the health seeking behaviors and health knowledge gaps in uninsured Hispanic populations in the United States, Cheong (2007) surveyed 737 Hispanics in Los Angeles. Cheong found that a significantly larger proportion of uninsured vs. insured Hispanics used ethnically targeted television and interpersonal communication networks as preferred sources of health information, the latter of which supports the "emphasis on social relations in Hispanic cultures, or *familialism*" (p. 160). Thus, while each of the studies detailed above explore culture in different ways,[3] together, they help us see the tight knit between Latino culture(s) and health communication. Similarly, the Reyes family experiences are deeply embedded in *familialism*; Claudia's focus on her family's health over her own mental and emotional concerns as an undocumented person powerfully illustrate these values. Further, Jose consoling his daughter suffering from chronic back pain through the use of religion with a hint of fatalism, "God has a plan," also bring out how culture intimates shape how this mixed status family negotiates the meanings of health, family and migration.

Agency

The third central concept of culture-centered approaches to health com-munication is agency or "the capacity of cultural members to enact their choices and to participate actively in negotiating the structures within which they find themselves" (Dutta, 2008, p. 7). Agency can come in the form of proactive healthcare seeking or perhaps consciously *not seeking care* for fear of negative ramifications. Unauthorized immigrants may not seek treatment in fear of provider questions about legal status; or immigrants with legal status protections may delay treatment due to their lack of economic resources or health knowledge gaps or limited lit-eracy skills: English language or health literacy (Greder & Reina, 2018). Particularly for low-income immigrants employed in hourly-wage work in the United States, economic resources for health care can be limited or insurance non-existent through their employers. Thus, not surprisingly, the majority of Latino voters in the United States (71%) believe that gov-ernment should be doing more to ensure healthcare for all Americans (Manuel et al., 2020).

It is at the intersection of health and agency where we also see in-tensely difficult choices in the lives of mixed status families. Decisions to cross geographic borders entering into the United States – or to return to countries of origin – may be inseparable from family health issues, particularly as seen in the case of the Reyes family. The ques-tion of returning to Honduras inherently was a question of health. Despite concerns about Claudia's unauthorized status, the Reyes fam-ily did not decide to return to Honduras because of the health and healthcare for Jose and Katherine, both suffering from polycystic kid-ney disease. Other immigrant families alternatively decide to separate across boundaries; one parent migrates (i.e., a mother to earn money as a domestic worker or a father to engage in farm labor) looking for work while other family members (i.e., spouse and/or children) stay behind in their home country causing a potentially different set of health and health related concerns (Elder, 2009). Further, the choices of individual members of mixed status often are shaped by fears of potential consequences to other family members. Bishop (2017) found that undocumented and DACA recipient young adults' narrative activ-ism may be constrained by fears of how speaking publicly might affect their families.

Encouraging agency through promoting positive health behaviors his-torically has been a valuable focus of health communication research (e.g., Davis et al., 2017; Hubbell, 2006); albeit from different perspec-tives on culture than advocated by culture-centered approaches (Dutta, 2008). Davis et al., for example, investigated the influence of message tailoring and emotional arousal on identification and message recall in health narratives about childhood obesity prevention shared with

Mexican American women. They found that mothers identified with the protagonists and were most interested in narratives framed around scripts focused on helping them to improve their own lives. Davis and colleagues hope that their research findings are used increase the efficacy of evidence-based narrative health interventions in underserved populations. Further, there exists a long history of research on the role of communities in developing health agency in work on entertainment education (e.g., Singhal & Roger, 2021).

Recommended Health Communication Strategies and Practices

Five health communication recommendations are detailed below based on gaps in research and reflecting the ethos of CCA to health communication. Recommendations are designed to intervene across structure, culture and agency (Dutta & Basu, 2011).

1   **Advocate for increased government assistance for immigrant health-care.** In agreement with recommendations provided by John P. Elder (2003) in the *American Journal of Health Behavior*, strategy at the level of healthcare structure must focus on continued immigrant health rights advocacy. Research documents low-levels of healthcare access, insurance and financing in uninsured populations as well as low-socioeconomic and legal or temporarily legal immigrant populations as well as their potential negative health outcomes (Artiga & Diaz, 2019; Elder et al., 2009; Manuel et al., 2020). Thus, what are the ways for political and health communication scholars and activists to engage in effective campaigns at the national and state level to increase awareness and, potentially, access and assistance for all immigrants seeking healthcare? One way health communication scholars can contribute to raising awareness is by lending their expertise to immigrant rights organizations developing messages and strategies to educate local, state or national lawmakers. Through writing op-eds for publication in outlets read lawmakers and other government policy influencers, communication experts also can lend their voice to educate publics about the health needs of undocumented and mixed status families.

2   **Develop increased opportunities for mixed status community health dialogue.** There exists a need for increased community dialogue about health and healthcare, specifically in the lives of mixed status immigrant families. Health, partly, is a family meaning making and negotiation process, not singularly an individual experience. Thus, intervening through communication to improve health and healthcare for mixed status families must take into consideration the

implications of the varying legal status of family members. Research shows fears of parental deportation not only cause unauthorized immigrant parents to avoid seeking healthcare, but also may lead to decreased parental healthcare seeking on behalf of their US born citizen children (Greder & Reina, 2019). Convening with community advocates, legal advisors, and members for safe conversations and information sharing in immigrant advocacy organizations might be a means of developing new, more effective health communication strategies for this unique immigrant population. These dialogues also must be undertaken with the knowledge that Latino populations are not homogeneous (Cheong, 2007) nor are their strategies for health information seeking. Community-based dialogues can help to uncover differences and develop effective and participative strategies and collective agency.

3   **Focus on engaging 'broker' immigrant children in dialogue to develop resources.** As noted by Katz (2014), the children of unauthorized or low-level English-speaking immigrants often take on stressful roles as 'brokers' or intermediaries between their elders and care professionals in health and healthcare interactions. While the criticality of their roles has been documented, opportunities for dialogue and participation in developing additional resources for these young family health advocates is essential. Balancing multiple roles in high pressure interactions as language, cultural and/or media brokers can create stressful situations for young. What are ways that community organizations can assist these children in their roles as intermediaries with emotional support, informational support and, at times, instrumental support such as support groups, health system knowledge, or rides to health appointments?

4   **Increase the focus on mental health communication for immigrant populations.** Non-profits such as the *Coalition for Immigrant Mental Health* and work done by organizations such as the *New York Immigrant Coalition* on issues of mental health must be expanded. Mental health issues, particularly for unauthorized immigrants and their families are well documented (Elder, 2003; Kia-Keating et al., 2016). To increase communication and community around these issues requires a focus on community dialogue with health care organizations as well as advocacy to raise awareness within immigrant communities about the negative effects of low-levels of mental health. Raising awareness and garnering resources will require development communication for fund raising and political advocacy for resources and support. For example, the work of advocacy organizations on mental health issues – i.e., community outreach, interpretation services, psychological services – requires significant financial and human resources. Health communication

scholars with expertise in designing messages for development campaigns can help raise needed capital. Or, scholars with significant grant writing experience can assist organization in the grant writing process or can collaborate with community partners in designing action-based research to improve immigrant mental health and health care access.

5   **Increase the use of social media, social networks, and ethnically targeted media.** Levels of agency to navigate health and healthcare systems within mixed status immigrant families varies greatly as do their information seeking strategies. According to Cheong (2007), it is important to find ways through social media, interpersonal networks, and ethnically targeted media to share health and health related information and success stories as means of closing family knowledge gaps. The use of online information campaigns and messages may be particularly useful in reaching out to second-generation immigrants, better educated, younger, employed Hispanic males who have health insurance (Cheong, 2007). Online disseminated bi-lingual materials, even if initially only accessed by younger, educated family members can be shared within mixed status immigrant families, church communities, and advocacy groups. For example, health communication scholars working in institutions of higher education, including community colleges in cities with high unauthorized immigrant populations, might work with student-immigrant and/or DACA student support groups to share information about healthcare access through their online networks such as Facebook, Instagram or Twitter. DACA students themselves and/or their peers may be serving in brokering roles for their families; this particular use of social media may provide additional channels for targeted dissemination of critical health information.

Notes

1   This case study is based on an oral history interview completed for a larger project exploring mixed status immigrant Latino families and work-family negotiations (see Bishop & Medved, 2020). In the course of sharing their life experiences, the Reyes family also recalled situations related to intergenerational health communication. Disfluencies in language remain to preserve and respect the authenticity of their narratives. The family name is a pseudonym to protect participant confidentiality.

2   For an explanation of the terms Hispanic, Latino/a, Latinx see Lopez et al. (2020).

3   In explaining the CCA approach, Dutta and Basu (2011) detail four different perspectives on culture in use in health communication scholarship: cultural sensitivity, ethnographic, structure-centered, and culture-centered; all of which vary in on two dimensions: (a) culture as dynamic vs. culture as static and (b) status quo/social change.

Recommended Readings

Artiga, S. & Diaz, M. (2019*). Issue brief: Health coverage and care for undocumented immigrants.* Washington, DC: Kaiser Family Foundation. https://www.kff.org/racial-equity-and-health-policy/fact-sheet/health-coverage-of-immigrants/

Budiman, A. (2020). Key findings about immigration. *Pew Center for Research.* https://www.pewresearch.org/fact-tank/2020/08/20/key-findings-about-u-s-immigrants/

Cheong, P. H. (2007). Health communication resources for uninsured and insured Hispanics. *Health Communication, 21*(2), 153–163. https://doi.org/10.1080/10410230701307188

Dutta, M. & Basu, A. (2011). Culture, communication and health: A guiding framework. In Thompson, T. L., Parrott, R. & Nussbaum, J. F. (Eds.). *The Routledge handbook of health communication* (pp. 320–334). New York: Taylor & Francis.

Elder, J. P. Ayala, G. X., Parra-Median, D. & Talavera, G. A. (2009). Health communication in the Latino community: Issues and approaches. *Annual Review of Public Health, 30,* 227–251. https://doi.org/10.1146/annurev.publhealth.031308.100300

References

American Medical Association. (2014). *Opposition to criminalization of medical care provided to undocumented immigrant patients H-440.876.* https://policysearch.ama-assn.org/policyfinder/detail/immigrants?uri=%2-FAMADoc%2FHOD.xml-0-3892.xml.

Artiga, S. & Diaz, M. (2019). *Issue brief: Health coverage and care for undocumented immigrants.* Kaiser Family Foundation. https://www.kff.org/racial-equity-and-health-policy/fact-sheet/health-coverage-of-immigrants/

Barnes, R. (2021, June 7). Supreme court unanimously backs limits on immigrants with temporary protective status seeking green cards. *Washington Post.* https://www.washingtonpost.com/politics/courts_law/supreme-court-tps-green-card/2021/06/07/6d9b104e-c793-11eb-81b1-34796c7393af_story.html

Bishop, S. C. (2017). (Un)documented immigrant media makers and the search for connection online. *Critical Studies in Media Communication, 34*(5), 415–431. https://doi.org/10.1080/15295036.2017.1351618

Bishop, S. C. & Medved, C. E. (2020). Relational tensions, narrative, and materiality: Intergenerational communication in families with undocumented immigrant parents. *Journal of Applied Communication Research, 48*(5), 227–247. https://doi.org/10.1080/00909882.2020.1735646

Budiman, A. (2020). Key findings about immigration. *Pew Center for Research.* https://www.pewresearch.org/fact-tank/2020/08/20/key-findings-about-u-s-immigrants/

Candeleria, J., Campbell, N., Lyons, G., et al., (1998). Strategies for health education: Community-based methods. In S. Louie (Ed.). *Handbook of immigrant health* (pp. 587–606). New York, NY: Plenum.

Center for Disease Control. (2004). *Health Disparities Experienced by Hispanics.* Office of Minority Health. https://www.cdc.gov/mmwr/preview/mmwrhtml/mm5340a1.htm

Cheong, P. H. (2007). Health communication resources for uninsured and insured Hispanics. *Health Communication*, *21*(2), 153–163. https://doi.org/10.1080/10410230701307188

Cohen, D., Passel, J. S., & Bialik, K. (2019). *Many immigrants with Temporary Protected Status face uncertain future in U.S. Pew Center for Research.* Washington D.C. https://www.pewresearch.org/fact-tank/2019/11/27/immigrants-temporary-protected-status-in-us/

Crenshaw, K. (1990). Mapping the margins: Intersectionality, identity politics, and violence against women of color. *Stanford Law Review*, *43*(6), 1241–1299. https://doi.org/10.2307/1229039

Davis, R. E., Dal Cin, S., Cole, S. M., Reyes, L. I., McKenney-Shubert, S. J., Fleischer, N. L., Densen, L. C. & Peterson, K. E. (2017). A tale of two stories: An exploration of identification, message recall, and narrative preferences among low-income, Mexican American women. *Health Communication*, *32*(11), 1409–1421. https://doi.org/10.1080/10410236.2016.1228029

Dutta, M. (2008). *Communicating health: A culture centered approach.* Malden, MA: Polity.

Dutta, M. & Basu, A. (2011). Culture, communication and health: A guiding framework. In Thompson, T. L., Parrott, R. & Nussbaum, J. F. (Eds.). *The Routledge handbook of health communication* (pp. 320–334). New York, NY: Taylor & Francis.

Elder, J. P. (2003). Reaching out to America's immigrants: Community health advisors and health communication. *American Journal of Health Behavior*, *27*(Supplement 3), S197–S205.

Elder, J. P. Ayala, G. X., Parra-Median, D. & Talavera, G. A. (2009). Health communication in the Latino community: Issues and approaches. *Annual Review of Public Health*, *30*, 227–251. https://doi.org/10.1146/annurev.publhealth.031308.100300

Gonzalez, K. A., Abreu, R. L., Capielo Rosario, C., Koech, J., M., Lockett, G. M. & Lindley, L. (2020, October 15): "A center for transwomen where they help you:" Resource needs of the immigrant Latinx transgender community, *International Journal of Transgender Health*. https://doi.org/10.1080/26895269.2020.1830222

Greder, K. & Reina, A. S. (2019). Procuring health: Experiences of Mexican immigrant women in rural Midwestern communities. *Qualitative Health Research*, *29*(9), 1334–1344. https://doi.org/10.1177/1049732318816676

Hacker, K., Aines, M., Folb, B. L. & Zallman, L. (2015). Barriers to health care for undocumented immigrants: A review of literature. *Risk Management and Health Care*, *8*, 175–183. https://doi.org/10.2147/RMHP.S70173

Hamari, L., Konttila, J., Merikukka, M., Tuomikoski, A. M., Kouvonen, P. & Kurki, M. (2021). Parent support programmes for families who are immigrants: A scoping review. *Journal of Immigrant and Minority Health*, 1–20. https://doi.org/10.1007/s10903-021-01181-z

Hubbell, A. P. (2006). Mexican American women in a rural area and barriers to their ability to enact protective behaviors against breast cancer. *Health Communication*, *20(1)*, 35–44. https://doi.org/10.1207/s15327027hc2001_4

Katz, V. S. (2014). *Kids in the middle: How children of immigrants negotiate community interactions for their families.* New Brunswick, NJ: Rutgers University Press.

Kia-Keating, M., Capous, D., Juang, L. & Bacio, G. (2016). Family factors: Immigrant families and intergenerational considerations. In S. Patel & Reicherter (Eds.) *Psychotherapy for immigrant youth* (pp. 49–70). Zurich: Springer International Publishing.

Lopez, M. H., Korgstad, J. M. & Passel, J. S. (2020). Who is Hispanic? *Pew Center for Research*. https://www.pewresearch.org/fact-tank/2020/09/15/who-is-hispanic/

Luhby, T. (2019, September 11). Democrats want to offer health care to undocumented immigrants. Here's what that means, *CNN*. https://www.cnn.com/2019/09/11/politics/undocumented-immigrants-health-care-democrats/index.html

Manuel, J., Krogstad, M. H. & Budiman, A. (2020). *Latino voters favor rising minimum wage, government involvement in healthcare, stricter gun laws.* Washington, DC: Pew Center for Research. https://www.pewresearch.org/fact-tank/2020/02/20/latino-voters-favor-raising-minimum-wage-government-involvement-in-health-care-stricter-gun-laws/

Mathema, S. (2017). *Keeping families together. Why all Americans should care about what happens to unauthorized immigrants.* Washington, DC: Center for American Progress. https://www.americanprogress.org/issues/immigration/reports/2017/03/16/428335/keeping-families-together/

National Immigration Law Center. (2021). *Medical assistance for immigrants in various states.* https://www.nilc.org/wp-content/uploads/2015/11/med-services-for-imms-in-states.pdf

Singhal, A. & Rogers, E. (2012). *Entertainment-education: A communication strategy for social change.* New York, NY: Lawrence Erlbaum Associates.

Sun, K. & Dutta, M. J. (2017). Meanings of care: A culture-centered approach to left-behind family members in the countryside of China. *Journal of Health Communication*, 21(11), 1141–1147. https://doi.org/10.1080/10810730.2016.1225869

2 Cultural Factors Influencing Health Literacy, Health Care Access, and Health Behaviors Among Korean-Americans

Kyeung Mi Oh, Kyungeh An, Moonju Lee, and Gary L. Kreps

According to the 2019 Census Bureau population estimate, approximately 18.9 million Asian Americans (hereafter AAs) live in the United States, and this population has been rapidly increasing. Korean Americans (hereafter KAs) comprise the fifth largest Asian American subgroup, with more than 1.9 million living in the United States in 2019 (Pew Research Center, 2019).

There have been several waves of KA immigrations which began before the turn of the 20th century. Since 1965, most Korean immigrants coming to the United States have been highly educated professionals or political refugees, while before 1965, most Korean immigrants coming to the United States were uneducated laborers (Shin, Shin, & Blanchette, n.d.;). However, since the US-amended immigration laws in the 1970s to restrict occupational preference admissions, Koreans have entered the United States primarily through family reunification preferences. Thus, the new immigrants represent a larger spectrum of education levels and occupational backgrounds reflective of the general South Korean population. A majority of KAs are relatively new immigrants, with 62% of Koreans were foreign-born in 2015 and 26% having arrived in the United States within the past ten years (Pew Research Center, 2019). As a recent immigrant group, KAs face many barriers to accessing relevant health information and health services, partly due to their low English language proficiency levels and their low rates of having health insurance (Oh, Kreps, & Jun, 2013).

Top Health Issues Among Korean Americans

Cancer is the leading cause of death for KAs (Chen Jr., 2005; Hastings et al., 2015; McCracken et al., 2007). KAs experience the highest mortality rates of any racial/ethnic group for several types of cancers, in particular those of infectious origins, such as cancers of the liver,

DOI: 10.4324/9781003230243-2

uterine, cervix, and stomach (Jemal et al., 2004; Lee et al., 2021; Miller et al., 2008). Despite their high cancer mortality rates, cancer screening rates among KAs are consistently lower than other ethnic groups, and the goals in Healthy People 2030 (Choi et al., 2010; Han et al., 2019; Jin et al., 2019; Lee & Lee, 2018; Maxwell et al., 2010; Pourat et al., 2010; Prevent Cancer Foundation, 2017; Tran et al., 2018; U.S. Department of Health and Human Services, 2011).

Cardiovascular disease (CVD) is the second leading cause of death following cancer in Asian Americans (AAs). Among them, the majority are foreign-born (Hastings, 2015). Heart disease is a significant cause of death in nearly every Asian subgroup and non-Hispanic White women (Hastings et al., 2015). Among the subgroups of AAs, KAs are no exception from the CVD risks and mortality: Heart disease is the second cause of death after cancer, and stroke is the third cause of death in KAs. Further, more KA men die from both heart disease and stroke than the KA men and women combined (21.6% vs. 19.2%, then 8.7% vs. 6.1%, respectively), when their mortality from cancer is lower than in KA men and women combined (30.3 vs. 34.2%) (Hastings et al., 2015). Moreover, previous studies have found a markedly higher prevalence of chronic health conditions (e.g. type 2 diabetes, high blood pressure, abnormal blood cholesterol, and metabolic syndrome) in KAs when compared with other same-aged Americans (Han et al., 2007; Kim et al., 2000, 2006; Shin et al., n.d.). The prevalence of diabetes has been more prevalent among KAs (16.8% in men, 12.6% in women) compared to non-Hispanic Whites (8.6% in men, 5.9% in women) after adjusting for age and body mass index (BMI) (Wang et al., 2011).

Nowadays, information and communication technology development has facilitated increasing dissemination of health-related information via many different communication channels that has led to information overload, especially for many immigrant populations (Kreps, 2012; Kreps & Neuhauser, 2015). Due to information overload, despite the growing body of health information available online, failure to use credible health information or understand health-related information may adversely impact an individual's health and could be a leading factor for health disparities (Custodio et al., 2009; Kreps, 2018). Health literacy was previously defined as "the degree to which individuals have the capacity to obtain, process, and understand basic health information and services needed to make appropriate health decisions", but it was updated in August 2020 with the release of the US government's Healthy People 2030 (CDC, 2021). The new definition emphasizes people's ability to *use* health information rather than just understand it and focuses on the ability to make "well-informed" decisions rather than "appropriate" ones. Health literacy issues that may limit understanding of relevant health information can be most problematic for those KA immigrants who are not native English speakers (Oh, Kreps, Jun, Chong, & Ramsey, 2012; Oh, Kreps, Jun, & Ramsey, 2011).

Health information seeking, the purposive acquisition of information from selected information carriers to guide health-related decision making (Freimuth et al., 1989; Kreps, 1988), has been increasingly examined in recent years (Brashers et al., 2002). Individuals who seek health information report that the information they acquire is highly influential in guiding their health behavior decisions (Freimuth et al., 1989; Niederdeppe & Levy, 2007). Also, health information seeking has been related to gains in knowledge and the adoption of recommended health behaviors such as adhering to cancer screening recommendations and healthy lifestyle behaviors (Shim et al., 2006). According to Ramanadhan and Viswanath (2006), ethnic groups experience reduced access to health-related information, leading to gaps in knowledge and widening health disparities. Despite evidence suggesting the importance of health information for promoting population health, there is little clarity about the unequal access to health information for KAs.

Due to the common practice of aggregating national health data for more than 60 Asian nationalities into one Asian American group, important cultural variables related to specific ethnicity have been missing from a major analysis of national data. Therefore, little is known about health and health information needs, barriers to health information seeking, communications and health care services of KAs. Therefore, this chapter reviews the study of KAs to describe the health information seeking behaviors and synthesize cultural and linguistic barriers to health literacy, health care access, and health behaviors among KAs. Based on synthesizing existing empirical evidence, we provide recommendations for strategies to promote proper health communication and optimize information seeking to meet the health priorities and demands in KAs.

Health Information Seeking Behaviors of Korean Americans

Sources of Health Information Seeking

In Lee et al.'s study (In Press), 72.5% of the participants sought health information from the internet and followed by health care providers (46.3%), and then family and friends (40%). These results were consistent with the Prevent Cancer Foundation (PCF) data that showed KA's most preferred source of health information is the internet, followed by health care providers, then ethnic newspapers (PCF, 2017). According to the results of a previous study (Oh et al., 2015), many participants have heard of cancer-related information often or very often from the Internet (35.2%), family or friends (31.6%), Korean TV (30.7%), and Korean newspaper/magazines (28.6%) in the past 12 months. On the other hand, the use of English language media, Korean radio, and doctors or other health care professionals as cancer information sources was limited. Many participants indicated that they had never obtained cancer information from US mainstream newspapers/magazines (45.7%) or US mainstream TV channels (40.2%). Interestingly, exposure to cancer information through doctors or health care professionals was also low – nearly 40% of participants had never received cancer information from health care professionals. Neither Korean radio (never = 46.8%) nor US mainstream radio (never = 58.8%) was used frequently for cancer information seeking. Although the Internet, family or friends, and Korean media were used more frequently than US mainstream media and doctors or other health care professionals, they were not necessarily the most trusted sources. Among survey participants, doctors and other health care professionals were the most trusted cancer information sources (47.2%), followed by Korean TV (22.6%), family or friends (20.3%), and Korean periodicals (17.3%). Meanwhile, a relatively high number of participants reported that they did not trust cancer information from the following sources at all: US radio (15.8%), US periodicals (14.3%), and US TV (12.0%). Correlation tests revealed mostly moderate to strong positive correlations between general exposure to and usage of cancer information sources. Overall, KAs were more likely to obtain cancer information from media that they have used frequently for general purposes. Relationships between usage frequency and trust in cancer information sources were mostly positive and weak to moderate in size. However, there was no significant correlation between use frequency and trust for doctor/health providers. Also, correlations for Korean radio and the Internet were significant, but negligible by conventional standards.

Use of and Trust in Health Information Sources

An important issue in the effective dissemination and reception of health information is trust (Gilson, 2003). Trust in health information has been found to play an important role in influencing health behaviors, such as vaccine acceptance (Nan et al., 2014), HIV and STI prevention (Veinot et al., 2013), and cancer screening (Ling et al., 2006). Communication research has long established trust as a fundamental dimension of source credibility (Pornpitakpan, 2004). Without a sufficient level of trust, factors such as expertise or quality of information are unlikely to generate meaningful influences on targeted audiences. Moreover, patients, caregivers, and the general public today are faced with vast amounts of cancer information from a wide variety of sources. To sift through the clutter of all this information and find the answers they need for cancer-related questions, users have to first ascertain the level of trust they can place in the information and its source (Hesse et al., 2005).

For these reasons and more, trust is often a critical determinant of the effectiveness of health communication efforts. Trust can be a particularly challenging problem when communicating with racial, ethnic, and other minority populations (Halbert et al., 2006).

Health Care Providers

Previous studies show that the most trusted source of health information among both KAs and native Koreans were health care providers (Oh et al., 2012, 2014). When comparing native Koreans with KAs, the levels of trust in health care providers as a source of health information were not significantly different. Doctors were a primary source of health information for the general population and other non-Asian minority groups (Hesse et al., 2005). In contrast, doctors or other health care professionals were the most trusted source for cancer information among KAs (Oh et al., 2012, 2014), but the Internet was their primary source for health, cancer, and stroke information (Oh et al., 2015; Song et al., 2013). Limited health care access, lack of familiarity with the US health care system, inadequate health insurance coverage, financial concerns, and language barriers all may lead individuals to be more active in seeking health information through available sources, such as online information (Kim, Kreps, & Shin, 2015; Kim & Yoon, 2012; Lee et al., 2018). The results of a mixed-methods study (Oh et al., 2015) also explored that health care professionals' health and cancer information was most highly trusted among the participants, but was also considered inaccessible or expensive. Moreover, the language barriers and cultural differences between KAs and most health care providers made it difficult for KA women to get health and cancer information from health professionals.

Internet

According to HINTS data collected in 2008, 55.3% of the US population reported that they searched the Internet first when they need cancer information, followed by 24.9% citing seeking information from their health care providers (National Cancer Institute [NCI]). In line with these findings from the general population, the Internet was most frequently used, but not highly trusted among KAs.

The Internet could be the only source for health and cancer information for some KAs, particularly if they do not have health insurance, and therefore, cannot visit a doctor, or if they are new immigrants with limited interpersonal networks in the United States. These consumers searched KA online communities where they could obtain advice and information from others. Consistently, a previous study (Kim & Yoon, 2012) found that married Korean women living in the United States commonly sought health information from online health forums. The most frequent questions asked in the forums were about recommendations for hospitals or doctors, including doctors who spoke Korean; potential causes of symptoms experienced, or treatment methods to consider before consulting a doctor. A multi-methodological study that triangulated both quantitative and qualitative data found that the use of online personal social support networks comprised of KA peers were important sources of both content and relational health information concerning cancer and other health issues for many KAs (Kim, Kreps, & Shin, 2015).

Numerous benefits to using the Internet have motivated KAs to use this important communication channel, including the ability to use the Internet as an easy and immediate information source to access, the ability to search Internet content, the easy collection and tracking of useful information on the Internet, and the Internet being a convenient gateway to accessing other forms of relevant health information and disease coping stories from current patients and survivors (Kreps, Beckjord, Atkinson, Saperstein, & Pleis, 2009; Oh et al., 2015). The explosion and proliferation of health information available online are on the promise that these online resources can confirm or broaden patients or families' understanding of diseases and treatment opinions that influence health care decisions and empower them to effectively self-manage health conditions (Du et al., 2016; Walsh & Volsko, 2008). Despite the various benefits of internet health information seeking, there are general concerns about the quality of online health information in terms of readability, suitability aspects, and trustworthiness (Lee et al., 2018). Particular concerns that KAs have are that online information may be biased, commercialized, and exaggerated (Oh et al., 2015).

Interpersonal Sources

Previous studies reported Asian Americans' heavy reliance on health information from families, friends, and ethnic/regional communities (Kim, Kreps, & Shin, 2015; Lee, 2010; Todd & Hoffman-Goetz, 2011). Consistent with these findings, a mixed methods study (Oh et al., 2015) indicated that interpersonal sources, including family and friends, are regarded as important sources for health and cancer information among KA women. Following the Internet, family or friends are the most frequently used sources of cancer information, but they are less trusted than health care professionals and Korean TV channels. Qualitative results also confirmed that word of mouth through family, friends and religious members is an important conduit for sharing health and cancer information among KA women (although information from interpersonal sources may not be relevant to their current information needs). Also, religious organizations, especially Korean churches, are an important channel for accessing cancer information for KA women. Beyond spiritual guidance and social support, Korean churches play an important role in providing health and cancer health information seminars, workshops, and free consulting from health professionals for KA women. About 80% of KAs are Christian and 63% participate in religious activities at least once a month (Lee et al., 2002; Suh, 2004). KAs' high level of participation in church activities may make Korean ethnic churches an especially important site for health communication.

Ethnic Media

When comparing native Koreans with KAs, the levels of trust in health care providers as a source of health information were not significantly different; however, KAs were three times more likely to trust health information from newspapers or magazines and 11 times more likely to read the health sections of newspapers or magazines (Oh et al., 2014). These findings suggest that immigration status can have profound influences on KAs' exposure to, and trust in, different health information sources (Oh et al., 2014). The reason for KAs heightened reliance on newspapers and magazines compared to native Koreans may be due to the limited health care access in the United States than a trust issue. Koreans in Korea have national health insurance and do not experience health care access issues, but in the United States, KAs have limited access to healthcare and it may lead to underutilization of health care services, although many factors can affect health care access. Availability of in-depth health or cancer information through specialized newspaper health sections was another merit of using Korean language newspapers. There are a number of KA periodicals available throughout the United States. Among the periodicals, the Korea Daily and the Korea Times are the most widely read Korean language daily newspapers in the United States and have online versions that can be searched for specific content (Jun & Oh, 2015). Also, Korean TV programs are beneficial to KAs to conveniently obtain entertaining, understandable, and reliable health and cancer information. Particularly, second-hand contact with health professionals and availability of culturally appropriate cancer information from both Western medicine and traditional Korean medicine perspectives (*Hanbang,* 漢方) was highly regarded as a merit of Korean TV programs. This positive perception towards cancer information provided by Korean ethnic media is also aligned with a previous study showing that Korean seniors described health care information on Korean mass media as diverse, comprehensive, and reachable (Lee et al., 2010).

KAs' health and cancer information-seeking behaviors are expected to be different from those of the general population as KAs are heavily dependent on ethnic Korean media (Oh et al., 2011, 2012, 2014, 2015;

Prevent Cancer Foundation, 2017). However, it also raises concerns about whether KAs are currently obtaining good-quality health information. Oh et al. (2011) examined cancer information seeking from and awareness of major national cancer information sources such as the NCI and NCI's Cancer Information Service among KAs. They found that KAs' frequency of US media use, including American TV, radio, newspaper, and the magazine, was significantly related to their awareness of cancer information resources, but their frequency of using Korean media was not related to such awareness. These findings suggest that ethnic media that KAs use frequently for general purposes may have limited effectiveness in providing them with credible cancer information and national efforts to convey health and cancer information to the overall US population that do not typically utilize Korean language messaging often fail to reach KAs (Oh et al., 2011).

Cultural and Linguistic Barriers to Health Literacy, Health Care Access, and Health Behaviors in Korean Americans

Limited health literacy is a critical barrier to health literacy and health care access (American Cancer Society [ACS], 2020; Lee et al., 2009). Limited health literacy is more likely to be associated with foreign-born, non-native speakers of English, and low level of acculturation (Berger et al., 2017; Kino & Kawachi, 2020).

Limited English Proficiency

Although more than half of Korean immigrants have a bachelor's degree or higher, the majority have limited proficiency in English (Lee & Lee, 2018; Terrazas, 2009). About 68% of KAs do not speak English at home, and 38% speak English less than "very well" (ACS, 2016). According to a state-wide public survey in California, 36% of KA respondents reported problems with understanding health information provided in their doctors' offices or clinics (New California Media, 2003). The majority of KAs with intermediate-level English skills do not feel comfortable communicating with English-speaking health care professionals (Oh, Kreps, Jun, & Ramsey, 2011; Oh, Kreps, Jun, Chong, & Ramsey, 2012).

In addition to language barriers, most mainstream healthcare providers are not familiar with the cultural perspectives that KAs have about health and healthcare services (Kim et al., 2002). These communication barriers may make it difficult for KAs to access healthcare services (Oh & Jacobsen, 2013). Limited English proficiency is highly relevant to low health literacy among KAs (Lee et al., 2018). The majority of foreign-born KAs with limited English skills are most likely to be isolated from communication. KAs who are recent immigrants may confront many barriers to accessing health information and services due to low levels of English language proficiency.

Limited Knowledge and Misperceptions about Specific Cancer and Cardiovascular Disease

Previous studies have linked limited literacy with challenges in health care, including lower health knowledge, misperceptions about specific cancers and chronic diseases, which are prevalent among KAs, lower receipt of preventive services, and poor chronic disease prevention and management. In general, socioeconomic status impacts health behaviors and CVD risk: people at lower socioeconomic status usually have increased CVD risks. However, in AAs who participated in National Health and Nutrition Examination Survey (NAHANES), the association between the socioeconomic status and an increase in CVD risks disappeared, different from other ethnic groups. Alternatively, some studies suggested that acculturation and perceived stress of KAs, particularly among foreign-born KAs, impact their health behaviors and subsequently affect the incidence of T2DM, hypertension, CVD, and stroke (An et al., 2008; Bhimla et al., 2019; Kim et al., 2007; Shin et al., 2018). According to a systematic review, the consumption of a high-sodium diet, physical inactivity, smoking, and higher incidence of hypertension and diabetes are higher among KAs than other ethnic groups (Shin et al., 2018). Nevertheless, a majority of KAs were not well informed about their chronic diseases and tended to depend on traditional medications according to studies conducted in the early 2000s (Kim, Han, Kim, & Duong, 2002; Shin et al., n.d.). A decade later, studies reported that KAs demonstrated their understanding of CVD, including the cause of the heart disease, symptoms of heart disease, yet lacked knowledge of stroke symptoms.

Moreover, KAs lack adequate information about cancer screening tests, and knowledge and perceptions play an important role in cancer screenings among KAs. Previous studies suggest that a lack of adequate information about cancer and cancer screening is one of the primary reasons why KAs have low cancer screening rates (Kim et al., 1999; Oh et al., 2011, 2015; Oh, Kreps et al., 2013). For instance, Maxwell et al. (2010) found that the leading reason for not receiving colorectal cancer screening among five different Asian American subgroups was not the cost, lack of insurance, or not having a doctor, but being unaware of colorectal cancer tests. Knowledge of general cancer warning signs or colorectal cancer information is associated with higher screening rates, as is specific knowledge about colorectal cancer screening tests, where to go for testing, and the age at which testing should begin (Jo et al., 2008; Kim et al., 1998; Maxwell et al., 2010; Oh, Jun, et al., 2013). Among KA women, those who are knowledgeable about screening guidelines

(Juon et al., 2004; Lee, Nandy, Szalacha, Park, Oh, Lee, & Menon, 2015) and have read printed health education materials (Wismer et al., 1998) have higher rates of mammography. Not knowing where to go for screening (Kim & Menon, 2009) and the perception that it is difficult to access mammography (Han et al., 2000; Kim, 2014; Kim et al., 2010; Lee et al., 2015; Maxwell et al., 1998) are barriers to cancer screening among KA women.

Also, cultural factors might be contributing to the lower-than-typical rates of colorectal cancer screening among KAs. The cultural barriers include the misperception that Korean diets and lifestyles reduce the likelihood of developing colorectal cancer, some aspects of fatalism that might downplay the perceived severity of cancer (Lee & Lee, 2018; Tran et al., 2018; Yun & Im, 2013), the common belief that only symptomatic people need cancer screening and routine testing may be of limited benefit (Jung et al., 2018), and a preference for traditional Korean approaches to medicine and healthcare that may be a barrier to following US recommendations for cancer screening (Kim et al., 2002). However, most mainstream health care providers are not familiar with the health needs of KA immigrants, the unique barriers they face, and their views about health (Kim, Cho, Cheon-Klessig, Gerace, & Camilleri, 2002). Therefore, 75% of KAs prefer to visit Korean-speaking doctors (Asian Pacific Islander American Health Forum [APIAHF], 2006; Shin & Robert, 2010). However, Korean speaking doctors tend not to recommend cancer screening tests at the same rates as other doctors. For example, surveys found that women who received care from Korean doctors were less likely to have had a recent Pap test, mammogram, or clinical breast examination than women who received care from a non-Korean doctor (Lew et al., 2003; Moskowitz et al., 2004). This disparity in receiving cancer screening tests could be related to the fact that many Korean doctors do not view cancer screening as a priority. However, a previous study indicated a contradictory finding. According to Maxwell et al. (2009), numerous Korean physicians state that "screening" or testing in the absence of symptoms is an unfamiliar concept to many KAs, especially among the elderly. They explained that although disease prevention and health maintenance are highly important in this population, the concept of "preventive medicine" is relatively new and unfamiliar. They insist that their patients generally equate having no symptoms with having good health or having no disease. Consistent with these findings, mammography is only believed to be necessary when symptoms are present (Maxwell et al., 1998).

Cultural Competence

Asian American immigrant patients' communication dissatisfaction with their doctors due to cultural incongruities was pointed out in previous studies (Chen et al., 2010). According to Ngo-Metzger et al. (2004), Asian American patients who place greater emphasis on their cultural values may often feel that their doctors do not understand their values and thus they often have lower satisfaction with their medical care. Such patients may also be less likely to seek information from health care professionals. Lee, Kearns, and Friesen (2010) reported that Korean patients experience more distrust and anxiety during communication with Western doctors who often appear to be less confident in their diagnosing practices in comparison with Korean doctors who tend to be authoritative and confident about their diagnoses. Among KA women, fear of embarrassment or concerns about modesty (Lee et al., 2009; Maxwell et al., 1998) are barriers to screening, along with discomfort with asking a physician for a referral for a mammogram (Maxwell et al., 1998). Kim, Kreps, and Shin (2015) found that social support was often sought online among KA peers to address both informational and emotional health concerns.

Social Support

Social support played a critical role in moderating the adverse effects of acculturation stress for KA immigrants. The results of a recent study (Sagong & Yoon, 2021) indicated that limited health literacy and lack of social support directly led to poor health. Social support and acculturation were identified to influence health literacy. Health literacy had a partial mediating effect in the relationship between social support and poor health and a complete mediating effect in the relationship between acculturation and poor health.

A variety of perceptions about social support are also influential, including being encouraged to seek screening by a family member, friend, or physician; discussing colorectal cancer screening with a family member or friend who has been tested for colorectal cancer; feeling that the family would be supportive if the test detected cancer; and believing that the usual healthcare provider is trustworthy (Jo et al., 2008). These findings address that it is necessary to consider enhancing immigrants' health literacy by elevating acculturation and access to social support to prevent negative health outcomes.

Discussions on Health Communication Needs and Priorities of Korean Americans

This review synthesized that KAs' employ unique health information-seeking behaviors as they adjust to their new environment as immigrants, health information needs, and cultural barriers to desirable health behaviors. This review also supports developing culturally sensitive health communication interventions using Korean language media including print, television, and the Internet for health promotion and cancer prevention targeting KAs to reduce health disparities.

Understanding patterns of media use and trust in health information sources are useful when designing health promotion campaigns (Clayman et al., 2010). There is no doubt that trust is an important factor in the selection of health information sources. However, there seem to be many other factors that can determine the actual use of sources of health and cancer information such as accessibility, affordability, language proficiency, cultural sensitivity, meeting immediate needs, understandability, convenience, and reliability (Oh et al., 2015). These factors may have played a role in the insignificant or negligible relationships between usage frequency and trust in the sources of health information. Our review identified that KAs are more likely to obtain health information from the specific media that they use frequently for general purposes. This communication behavior has important implications for developing communication interventions for health promotion and disease prevention. However, it also raises concerns about whether KAs are currently obtaining good-quality health information. The findings of previous studies indicated that ethnic media that KAs use frequently for general purposes may have limited effectiveness in providing them with credible health information (Oh et al., 2011; Oh, Kreps, Jun, Chong, & Ramsey, 2012). However, the importance of Korean ethnic media is undeniable as a potential channel for providing relevant health information to this population.

Although doctors and other health care professionals were the most trusted health information sources, the frequently used health information resources for KAs are the internet, newspaper/magazines, and family/friends (Oh, Zhou, Kreps, & Kim, 2014; Lee et al., in press; Oh, 2015a). This tendency was also significantly higher compared to those of Koreans in Korea. KAs' health information seeking behavior might be influenced by the lack of access to health care services. Koreans in Korea have national health insurance, and it covers mandatory preventive care services with major cancer screening (National Health Insurance Service, 2020). However, KAs have limited healthcare access and English proficiency in the United States as immigrants, leading to healthcare services underutilization. Although rates of health insurance coverage increased in KAs after the passage of the Affordable Care Act (Jin et al., 2019; Jung et al., 2018; Lee & Lee, 2018; Park et al., 2019), little has been studied concerning the impact of improved health insurance on healthcare service utilization. According to the Lee et al. study (2021, in press), Asian Americans had marginal health literacy, poor understanding of health insurance and insurance coverage, underutilize of health care services, and engaged in undesirable health behaviors.

Online health information has become increasingly common as a source of health information by connecting individuals with health content, experts, and support among those who use the internet, particularly underserved immigrants with low level of English proficiency and acculturation including KA immigrants (Islam et al., 2016; Kim & Yoon, 2012; Oh et al., 2011, 2012). The Internet may serve an important role for individuals preventing disease and managing chronic illness. Nowadays, health professionals have contributed to online health information, however a large amount of online health information originates from individuals sharing health experiences. For example, online social media, which is increasingly popular, such as online health forums and support groups, allow a growing number of people to find peers who experience similar health conditions or concerns or to follow others' health related experience (Kreps, 2017). However, the quality of such online health information remains questionable, and the trustworthiness of online health information has been a concern. Questionable health information may have an adverse impact on lifestyle behavior and health-related decisions of KAs. With pervasive mobile technologies and the popularity of social media, future research focusing on the development of culturally and linguistically competent mobile health interventions to improve health literacy and overcome identified barriers of health promoting behavior such as early disease detection and prevention and chronic disease self-care management. Culturally competent information and education program may offer a way to improve health litracy and ultimately health outcomes of underserved KA immigrants. Finally, customized public health and health communication programs will meet the needs by addressing cultural and linguistic barriers related to health and health communication among KA immigrants.

References

American Cancer Society. (2016). California cancer facts and figures 2016. Special section: Cancer in Asian Americans, Native Hawaiians, and Pacific Islanders.

American Cancer Society. (2020). Cancer Facts & Figures 2020. https://www.cancer.org/content/dam/cancer-org/research/cancer-facts-and-statistics/annual-cancer-facts-and-figures/2020/cancer-facts-and figures-2020 pdf

An, N., Cochran, S. D., Mays, V. M., & McCarthy, W. J. (2008). Influence of American acculturation on cigarette smoking behaviors among Asian American subpopulations in California. *Nicotine & Tobacco Research: Official Journal of the Society for Research on Nicotine and Tobacco*, 10(4), 579–587.

Asian Pacific Islander American Health Forum (APIAHF). (2006). Asian and Pacific Islander American Health Forum, Health Brief: Koreans in the United States. Asian and Pacific Islander American Health Forum. http://www.api-cat.org/wp-content/uploads/2010/09/Tobacco-Brief-APIAHF.pdf

Berger, S., Huang, C.-C., & Rubin, C. L. (2017). The role of community education in increasing knowledge of breast health and cancer: Findings from the Asian Breast Cancer Project in Boston, Massachusetts. *Journal of Cancer Education*, 32(1), 16–23.

Bhimla, A., Gadegbeku, C. A., Tan, Y., Zhu, L., Aczon, F., & Ma, G. X. (2019). A study of physical activity determinants among high-risk hypertensive Filipino and Korean Americans. *International Journal of Environmental Research and Public Health*, 16(7), 1156.

Brashers, D. E., Goldsmith, D. J., & Hsieh, E. (2002). Information seeking and avoiding in health contexts. *Human Communication Research*, 28(2), 258–271.

Centers for Disease Control and Prevention. (2021, January 28). What is health literacy? https://www.cdc.gov/healthliteracy/learn/index.html

Chen, C.-J., Kendall, J., & Shyu, Y.-I. L. (2010). Grabbing the rice straw: Health information seeking in Chinese immigrants in the United States. *Clinical Nursing Research*, 19(4), 335–353.

Chen Jr., M. S. (2005). Cancer health disparities among Asian Americans. *Cancer*, 104(S12), 2895–2902.

Choi, K. S., Lee, S., Park, E., Kwak, M., Spring, B. J., & Juon, H. (2010). Comparison of breast cancer screening rates between Korean women in America versus Korea. *Journal of Women's Health* (15409996), 19(6), 1089–1096.

Clayman, M. L., Manganello, J. A., Viswanath, K., Hesse, B. W., & Arora, N. K. (2010). Providing health messages to Hispanics/Latinos: understanding the importance of language, trust in health information sources, and media use. *Journal of Health Communication*, 15(Suppl 3), 252–263.

Custodio, R., Gard, A. M., & Graham, G. (2009). Health information technology: Addressing health disparity by improving quality, increasing access, and developing workforce. *Journal of Health Care for the Poor and Underserved*, 20(2), 301–307.

Du, H.-S., Ma, J.-J., & Li, M. (2016). High-quality health information provision for stroke patients. *Chinese Medical Journal*, 129(17), 2115–2122.

Freimuth, V. S., Stein, J. A., & Kean, T. J. (1989). *Searching for health information: The cancer information service model.* University of Pennsylvania Press.

Gilson, L. (2003). Trust and the development of health care as a social institution. *Social Science & Medicine* (1982), 56(7), 1453–1468.

Halbert, C. H., Armstrong, K., Gandy, O. H., & Shaker, L. (2006). Racial differences in trust in health care providers. *Archives of Internal Medicine*, 166(8), 896–901.

Han, H.-R., Kim, K., Cudjoe, J., & Kim, M. T. (2019). Familiarity, navigation, and comprehension: Key dimensions of health literacy in pap test use among Korean American women. *Journal of Health Communication*, 24(6), 585–591.

Han, H.-R., Kim, K. B., & Kim, M. T. (2007). Evaluation of the training of Korean community health workers for chronic disease management. *Health Education Research*, 22(4), 513–521.

Han, Y., Williams, R., & Harrison, R. (2000). Breast cancer screening knowledge, attitudes, and practices among Korean American women. *Oncology Nursing Forum*, 27(10), 1585–1591.

Hastings, K. G., Jose, P. O., Kapphahn, K. I., Frank, A. T. H., Goldstein, B. A., Thompson, C. A., Eggleston, K., Cullen, M. R., & Palaniappan, L. P. (2015). Leading causes of death among Asian American Subgroups (2003–2011). *PLoS One*, 10(4), e0124341.

Hesse, B. W., Nelson, D. E., Kreps, G. L., Croyle, R. T., Arora, N. K., Rimer, B. K., & Viswanath, K. (2005). Trust and sources of health information: The impact of the Internet and its implications for health care providers: Findings from the first Health Information National Trends Survey. *Archives of Internal Medicine*, 165(22), 2618–2624.

Islam, N. S., Patel, S., Wyatt, L. C., Sim, S.-C., Mukherjee-Ratnam, R., Chun, K., Desai, B., Tandon, S. D., Trinh-Shevrin, C., Pollack, H., & Kwon, S. C. (2016). Sources of health information among select Asian American immigrant groups in New York City. *Health Communication*, 31(2), 207–216.

Jemal, A., Tiwari, R. C., Murray, T., Ghafoor, A., Samuels, A., Ward, E., Feuer, E. J., & Thun, M. J. (2004). Cancer statistics, 2004. *CA: A Cancer Journal For Clinicians*, 54(1), 8–29.

Jin, S. W., Lee, H. Y., & Lee, J. (2019). Analyzing factors of breast cancer screening adherence among Korean American Women using Andersen's behavioral model of healthcare services utilization. *Ethnicity & Disease*, 29(Suppl 2), 427–434.

Jo, A., Maxwell, A., Wong, W., & Bastani, R. (2008). Colorectal cancer screening among underserved Korean Americans in Los Angeles County. *Journal of Immigrant & Minority Health*, 10(2), 119–126.

Jun, J., & Oh, K. M. (2015). Framing risks and benefits of medical tourism: A content analysis of medical tourism coverage in Korean American community newspapers. *Journal of Health Communication*, 20(6), 720–727.

Jung, M. Y., Holt, C. L., Ng, D., Sim, H. J., Lu, X., Le, D., Juon, H.-S., Li, J., & Lee, S. (2018). The Chinese and Korean American immigrant experience: A mixed-methods examination of facilitators and barriers of colorectal cancer screening. *Ethnicity & Health*, 23(8), 847–866.

Juon, H.-S., Kim, M., Shankar, S., & Han, W. (2004). Predictors of adherence to screening mammography among Korean American women. *Preventive Medicine*, 39(3), 474–481.

Kim, J. H., & Menon, U. (2009). Pre- and postintervention differences in acculturation, knowledge, beliefs, and stages of readiness for mammograms among Korean American women. *Oncology Nursing Forum*, 36(2), E80–E92.

Kim, J. H., Menon, U., Wang, E., & Szalacha, L. (2010). Assess the effects of culturally relevant intervention on breast cancer knowledge, beliefs, and mammography use among Korean American women. *Journal of Immigrant and Minority Health*, 12(4), 586–597.

Kim, J. K. (2014). Effects of acculturation on mammography utilization among Korean American women. (UMI Order AAI3578854.) [University of San Diego].

Kim, K., Yu, E., Chen, E., Kim, J., & Brintnall, R. A. (1998). Colorectal Cancer Screening knowledge and practices among Korean Americans. *Cancer Practice*, 6(3), 167–175.

Kim, K., Yu, E. S. H., Chen, E. H., Kim, J., Kaufman, M., & Purkiss, J. (1999). Cervical cancer screening knowledge and practices among Korean-American women. *Cancer Nursing*, 22, 297–302.

Kim, M., Han, H.-R., Kim, K. B., & Duong, D. N. (2002). The use of traditional and Western medicine among Korean American elderly. *Journal of Community Health*, 27(2), 109–120.

Kim, M. J., Cho, H.-I., Cheon-Klessig, Y. S., Gerace, L. M., & Camilleri, D. D. (2002). Primary health care for Korean immigrants: Sustaining a culturally sensitive model. *Public Health Nursing*, 19(3), 191–200.

Kim, M. J., Lee, S. J., Ahn, Y.-H., Bowen, P., & Lee, H. (2007). Dietary acculturation and diet quality of hypertensive Korean Americans. *Journal of Advanced Nursing*, 58(5), 436–445.

Kim, M. T., Kim, K. B., Juon, H. S., & Hill, M. N. (2000). Prevalence and factors associated with high blood pressure in Korean Americans. *Ethnicity & Disease*, 10(3), 364–374.

Kim, S. M., Lee, J. S., Lee, J., Na, J. K., Han, J. H., Yoon, D. K., Baik, S. H., Choi, D. S., & Choi, K. M. (2006). Prevalence of diabetes and impaired fasting glucose in Korea: Korean National Health and Nutrition Survey 2001. *Diabetes Care*, 29(2), 226–231.

Kim, S., & Yoon, J. (2012, June 15). The use of an online forum for health information by married Korean women in the United States. *Information Research*, 17(2), 1–18.

Kim, W., Kreps, G. L., & Shin, C-N. (2015). The role of social support and social networks in health information-seeking behavior among Korean Americans: A qualitative study. *International Journal of Equity in Health*, 14(40). DOI 10.1186/s12939-015-0169-8.

Kino, S., & Kawachi, I. (2020). Can health literacy boost health services utilization in the context of expanded access to health insurance? *Health Education & Behavior: The Official Publication of the Society for Public Health Education*, 47(1), 134–142.

Kreps, G. L. (1988). The pervasive role of information in health and health care: Implications for health communication policy. In J. Anderson (Ed.), *Communication yearbook* (Vol. 11, pp. 238–276). Sage.

Kreps, G. L. (2012). Strategic communication for cancer prevention and control: Reaching and influencing vulnerable audiences. In A. Georgakilas (Ed). *Cancer prevention* (pp. 375–388). Vienna: Intech Publishers.

Kreps, G. L. (2017). Online information and systems to enhance health outcomes through communication convergence. *Human Communication Research*, 43(4), 518–530.

Kreps, G. L. (2018). Promoting patient comprehension of relevant health information. *Israel Journal of Health Policy Research*, 7, 56, https://doi.org/10.1186/s13584-018-0250-z

Kreps, G. L., Beckjord, E. B., Atkinson, N. L., Saperstein, S. L., & Pleis, J. R. (2009). Using the Internet for health-related activities: Findings from a national probability sample. *Journal of Medical Internet Research*. DOI:10.2196/jmir.1035

Kreps, G. L., & Neuhauser, L. (2015). Designing health information programs to promote the health and well-being of vulnerable populations: The benefits of evidence-based strategic health communication. In C. A. Smith & A. Keselman (Eds.), *Meeting health information needs outside of healthcare: Opportunities and challenges* (pp. 3–17). Waltham, MA: Chandos Publishing.

Lee, E. E., Nandy, K., Szalacha, L., Park, H., Oh, K. M., Lee, J., & Menon, U. (2015). Korean American women and mammogram uptake. *Journal of Immigrant And Minority Health*, 18(10), 179–186.Lee, H., Kim, J., & Han, H.-R.

(2009). Do cultural factors predict mammography behaviour among Korean immigrants in the USA? *Journal of Advanced Nursing*, 65(12), 2574–2584.

Lee, H. J., Kazinets, G., & Moskowitz, J. (2002). *Korean American community health survey: Alameda and Santa Clara Counties, CA*. Center for Family and Community Health, University of California at Berkeley.

Lee, H. Y., Stange, M. J., & Ahluwalia, J. S. (2015). Breast cancer screening behaviors among Korean American immigrant women: Findings from the health belief model. *Journal of Transcultural Nursing: Official Journal of the Transcultural Nursing Society / Transcultural Nursing Society*, 26(5), 450–457.

Lee, J. S. (2010). Channels of health communications used among Korean and Asian Indian older adults. *Social Work in Health Care*, 49(2), 165–175.

Lee, J. Y., Kearns, R. A., & Friesen, W. (2010). Seeking affective health care: Korean immigrants' use of homeland medical services. *Health & Place*, 16(1), 108–115.

Lee, M., Lee, M. A., Ahn, H., Ko, J., Yon, E., Lee, J., Kim, M. T., & Braden, C. J. (In Press). *Health literacy and access to care on cancer screening among Korean Americans*. Health Literacy Research and Practice.

Lee, M. A., Shin, C.-N., & An, K. (2018). Trustworthiness, readability, and suitability of web-based information for stroke prevention and self-management for Korean Americans: Critical evaluation. *Interactive Journal of Medical Research*, 7(2). https://doi.org/10.2196/10440

Lee, R. J., Madan, R. A., Kim, J., Posadas, E. M., & Yu, E. Y. (2021). Disparities in cancer care and the Asian American population. *The Oncologist*, 26, 453–460.

Lee, S. Y., & Lee, E. E. (2018). Access to health care, beliefs, and behaviors about colorectal cancer screening among Korean Americans. *Asian Pacific Journal Of Cancer Prevention: APJCP*, 19(7), 2021–2027.

Lee, T. W., Kang, S. J., Lee, H. J., & Hyun, S. I. (2009). Testing health literacy skills in older Korean adults. *Patient Education and Counseling*, 75(3), 302–307.

Lew, A. A., Moskowitz, J. M., Ngo, L., Wismer, B. A., Wong, J. M., Ahn, Y., & Tager, I. B. (2003). Effect of provider status on preventive screening among Korean-American women in Alameda County, California. *Preventive Medicine*, 36(2), 141–149.

Ling, B. S., Klein, W. M., & Dang, Q. (2006). Relationship of communication and information measures to colorectal cancer screening utilization: Results From HINTS. *Journal of Health Communication: International Perspectives*, 11(1 supp 1), 181–190.

Maxwell, A. E., Bastani, R., & Warda, U. S. (1998). Misconceptions and mammography use among Filipino-and Korean-American women. *Ethnicity & Disease*, 8(3), 377–384. mnh.

Maxwell, Annette E., Crespi, C. M., Antonio, C. M., & Peiyun Lu. (2010). Explaining disparities in colorectal cancer screening among five Asian ethnic groups: A population-based study in California. *BMC Cancer*, 10, 214–222.

McCracken, M., Olsen, M., Chen, M. S., Jemal, A., Thun, M., Cokkinides, V., Deapen, D., & Ward, E. (2007). Cancer incidence, mortality, and associated risk factors among Asian Americans of Chinese, Filipino, Vietnamese, Korean, and Japanese ethnicities. *CA: A Cancer Journal for Clinicians*, 57(4), 190–205.

Miller, B. A., Chu, K. C., Hankey, B. F., & Ries, L. A. G. (2008). Cancer incidence and mortality patterns among specific Asian and Pacific Islander populations in the U.S. *Cancer Causes & Control*, 19(3), 227–256.

Moskowitz, J. M., Kazinets, G., Tager, I. B., & Wong, J. M. (2004). Breast and cervical cancer screening among Korean women, Santa Clara County, California, 1994 and 2002. *Morbidity and Mortality Weekly Report*, 53(33), 765–767.

Nan, X., Zhao, X., & Briones, R. (2014). Parental cancer beliefs and trust in health information from medical authorities as predictors of HPV vaccine acceptability. *Journal of Health Communication*, 19(1), 100–114.

National Health Insurance Service. (2020). National Health Insurance Program. https://www.nhis.or.kr/static/html/wbd/g/a/wbdga0401.html

New California Media. (2003). *Bridging language barriers in health care: Public opinion survey of California immigrants from Latin America, Asia and the Middle East*. New California Media. http://bendixenandamandi.com/wp-content/uploads/2010/08/NCM-Health-Care-Presentation-2003.pdf

Ngo-Metzger, Q., Legedza, A. T. R., & Phillips, R. S. (2004). Asian Americans' reports of their health care experiences: Results of a National Survey. *Journal of General Internal Medicine*, 19(2), 111–119.

Niederdeppe, J., & Levy, A. G. (2007). Fatalistic beliefs about cancer prevention and three prevention behaviors. *Cancer Epidemiology, Biomarkers & Prevention: A Publication of the American Association For Cancer Research, Cosponsored By The American Society Of Preventive Oncology*, 16(5), 998–1003.

Oh, K., Kreps, G., Jun, J., & Ramsey, L. (2011). Cancer information seeking and awareness of cancer information sources among Korean Americans. *Journal of Cancer Education*, 26(2), 355–364. h

Oh, K. M., & Jacobsen, K. H. (2013). Colorectal cancer screening among Korean Americans: A systematic review. *Journal of Community Health*, 39(2), 193–200.

Oh, K. M., Jun, J., Zhao, X., Lee, E., & Kreps, G. (2015). Cancer information seeking behaviors of Korean American women: A mixed methods study using surveys and focus group interviews. *Journal of Health Communication*, 20(10), 1–12.

Oh, K. M., Kreps, G. L., & Jun, J. (2013). Colorectal cancer screening knowledge, beliefs, and practices of Korean Americans. *American Journal of Health Behavior*, 37(3), 381–394.

Oh, K. M., Kreps, G. L., Jun, J., Chong, E., & Ramsey, L. (2012). Examining the health information-seeking behaviors of Korean Americans. *Journal of Health Communication*, 17(7), 779–801.

Oh, K. M., Kreps, G. L., Jun, J., & Ramsey, L. (2011). Cancer information seeking and awareness of cancer information sources among Korean Americans. *Journal of Cancer Education: The Official Journal of the American Association for Cancer Education*, 26(2), 355–364.

Oh, K. M., Zhou, Q. (Pearl), Kreps, G., & Kim, W. (2014). The influences of immigration on health information seeking behaviors among Korean Americans and Native Koreans. *Health Education & Behavior*, 41(2), 173–185.

Park, S., Stimpson, J. P., Pintor, J. K., Roby, D. H., McKenna, R. M., Chen, J., & Ortega, A. N. (2019). The effects of the affordable care act on health care access and utilization among Asian American subgroups. *Medical Care*, 57(11), 861–868.

Pew Research Center. (2019). Koreans in the U.S. Fact Sheet. https://www.pewresearch.org/social-trends/fact-sheet/asian-americans-koreans-in-the-u-s/

Pornpitakpan, C. (2004). The persuasiveness of source credibility: A critical review of five decades' evidence. *Journal of Applied Social Psychology*, 34(2), 243–281.

Pourat, N., Kagawa-Singer, M., Breen, N., & Sripipatana, A. (2010). Access versus acculturation: Identifying modifiable factors to promote cancer screening among Asian American women. *Medical Care*, 48(12), 1088–1096.

Prevent Cancer Foundation. (2017). 80% by 2018. Recommended messages to reach Asian Americans. Asian Americans and Colorectal Cancer Companion Guide. https://nccrt.org/resource/asian-americans-colorectal-cancer-companion-guide/

Ramanadhan, S., & Viswanath, K. (2006). Health and the information non-seeker: A profile. *Health Communication*, 20(2), 131–139.

Sagong, H., & Yoon, J. Y. (2021). Pathways among frailty, health literacy, acculturation, and social support of middle-aged and older Korean immigrants in the USA. *International Journal of Environmental Research and Public Health*, 18(3). https://doi.org/10.3390/ijerph18031245

Shim, M., Kelly, B., & Hornik, R. (2006). Cancer information scanning and seeking behavior is associated with knowledge, lifestyle choices, and screening. *Journal of Health Communication*, 11(Suppl 1), 157–172.

Shin, C.-N., Keller, C., An, K., & Sim, J. (2018). Cardiovascular disease in Korean Americans: A systematic review. *Journal of Cardiovascular Nursing*, 33(1), 82–93.

Shin, H. B., & Robert, A. K. (2010). *Language use in the United States: 2007, American community survey reports, ACS-12*. Washington, DC: U.S. Census Bureau.

Shin, K. R., Shin, C., & Blanchette, P. L. (n.d.). Health and health care of Korean-American elders. http://www.stanford.edu/group/ethnoger/korean.html

Song, S., Son, J., Park, H., Park, H., Chung, J., Panel, T. S.-C. C. A., Ryan, G., & Vickrey, B. (2013). Exploring stroke knowledge in Korean-American Seniors: The strengthening our korean elders through community-partnered education (STROKE-COPE) project (P05.237). *Neurology*, 80(7 Supplement), P05.237–P05.237.

Suh, S. A. (2004). *Being Buddhist in a Christian World: Gender and community in a Korean American temple – Sharon A. Suh*. University of Washington Press.

Terrazas, A. (2009). *Migration Information source—Korean immigrants in the United States*. Migration Policy Institute. http://www.migrationinformation.org/usfocus/display.cfm?ID=716

Todd, L., & Hoffman-Goetz, L. (2011). A qualitative study of cancer information seeking among English-as-a-second-Language older Chinese immigrant women to canada: Sources, barriers, and strategies. *Journal of Cancer Education: The Official Journal of the American Association for Cancer Education*, 26(2), 333–340.

Ton, T. G. N., Steinman, L., Yip, M.-P., Ly, K. A., Sin, M.-K., Fitzpatrick, A. L., & Tu, S.-P. (2011). Knowledge of cardiovascular health among Chinese,

Korean and Vietnamese immigrants to the US. *Journal of Immigrant and Minority Health*, 13(1), 127–139.

Tran, M. T., Jeong, M. B., Nguyen, V. V., Sharp, M. T., Yu, E. P., Yu, F., Tong, E. K., Kagawa-Singer, M., Cuaresma, C. F., Sy, A. U., Tsoh, J. Y., Gildengorin, G. L., Stewart, S. L., & Nguyen, T. T. (2018). Colorectal cancer beliefs, knowledge, and screening among Filipino, Hmong, and Korean Americans. *Cancer*, 124(Suppl 7), 1552–1559.

U.S. Department of Health and Human Services. (2011). *Healthy people 2020 topics and objectives: Cancer.* http://www.healthypeople.gov/2020/topicsobjectives2020/objectiveslist.aspx?topicId=5

Veinot, T. C., Campbell, T. R., Kruger, D. J., & Grodzinski, A. (2013). A question of trust: User-centered design requirements for an informatics intervention to promote the sexual health of African-American youth. *Journal of the American Medical Informatics Association: JAMIA*, 20(4), 758–765.

Walsh, T. M., & Volsko, T. A. (2008). Readability assessment of internet-based consumer health information. *Respiratory Care*, 53(10), 1310–1315.

Wang, E. J., Wong, E. C., Dixit, A. A., Fortmann, S. P., Linde, R. B., & Palaniappan, L. P. (2011). Type 2 diabetes: Identifying high risk Asian American subgroups in a clinical population. *Diabetes Research and Clinical Practice*, 93(2), 248–254.

Wismer, B. A., Moskowitz, J. M., Chen, A. M., Kang, S. H., Novotny, T. E., Min, K., Lew, R., & Tager, I. B. (1998). Mammography and clinical breast examination among Korean American women in two California counties. *Preventive Medicine*, 27(1), 144–151.

Yun, L. H., & Im, H. (2013). Colorectal cancer screening among Korean American immigrants: Unraveling the influence of culture. *Journal of Health Care for the Poor & Underserved*, 24(2), 579–598.

3 Addressing the Health Communication Challenges facing Chinese American Immigrants

Xuewei Chen, Ming Li, and Gary L. Kreps

Accoridng to the Pew Research Center analysis of US Census Bureau population estimates, the Asian American population (including all national subgroups) was the fastest growing racial/ethinic minority group in the United States between the years 2000 and 2019, with total population estimates ranging from 10.5 million to 18.9 million people (Pew Research Center, 2021a). The Chinese American (C-A) subgroup comprises the largest subpopuation (23%) of Asian people living in the United States (Pew Research Center, 2012). Demographic data that was reported in 2019 estimated that there were 5.4 million Chinese living in the United States and that C-As were the fastest growing immigrant population living in the United States (Pew Research Center, 2021b). Also according to a report by the Pew Research Center (2021b), about 76% of C-As living in the United States who are 18 years old or above were born outside of the United States and only 39% of Chinese immigrants living in the United States speak Enlgish very well. The majority of C-As (81%) speak Mandarin or Cantonese at home, and the median annual household income of Chinese living in the United States was $65,050, with a poverty rate of 13% (Pew Research Center, 2021b).

The earliest groups of C-A immigrants migrated to the United States during the California gold rush in the 1850s, often as construction workers to help build railroads and to construct other parts of the physical infrastructure of the rapidly develping West coast of America (Office of the Historian, 2021; Pew Research Center, 2021c; Voss, 2018). These early Chinese immigrants were primarily men who worked long hours of back-breaking work as laborers, often in very poor work and living conditions, and for minimal pay, while leaving most of their families back in China (Black, 1963; Office of the Historian, 2021). Eventually many of these C-A laborers were able to bring some members of their trailing families to the United States once they had earned adequate funds to repatriate with them (Black, 1963; Chen, 2019). The newer C-A arrivals often found work as house servants, cooking, cleaning, and taking care of children, adding a more domesticated employment path to the established construction laborer vocation for new C-As. Importantly, these C-A immigrants were often quite industrious, thrifty,

DOI: 10.4324/9781003230243-3

and entrepreneurial people who eventually began to start their own businesses, stores, and restaurants in America (Zhou & Liu, 2017). Over the past four decades, there have been increasing numbers of well-educated professionals among the Chinese immigrants, reflecting a high priority for educational attainment among members of this cultural group (Hooper & Batalova, 2015). Due to the high cultural value that many C-A immigrants placed on educational attainment, strong work ethic, and commitment to family, CAs have made significant contrbutions to their adopted country (Yung, Chang, & Lai, 2006; Zhou & Liu, 2017). Unfortunately, this has not always translated into the best health care for Chinese immigrants in the United States.

Sadly, there have been many serious challenges that C-A immigrants have faced with efforts to acculturate to life in the United States due to a complex confluence of serious, and often insidious, cultural factors, including relatively low levels of English language proficiency among many new C-A immigrants, difficulties in adapting to unfamiliar cultural norms and regulations in American, and a history of serious problems with prejudice against the Chinese people in America (Tang & Merrilees, 2021; Voss, 2018). There has been a long-standing problem with discrimination and often violent forms of prejudice against Chinese immigrants, with C-As too often being treated like slaves in America, being called unsavory names like Coolies, and being widely villanised in America as part of the fearful "Yellow Peril" conspriacy theory (Lew-Williams, 2021; Voss, 2018; Zhou & Liu, 2017). These problems with bias have not abated in America, and in recent years Chinese (and other Asian people) in the United States have faced serious discrimination and violence as scapegoats for the deadly COVID-19 pandemic, especially with former President Trump, breeding prejudice against the Chinese people by referring to the virus as the "China Flu" (Roberto, Johnson, & Rauhaus, 2020). This recent wave of anti-Chinese bias has resulted in high levels of stress and mental health problems for many C-A immigrants and has often made it difficult for C-As to get the best health care and to experience optimal health outcomes in the United States (Cheah, Wang, Ren, Zong, Cho, & Xue, 2020).

Top Health Issues among Chinese Americans

Cancer is the leading cause of death for C-As (Hastings et al., 2015). The top five cancers-related mortality in Chinese men are lung cancer, liver cancer, colorectal cancer, stomach cancer, and pancreas cancer; the top five cancer-related motality in Chinese women are lung cancer, breast cancer, colonrectal cancer, pancreas cancer, and stomach cancer (Thompson et al., 2016). However, C-As have low uptake rates of cancer screenings (Chen, Diamant, Kagawa-Singer, Pourat, & Wold, 2004; Kagawa-Singer & Pourat, 2000; Sentell, Tsoh, Davis, Davis, &

Braun, 2015). For example, colorectal cancer screening is significantly underutilized by C-As (Sentell et al., 2015; Tang, Solomon, & McCracken, 2001). C-A women are less likely to report having Pap smears or mamograms than other Asian American and Pacific Islander women (Chen et al., 2004; Kagawa-Singer & Pourat, 2000; Sentell et al., 2015). The reported factors associated with lower cancer screening uptake among this population include having no time, having no symptoms, low empahsis on preventive primary care, perceived lower susceptibility to cancer, lack of knowledge about cancer screening, having concerns about pain/discomfort from the screening, fear of obtaining unwanted screening findings, limited English proficiency (LEP), low health literacy (LHL), cultural beliefs about modesty, fatalism, stigma towards cancer, and access barriers (Jung et al., 2018; Lee-Lin et al., 2007; Ma et al., 2009; Sentell et al., 2015).

Cardiovascular disease (CVD) is another leading cause of death among C-As in the United States (Hastings et al., 2015). Compared to Chinese living in Asia, Chinese living in the United States have higher CVD mortality rates. This may be related to their significant dietary changes when they migrate to the United States (Wong, Dixon, Gilbride, Kwan, & Stein, 2013). For example, Chinese immigrants may have increased consumption of fast food, processed meat, refined grains, dairy products, high fat and high sugar foods that are popular in the United States (Fung, Schulze, Manson, Willett, & Hu, 2004; Lv & Cason, 2004; Pan, Dixon, Himburg, & Huffman, 1999; Yang & Read, 1996); they may also have increased frequency of engaging in sedentary activity in the United States. These changes in diet and sedentary activity increase C-As' risks for developing CVD (Diez Roux et al., 2005; Wong et al., 2013).

Health Communication Behaviors of Chinese Americans

Effective health communication is important to deliver high quality health care (Kreps, 2018). Poor patient-provider communication leads to lower patient satisfaction, lower adherence, reduced patient education, and decreased health information seeking behaviors (Ferguson & Candib, 2002; Ngo-Metzger et al., 2007; Paternotte, van Dulmen, van der Lee, Scherpbier, & Scheele, 2015; Simon, Tom, Taylor, Leung, & Vicencio, 2019). Due to the complexities of health information and numerous barriers to communicating health information to members of this population, it has been challenging for Chinese Americans to access and understand the relevant health information they need to make informed health decisions (Kreps & Sparks, 2008). Previous research studies have shown that Chinese immigrants experience numerous barriers in health communication (Chen, Li, Talwar, Xu, & Zhao, 2016; Simon et al., 2019; Tsoh et al., 2016). For example, a qualitative study with 49 Chinese Americans showed that Chinese Americans rarely communicated with their health care providers regarding family health history, which is an essential part of establishing accurate diagnoses and treatment plans) due to culturally-based interpersonal communication barriers (Chen et al., 2016).

Barriers affecting Effective Health Communication in Chinese Americans

Language

Health messages should be disseminated in the appropriate and preferred languages to members of immigrant populations (Kreps & Sparks, 2008). In the United States, less than 40% of Chinese immigrants speak English very well; approximately 60% of C-As have low English language proficiency (LEP) (Chen, Goodson, Acosta, Barry, & McKyer, 2018; Gambino, Acosta, & Grieco, 2014). Previous research has indicated that compared to those with adequate English proficiency, people with LEP were more likely to experience poor communication with their health care providers and are also likely to experience difficulty understanding health information (Chen, Acosta, & Barry, 2016, 2017; Chen et al., 2018; Lindholm, Hargraves, Ferguson, & Reed, 2012). Even for those C-As who have achieved high levels of education and are fluent in using English, they often prefer using their native language (Chinese) instead of using English for health communication due to the complexity of medical terms. In addition, Chinese immigrants have dialect preferences in both oral communication (to use either Mandarin or Cantonese), and in written communication (to use either traditional or simplified written characters). Chinese immigrants' dialect preferences may also influence their effectiveness as health communicators and their willingness to participate in health interventions (Ho, Chesla, & Chun, 2012; Wang & Chan, 2005).

Low Health Literacy

In addition to English language barriers, many Chinese Americans have low levels of health literacy (LHL). Many immigrants experience problems with LHL, especially when they need to communicate about frightening and debilitating health problems (Chen, Li, & Kreps, 2021; Kreps, Neuhauser, Sparks, & Labelle, 2020; Kreps & Sparks, 2008). Health literacy is defined as "the degree to which individuals have the capacity to obtain, process and understand basic health information and services needed to make appropriate health decisions" (Nielsen-Bohlman, Panzer, & Kindig, 2004). The definition includes four important components of LHL, as illustrated in Figure 3.1. People with

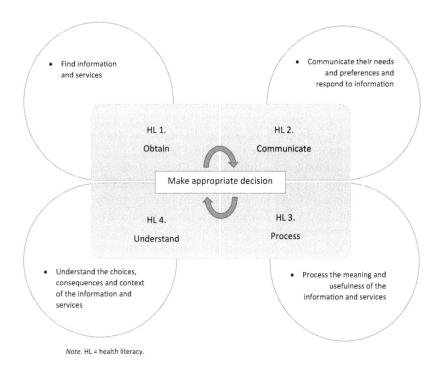

Note. HL = health literacy.

Figure 3.1 Health literacy (source from Leung, Bo, Hsiao, Wang, & Chi. (2014). Health literacy issues in the care of Chinese American immigrants with diabetes: a qualitative study BMJ Open 2014;4:e005294. doi: 10.1136/bmjopen-2014–005294)

LEP are more likely to have LHL (Institute of Medicine, 2004). However, there have been efforts to translate health educational materials into Chinese, but many Chinese immigrants cannot read or get access to such translated information (Ho, Tran, & Chesla, 2015). For instance, although Chinese translators are available in many clinics and hospitals, Chinese patients are less likely to receive diabetes related information from health professionals in comparison to White patients (Gucciardi, Smith, & DeMelo, 2006).

Cultural Factors

Along with LEP and LHL, Chinese cultural beliefs and norms significantly influence the health communication of Chinese immigrants living in the United States. For example, a qualitative study with 49 C-As showed that some participants were reluctant to discuss their family health history with physicians because of Chinese taboos and stigma (Chen et al., 2016). Due to a collectivist culture, disclosing private family information (secrets), especially about stigmatized health problems such as genetic-related diseases and mental disorders, may be considered as disloyal to the C-A family (Chen et al., 2016; Xu, 2004). Additionally, some C-As are afraid that disclosing health information to others may cause them to be stigmatized by people in their community (Warmoth, Cheung, You, Yeung, & Lu, 2017). Many Chinese immigrants even avoid talking with their own family members about diseases that run in the family (Cheng, Guerra, Pasick, Schillinger, Luce, & Joseph, 2018). In Chinese culture, people believe that talking about diseases or deaths, especially during festivals, may bring "bad luck."

Most Chinese immigrants living in the United States are foreign-born and are strongly influenced by Chinese cultural values. Traditional Chinese medicine (TCM) is popularly utilized by many members of this population. Under this cultural practice, *yin-yang* balance, *qi* (vital energy), and holism are emphasized in health promotion and disease management (Ma, 1999). A study that investigated the use of traditional and Western health services by Chinese Americans found that almost all respondents had used TCM, such as herbal medicines, herbal teas, cooking foods with herbs, acupuncture, massage, and Zhen Jiu (Ma, 1999). However, while seeking Western medical help, many C-As may withhold disclosing their culturally based practice of TCM. Meanwhile, Western health care providers often lack a basic understanding about the use of TCM, which lead to a challenge for them to understand this ethnic health belief, thus failing to effectively communicate with their Chinese patients and providing them with the best medical recommendations (Ma, 1999).

Many C-As may feel too much respect for the authority of health care providers to feel comfortable even asking them questions (Ho et al., 2012). Many of them may not challenge health care providers' decisions even if they disagree with these decisions. A survey study with 405 Chinese immigrants living in the United States with limited English proficiency found that participants were unlikely to question their physicians' and nurses' advice, regardless of which language (Chinese or English) they used to communicate with the health providers (Chen, Goodson, Acosta, Barry, & McKyer, 2018). This is a serious barrier to effective consumer-provider health communication. Due to this Chinese cultural norm, openly disagreeing with health care providers may be considered as offensive and be seen as a serious "loss of face." Previous research also showed that C-As limited their health information seeking activities because of an over-abundance concern about challenging or even questioning their health care providers (Simon et al., 2019). For example, they may not ask questions to clarify the things they don't understand because they think the doctor may be very busy. They may feel bad and "lose face" if they ask their health care providers too many questions (Simon et al., 2019).

Structural Barriers

C-As often encounter structural barriers when the try to seek health information and communicate with health care providers. For example, long wait times, difficult in scheduling apointments, lack of opportunities (and reluctance) to make inquiries with their doctors (and other health care providers) regarding relevant health information, never/ rarely visiting doctors in the United States, health insurance issues, financial concerns, issue with transportations, and lack of familiarity and mistrust of US health care systems are often major obstacles for Chinese immigrants to engaging in effective health communication and receiving high-quality health services in the United States (L. S. Chen et al., 2016; Simon et al., 2019). Due to these reasons, a large number of Chinese immigrant may prefer home remedies, self-treatments, and even may travel to other counties to access reproductive, surgical, dental, and other forms of health care.

Personal Factors

Personal factors, such as age, gender, educational levels, and acculturation levels, may also influence the effectiveness of health communication for C-As (Leung, Bo, Hsiao, Wang, & Chi, 2014). For example, in a survey study with 405 C-As, Chen et al. found that participants with higher levels of US acculturation were more likely to have higher English functional health literacy and higher English information appraisal (Chen, Li, & Kreps, 2021). This suggests that only those C-As with high levels of acculturation in the United States are likely to receive the best health care services.

Future Directions to Improve Health Communication among Chinese Americans

Due to serious language and cultural barriers, Chinese immigrants (and other immigrant groups in the United States) often seek health care providers who share similar cultural backgrounds and health beliefs as their own (Kreps & Sparks, 2008; Pecchioni, Ota, & Sparks, 2004). Many C-As prefer to seek Chinese-speaking health care providers or go to Chinese private clinics that may be located in Chinatowns. However, the high clinical demand of Chinatown clinics and the shortage of Chinese-speaking health care providers can make it difficult for establishing active patient-provider communication interactions. These health communication problems can lead to receiving poor quality health care services and lower levels of patient satisfaction among members of this immigrant population (Simon et al., 2019). Thus, the high demand and short supply of Chinese-speaking health care providers should be addressed within the US health care system.

Since LEP is a significant barrier for effective health communication among Chinese immigrants in the United States, there is a tremendous need for more well-designed language appropriate health information matierals and interventions in the United States. Effective health messages should be designed using familiar and preferred language, images, examples, and delivered through accessible channels for Chinese Americans (Kreps & Sparks, 2008). Meanwhile, translators are needed to provide language assistance for many C-A patients (Ho, Tran, & Chesla, 2015). Both the oral and written aspects of translated health materials need to meet C-As' dialect preferences. Furthermore, studies show that Chinese American participants report that although the translated health matierals were accurate, they were too simple and do not provide enough detailed information (Ho, Tran, & Chesla, 2015). Thus, future translated health information materials in Chinese need to provide more detailed and in-depth health information (Chun, Chesla, & Kwan, 2011; Ho et al., 2012).

Besides providing language-appropriate health information, it is important for health care providers to enhance their cultural competencies when communicating with C-A patients (Chen, Li, & Kreps, 2021). The US health care system needs to adapt the the health care practices of Chinese immigrants who have their own unique health beliefs, food preferences, and often use TCM. In addition, health care providers in the United States must be aware of how Chinese culture taboos and forms of stigma are likely to influence the health beliefs and behaviors of CA patients. Health care providers must consider these factor when working with Chinese patients to promote the best health oucomes.

Additionally, multi-level interventions to address patients, providers, and systems are imperative for improving health communications among C-As. Since many Chinese patients may feel uncomfortable speaking openly and assertively with their doctors, culturally and linguistically appropriate interventions are needed to improve C-As' awareness and capacity to ask questions and express doubts in decision-making with their doctors. Interventions for other non-physician healthcare professionals (such as front desk staff, nurses, health educators, and community health workers) are also needed for bridging language and cultural gaps in consumer-provider health communication (Simon et al., 2019). At the health care system level, it is urgent to create a friendly health care system for racial/ethnic minorities, especially for those with low English proficiency like many Chinese immigrants. For example, since many health information relevant webpages only have English and Spanish versions, developing Chinese versions is important for health care systems that serve many C-As to help these consumers get access to relevant health information. Since C-As comprise a large, productive, and growing segment of the US population, it is imperative to improve health communication programs, practices, and policies to better serve this important immigrant group.

Recommended Readings

Chen, X., Goodson, P., Acosta, S., Barry, A. E., & McKyer, L. E. (2018). Assessing Health Literacy Among Chinese Speakers in the US with Limited English Proficiency. *Health literacy research and practice, 2*(2), e94-e106. doi:10.3928/24748307-20180405-01

Chen, X., Li, M., & Kreps, G. L. (2021). Acculturation and Health Literacy Among Chinese Speakers in the USA with Limited English Proficiency. *J Racial Ethn Health Disparities*. doi:10.1007/s40615-021-00979-9

Ho, E. Y., Chesla, C. A., & Chun, K. M. (2012). Health communication with Chinese Americans about type 2 diabetes. *Diabetes Educ, 38*(1), 67–76. doi:10.1177/0145721711428774

Ho, E. Y., Tran, H., & Chesla, C. A. (2015). Assessing the cultural in culturally sensitive printed patient-education materials for Chinese Americans with type 2 diabetes. *Health communication, 30*(1), 39–49.

Kreps, G. L., & Sparks, L. (2008). Meeting the health literacy needs of immigrant populations. *Patient Educ Couns, 71*(3), 328–332. doi:10.1016/j.pec.2008.03.001

Xu, Y. (2004). When East and West Meet: Cultural Values and Beliefs and Health Behaviors. *Home Health Care Management & Practice, 16*(5), 433–435. doi:10.1177/1084822304264659

References

Black, I. (1963). American labour and Chinese immigration. *Past & Present, 25*, 59–76.

Cheah, C. S., Wang, C., Ren, H., Zong, X., Cho, H. S., & Xue, X. (2020). COVID-19 racism and mental health in Chinese American families. *Pediatrics, 146*(5), 1–10.

Chen, J. (2019). *The Chinese of America.* Lexington, MA: Plunkett Lake Press.

Chen, J. Y., Diamant, A. L., Kagawa-Singer, M., Pourat, N., & Wold, C. (2004). Disaggregating data on Asian and Pacific Islander women to assess cancer screening. *American Journal of Preventive Medicine, 27*(2), 139–145. doi:10.1016/j.amepre.2004.03.013

Chen, L. S., Li, M., Talwar, D., Xu, L., & Zhao, M. (2016). Chinese Americans' views and use of family health history: A qualitative study. *PLoS One, 11*(9), e0162706. doi:10.1371/journal.pone.0162706

Chen, X., Acosta, S., & Barry, A. E. (2016). Evaluating the accuracy of google translate for diabetes education material. *JMIR Diabetes, 1*(1), e3. doi:10.2196/diabetes.5848

Chen, X., Acosta, S., & Barry, A. E. (2017). Machine or human? Evaluating the quality of a language translation mobile app for diabetes education material. *JMIR Diabetes, 2*(1), e13. doi:10.2196/diabetes.7446

Chen, X., Goodson, P., Acosta, S., Barry, A. E., & McKyer, L. E. (2018). Assessing health literacy among Chinese speakers in the US with limited

English proficiency. *Health Literacy Research and Practice, 2*(2), e94–e106. doi:10.3928/24748307-20180405-01

Chen, X., Li, M., & Kreps, G. L. (2021). Acculturation and health literacy among Chinese speakers in the USA with limited English Proficiency. *Journal of Racial Ethnic Health Disparities.* doi:10.1007/s40615-021-00979-9

Cheng, J. K. Y., Guerra, C., Pasick, R. J., Schillinger, D., Luce, J., & Joseph, G. (2018). Cancer genetic counseling communication with low-income Chinese immigrants. *Journal of Community Genetics, 9*(3), 263–276.

Chun, K. M., Chesla, C. A., & Kwan, C. M. (2011). "So we adapt step by step": Acculturation experiences affecting diabetes management and perceived health for Chinese American immigrants. *Social Science Medicine, 72*(2), 256–264. doi:10.1016/j.socscimed.2010.11.010

Diez Roux, A. V., Detrano, R., Jackson, S., Jacobs, D. R., Jr., Schreiner, P. J., Shea, S., & Szklo, M. (2005). Acculturation and socioeconomic position as predictors of coronary calcification in a multiethnic sample. *Circulation, 112*(11), 1557–1565. doi:10.1161/circulationaha.104.530147

Ferguson, W. J., & Candib, L. M. (2002). Culture, language, and the doctor-patient relationship. *Family Medicine, 34*(5), 353–361.

Fung, T. T., Schulze, M., Manson, J. E., Willett, W. C., & Hu, F. B. (2004). Dietary patterns, meat intake, and the risk of type 2 diabetes in women. *Archives of Internal Medicine, 164*(20), 2235–2240. doi:10.1001/archinte.164.20.2235

Gambino, C. P., Acosta, Y. D., & Grieco, E. M. (2014). English-speaking ability of the foreign-born population in the United States: 2012. Retrieved from https://www.census.gov/content/dam/Census/library/publications/2014/acs/acs-26.pdf

Gucciardi, E., Smith, P. L., & DeMelo, M. (2006). Use of diabetes resources in adults attending a self-management education program. *Patient Education and Counselling, 64*(1–3), 322–330. doi:10.1016/j.pec.2006.03.012

Hastings, K. G., Jose, P. O., Kapphahn, K. I., Frank, A. T. H., Goldstein, B. A., Thompson, C. A., . . . Palaniappan, L. P. (2015). Leading causes of death among Asian American subgroups (2003–2011). *PLoS One, 10*(4), e0124341. doi:10.1371/journal.pone.0124341

Ho, E. Y., Chesla, C. A., & Chun, K. M. (2012). Health communication with Chinese Americans about type 2 diabetes. *Diabetes Education, 38*(1), 67–76. doi:10.1177/0145721711428774

Ho, E. Y., Tran, H., & Chesla, C. A. (2015). Assessing the cultural in culturally sensitive printed patient-education materials for Chinese Americans with type 2 diabetes. *Health Communication, 30*(1), 39–49.

Hooper, K., & Batalova, J. (2015). Chinese immigrants in the United States. *Migration Policy Institute, 28.* Retrieved from https://www.immigrationre-search.org/system/files/Chinese_Immigrants_in_the_United_States.pdf

Institute of Medicine. (2004). *Health literacy: A prescription to end confusion.* Washington, DC: The National Academies Press.

Jung, M. Y., Holt, C. L., Ng, D., Sim, H. J., Lu, X., Le, D., . . . Lee, S. (2018). The Chinese and Korean American immigrant experience: a mixed-methods examination of facilitators and barriers of colorectal cancer screening. *Ethnic Health, 23*(8), 847–866. doi:10.1080/13557858.2017.1296559

Kagawa-Singer, M., & Pourat, N. (2000). Asian American and Pacific Islander breast and cervical carcinoma screening rates and healthy people 2000 objectives. *Cancer, 89*(3), 696–705. doi:10.1002/1097-0142(20000801)89:3<696::aid-cncr27>3.0.co;2-7

Kreps, G. L. (2018). Promoting patient comprehension of relevant health information. *Israel Journal of Health Policy Research, 7*(1), 56. doi:10.1186/s13584-018-0250-z

Kreps, G. L., Neuhauser, L., Sparks, L., & Labelle, S. (2020). Promoting convergence between health literacy and health communication. *Studies in Health Technology and Informatics, 269,* 526–543.

Kreps, G. L., & Sparks, L. (2008). Meeting the health literacy needs of immigrant populations. *Patient Educcation and Counseling, 71*(3), 328–332. doi:10.1016/j.pec.2008.03.001

Lee-Lin, F., Pett, M., Menon, U., Lee, S., Nail, L., Mooney, K., & Itano, J. (2007). Cervical cancer beliefs and pap test screening practices among Chinese American immigrants. *Oncology Nursing Forum, 34*(6), 1203–1209. doi:10.1188/07.onf.1203-1209

Leung, A. Y. M., Bo, A., Hsiao, H.-Y., Wang, S. S., & Chi, I. (2014). Health literacy issues in the care of Chinese American immigrants with diabetes: A qualitative study. *BMJ Open, 4*(11), e005294. doi:10.1136/bmjopen-2014-005294

Lew-Williams, B. (2021). The Chinese must go: Violence, exclusion, and the making of the Alien in America (2018). In *Racism in America* (pp. 153–162). Cambridge, MA: Harvard University Press.

Lindholm, M., Hargraves, J. L., Ferguson, W. J., & Reed, G. (2012). Professional language interpretation and inpatient length of stay and readmission rates. *Journal of General Internal Medicine, 27*(10), 1294–1299. doi:10.1007/s11606-012-2041-5

Lv, N., & Cason, K. L. (2004). Dietary pattern change and acculturation of Chinese Americans in Pennsylvania. *Journal of American Dietetic Association, 104*(5), 771–778. doi:10.1016/j.jada.2004.02.032

Ma, G. X. (1999). Between two worlds: the use of traditional and Western health services by Chinese immigrants. *Journal of Community Health, 24*(6), 421–437. doi:10.1023/a:1018742505785

Ma, G. X., Toubbeh, J. I., Wang, M. Q., Shive, S. E., Cooper, L., & Pham, A. (2009). Factors associated with cervical cancer screening compliance and noncompliance among Chinese, Korean, Vietnamese, and Cambodian women. *Journal of National Medicine Association, 101*(6), 541–551. doi:10.1016/s0027-9684(15)30939-1

Ngo-Metzger, Q., Sorkin, D. H., Phillips, R. S., Greenfield, S., Massagli, M. P., Clarridge, B., & Kaplan, S. H. (2007). Providing high-quality care for limited English proficient patients: the importance of language concordance and interpreter use. *Journal of General Internal Medicine, 22*(Suppl 2), 324–330. doi:10.1007/s11606-007-0340-z

Nielsen-Bohlman, L., Panzer, A. M., & Kindig, D. A. (2004). *Health Literacy: A Prescription to End Confusion*. Washington, DC: National Academies Press.

Office of the Historian. (2021). Chinese immigration and the Chinese exclusion acts. Retrieved from https://history.state.gov/milestones/1866-1898/chinese-immigration

Pan, Y. L., Dixon, Z., Himburg, S., & Huffman, F. (1999). Asian students change their eating patterns after living in the United States. *Journal of American Dietetic Association, 99*(1), 54–57. doi:10.1016/s0002-8223(99)00016-4

Paternotte, E., van Dulmen, S., van der Lee, N., Scherpbier, A. J., & Scheele, F. (2015). Factors influencing intercultural doctor-patient communication:

a realist review. *Patient Educ Couns, 98*(4), 420–445. doi:10.1016/j. pec.2014.11.018

Pecchioni, L. L., Ota, H., & Sparks, L. (2004). Cultural issues in communication and aging. In J. F. Nussbaum, & J. Coupland (Eds.), *Handbook of Communication and Aging Research*, 167–207. Mahwah, NJ: Erlbaum.

Pew Research Center. (2012). *The Rise of Asian Americans.* Retrieved from https://www.pewresearch.org/social-trends/2012/06/19/chapter-1-portrait-of-asian-americans/

Pew Research Center. (2021a). *Asian Americans are the fastest-growing racial or ethnic group in the US.* Retrieved from https://www.pewresearch.org/fact-tank/2021/04/09/asian-americans-are-the-fastest-growing-racial-or-ethnic-group-in-the-u-s/.

Pew Research Center. (2021b). *Chinese in the US fact sheet.*

Pew Research Center. (2021c). *Key facts about Asian Americans, a diverse and growing population.* Retrieved from: https://www.pewresearch.org/fact-tank/2021/04/29/key-facts-about-asian-americans/

Roberto, K. J., Johnson, A. F., & Rauhaus, B. M. (2020). Stigmatization and prejudice during the COVID-19 pandemic. *Administrative Theory & Praxis, 42*(3), 364–378.

Sentell, T. L., Tsoh, J. Y., Davis, T., Davis, J., & Braun, K. L. (2015). Low health literacy and cancer screening among Chinese Americans in California: A cross-sectional analysis. *BMJ Open, 5*(1), e006104. doi:10.1136/bmjopen-2014-006104

Simon, M. A., Tom, L. S., Taylor, S., Leung, I., & Vicencio, D. (2019). 'There's nothing you can do … it's like that in Chinatown': Chinese immigrant women's perceptions of experiences in Chicago Chinatown healthcare settings. *Ethnic Health*, 1–18. doi:10.1080/13557858.2019.1573973

Tang, M., & Merrilees, S. (2021). Understanding the multifaceted acculturation process of Chinese immigrants. *International Journal for the Advancement of Counselling, 43*, 1–16.

Tang, T. S., Solomon, L. J., & McCracken, L. M. (2001). Barriers to fecal occult blood testing and sigmoidoscopy among older Chinese-American women. *Cancer Practice, 9*(6), 277–282. doi:10.1046/j.1523-5394.2001.96008.x

Thompson, C. A., Gomez, S. L., Hastings, K. G., Kapphahn, K., Yu, P., Shariff-Marco, S., . . . Palaniappan, L. P. (2016). The burden of cancer in Asian Americans: A report of national mortality trends by Asian Ethnicity. *Cancer Epidemiology Biomarkers and Prevention, 25*(10), 1371–1382. doi:10.1158/1055-9965.EPI-16-0167

Tsoh, J. Y., Sentell, T., Gildengorin, G., Le, G. M., Chan, E., Fung, L. C., . . . Nguyen, T. T. (2016). Healthcare communication barriers and self-rated health in older Chinese American immigrants. *Journal of Community Health, 41*(4), 741–752. doi:10.1007/s10900-015-0148-4

Voss, B. L. (2018). The archaeology of precarious lives: Chinese railroad workers in nineteenth-century North America. *Current Anthropology, 59*(3), 287–313.

Wang, C. Y., & Chan, S. M. (2005). Culturally tailored diabetes education program for Chinese Americans: a pilot study. *Nursing Research, 54*(5), 347–353. doi:10.1097/00006199-200509000-00009

Warmoth, K., Cheung, B., You, J., Yeung, N. C., & Lu, Q. (2017). Exploring the social needs and challenges of Chinese American immigrant breast cancer survivors: A qualitative study using an expressive writing approach. *International Journal of Behavioral Medicine, 24*(6), 827–835.

Wong, S. S., Dixon, L. B., Gilbride, J. A., Kwan, T. W., & Stein, R. A. (2013). Measures of acculturation are associated with cardiovascular disease risk factors, dietary intakes, and physical activity in older Chinese Americans in New York City. *Journal of Immigrant and Minority Health, 15*(3), 560–568. doi:10.1007/s10903-012-9669-4

Xu, Y. (2004). When east and west meet: Cultural values and beliefs and health behaviors. *Home Health Care Management & Practice, 16*(5), 433–435. doi:10.1177/1084822304264659

Yang, W., & Read, M. (1996). Dietary pattern changes of Asian immigrants. *Nutrition Research, 16*(8), 1277–1293. doi.org/10.1016/0271-5317(96)00137-6

Yung, J., Chang, G., & Lai, H. M. (Eds.). (2006). *Chinese American voices: From the gold rush to the present.* Oakland: University of California Press.

Zhou, M., & Liu, H. (2017). Immigrant entrepreneurship and diasporic development: The case of new Chinese migrants in the USA. In *Contemporary Chinese diasporas* (pp. 403–423). Singapore: Palgrave.

4 Survival Against Odds

Undocumented Immigrants and Communication about Policies and Access to Health Care in the United States

Jaime S. Robb and Ambar Basu

Survival Against Odds: Undocumented Immigrants[1] and Communication about Access to Health Care in the United States

On January 25, 2017, then U.S. President Donald J. Trump signed into law an executive order for "enhancing public safety in the interior of the United States," his first act as president.[2] While the implementation of this policy had minimal effect on the day-to-day rituals of most American citizens, it was a marked moment for individuals in the United States (U.S.) who had an undocumented status. As has been the case historically, undocumented immigrants face multiple structural and social challenges when attempting to access various social services. When representatives in power engage in anti-immigration rhetoric and enact policies that target undocumented people, it fosters a culture of fear that restricts their ability to survive, particularly with regard to accessing health care services (Passel & Cohn, 2009).

In the U.S., undocumented immigrants are not covered by government health programs at the state and federal levels because they lack documentation, such as a social security number, which is necessary for enrollment in a health care plan. Even if these individuals manage to find affordable healthcare providers, they may struggle with the decision to use such services because of fears associated with deportation (Kullgren, 2003). President Trump's abovementioned policy signaled to undocumented immigrants they should be wary of accessing public spaces, which meant that avenues for accessing health services were limited or even eliminated. The president's policy is just one instance, among many, that highlights how dominant anti-immigrant discourse influences decision making among undocumented immigrants.

DOI: 10.4324/9781003230243-4

Undocumented Immigration and Policy in the United States

According to Passel (2005) of the Pew Research Center, "Undocumented immigrants are those who entered the country without 'valid' documents, and those who entered the country with a valid visa but overstayed the time allocated via the visa" (p. 35). Contemporary media accounts of undocumented immigrants typically position this group as competing with citizens for resources. This has the effect of presenting to the public an image of the immigrant as having the same types of access as citizens, which is not the case. This means that most undocumented individuals lack the symbolic identifiers of citizenship (typically a social security number) needed to compete with citizens for most, if not all, of the country's resources. Additionally, by framing undocumented individuals as competing with citizens, political agents weaponize immigrants/immigration to create agendas that further limit the social support systems available to noncitizens (Newton, 2009).

Newton (2009) compares two moments when Congressional policies shifted our understanding of immigration in the U.S. The 1986 Immigration Reform and Control Act (IRCA) provided amnesty for thousands of immigrants that were illegally living in the U.S. at the time (Newton, 2009). Though the policy provided an avenue for individuals to gain legal status, it also created increased border enforcement to deter future illegal immigration. This act aimed to increase the American labor force by offering immigrants a path to inclusion if they were willing to work long enough to "earn" it (Newton, 2009). According to Newton, the IRCA of 1986 created the conditions needed for the formulation of the Illegal Immigration Reform and Immigrant Responsibility Act (IIRAIRA), which was enacted in 1996. This Act introduced the category of the "illegal" characterized as "usurpers of government munificence, undeserving recipients of public benefits, and in need of regulation and restriction" (Newton, 2009, p. 23). The language of both Acts created the conditions for presenting undocumented immigrants as plunderers in American communities.

The legality involved with entering and residing in a national space has become a contentious topic given the globalized society we live in today (Eriksen, 1998). The policing of borders can be argued for given the fears associated with foreign acts of terrorism and potential environmental contamination. However, the creation of policies and legislations that restrict social, economic, and political access for those who are already residing within these borders becomes problematic. Such restrictions create challenges associated with survival in an advanced society, whereby groups of undocumented immigrants likely need to circumvent rules to maintain a livelihood. Legislation like California's Proposition 187, passed in 1994, was designed to curtail illegal immigration by depriving undocumented immigrants of welfare, public education, and any kind of social support except for emergency medical service. This Act also forced teachers and police officers to report any suspected undocumented immigrants to the Immigration and Naturalization Services (INS) for deportation. Consequent to the passing of Proposition 187, many undocumented individuals were forced to leave their occupations and find other means of survival. Crime rates associated rose significantly during this time, leading to the state forging an inherent correlation between the rise in crime and undocumented immigrants, creating the conditions for framing this group as deviants with criminal intent.

Undocumented Immigrants and Healthcare

According to the U.S. Census (2016), there are over 11 million individuals living in the U.S. as undocumented immigrants. An additional 9 million immigrants travel back and forth to and from the country annually (U.S. Census, 2016). This includes women, children and the elderly who make up over 60% of this population. For those living in the U.S. as undocumented immigrants, access to the health marketplace is limited, if at all available. Government programs like Medicaid and Medicare fail to cover those who do not have a social security number to put on file (Edwards, 2014). In many ways, a costly trip to the emergency room is the only option available to undocumented immigrants when faced with health-related issues, but only if they are able to deal with the fears associated with having to provide official information to healthcare providers (Edwards, 2014). This likely indicates that a sizable portion of individuals in the U.S. lacks the access and coverage needed to address health-related issues.

Derose, Escarce, and Lurie (2007) suggest "65% of undocumented immigrants lack health insurance, compared with 32% of permanent residents," noting that policies created the difference in access among these groups (Derose et al., 2007, p. 1260). There are numerous factors that complicate undocumented immigrants' lack of access to health services. These range from limited knowledge about the health system, bureaucratic obstacles, general confusion about rules and restrictions, and fears of discrimination (Karp et al., 2007). Official policies like the Affordable Care Act explicitly exclude undocumented immigrants from obtaining health insurance while presenting itself as a "universal" health reform program (Biswas et al., 2012). Due to the exorbitant cost of medical services in the U.S., insurance is typically needed for affordable care and sometimes even required as a precursor to service (Edwards, 2014). National policies including the act of asking for any type of personal identification as a prerequisite for health services are the most salient barriers to undocumented immigrants' health care experiences in the U.S.

The Patient Protection and Affordable Care Act (PPACA) restricts access to health care for undocumented immigrants as does the Deficit Reduction Act passed in 2006, which requires both state and local Medicaid agencies to gain proof of citizenship for those who apply to the program (Edwards, 2014).The difficult circumstances under which undocumented individuals enter the country, and the potential precarious socio-economic conditions they live in can only compound poor health outcomes for this group (Kullgren, 2003).

Negative health outcomes for undocumented immigrants can create public health challenges for all (Passel, 2005). About 40% of undocumented immigrants are parents to children who are born as American citizens; often these parents fail to seek out service for their children due to an inability to provide documents for themselves. According to The Migration Policy Institute, in 2007, at least 59% of undocumented adults lacked health insurance, while 55% of children of undocumented individuals were uninsured (Capps et al., 2007). The implementation of policies that require medical professionals to act as gatekeepers to health services creates additional barriers in a health system that is largely inaccessible for undocumented immigrants. In this context, it becomes important from a critical health communication perspective to understand how undocumented immigrants, given their marginalized status, navigate limited access to healthcare. The culture-centered approach to health communication provides a theoretical umbrella to do this type of work.

Culture-Centered Approach to Health Communication

Prior research on undocumented immigrants and health care tends to focus heavily on barriers to accessing adequate health services (Kullgren, 2003; Cheong, 2007). Most of this type of research fails to account for how undocumented immigrants interpret and maneuver around structural/discursive limitations when seeking health care, how undocumented immigrants story their health, survival, resilience, and creativity.

The culture-centered approach (CCA) aligns with the goals of critical health communication (Dutta & Basu, 2009), examining the interrelationships between structure, culture, and agency in the lived experiences of marginalized group members. As such, it offers a viable lens to understand and document undocumented immigrant narratives of health. *Structure* deals with the formation and operations of social systems, means of distributing resources, and ways of controlling resources that work to sustain social inequities. Examples include policies, law, jobs, education, etc. (Basu, 2011). *Culture* can be explained as webs of meanings that shape social systems (Dutta, 2008). Structures mirror dominant cultural beliefs, values, and meanings, becoming the systems that "constrains, limits, and defines what is available to cultural members and what is not" (Dutta, 2008, p. 35). At the intersection of structure and culture also lies *agency*, which refers to a cultural group's ability to react and respond to shifting structures in their socio-cultural contexts (Basu & Dutta, 2009). To be an agent is to participate in everyday acts in a manner that highlights ones' awareness of the structural elements impacting choice and to navigate the limitations of a structure in nuanced ways (Dutta & Basu, 2009).

The CCA tries to reverse the logic that cultural members are passive receivers of information and resources (Dutta, 2008), and instead advocates listening to the ways local cultural members define, narrate, and understand their lived experiences. According to the CCA, local meanings are critical to interrupting health discourses that suggest one cultural understanding of health is best, while limiting the value of other cultural ways of knowing (Lupton, 1994; Dutta & Zoller, 2008). In the context of this project, the CCA helps us frame the following guiding research question: How does a group of undocumented immigrants in the U.S. communicate about negotiating access to healthcare?

Method

Conceptually framed within the CCA, this project focuses on the voice and agency of undocumented immigrants from the South Florida region as they narrate their experiences regarding healthcare. The first author interviewed 16 undocumented immigrants from the South Florida region about how they navigate the U.S. healthcare system, given their social status and the prevalence of anti-immigrant policies and rhetoric. Most research participants were identified based on their relationships with the first author who grew up in their communities as an undocumented immigrant. Participants included the first author's high school friends, neighbors, former teammates, former work colleagues, and family members. No identifying information (such as gender, race, and nationality) was collected from participants, partly for their safety, and partly to centralize their residency status as their unifying identity. However, nearly every participant spoke about their ethnic/national cultural identities, particularly about how important it was for survival in the U.S. to find others who shared these identities.

Semi-structured interviews were conducted with pre-constructed questions used to start conversations; impromptu prompts and queries were used during the interview process to better connect with participants and further explore their specific experiences. After transcribing and coding the interview data, a thematic analysis strategy was adopted to locate themes that emerged in the data. The idea was to have individual stories and experiences be the tool for generating critical insights into how undocumented immigrants in the U.S. communicate about and negotiate access to health care services. The three broad themes that we developed from the interviews are: a) Policy as rhetorical communication that influences undocumented immigrants' distrust of official spaces; b) Fear and distrust as health disparities for undocumented immigrants; and c) Resistance through solidarity.

Policy as Rhetoric

Several research participants suggested that the terms mainstream media uses to describe them as a group (undocumented, illegal) frame them negatively. One participant, Nancy, said she hears the word "undocumented" used to describe her situation and "it brings fear, lots of fear, you are not comfortable, that word does not allow you to feel comfortable." Her neighbor, Maxine, noted that using such terms to describe their situation creates a false sense of who they are and what they are trying to do in this country. She mentioned that being "undocumented," does not allow her to feel human: "When you hear it, you feel bad, it does not make you sound welcome, I wish they could have another name, you know, find a more decent term to use because we are all humans." When asked about the term "illegal" Nancy added, "oh my goodness, that's way worse, lots and lots of fear, that one really causes you to think about looking over your shoulder every time you leave the house." Both Nancy and Maxine have lived in the U.S. for over a decade now, and both suggested that the stigma towards undocumented immigrants has worsened over the years.

It is clear that research participants like Nancy and Maxine are aware of the rhetorical effects of the labels that are ascribed to them and the marginalization that follows. Serina expressed her feelings regarding the stereotypes and the impact of such language on the lives of those who must survive with such labels:

> Those words, it, it makes you feel like, as if you are not counted. If you are undocumented there is not accountability for you, so it is easier for things to happen outside of your control. It is hard for you to report if something goes wrong with you, because there is just so much fear. Things are so much harder for you, your circumstances are harder, you do not know where to turn to for help at times. You never know what you can get into, because you are undocumented, the fear that you have makes you wonder if someone might instigate something with you just because you look or sound a certain way, you don't want to get in anything that can prevent you from moving forward, so in a lot of ways you really become stuck.

Serina's dislocation from mainstream discourse, her not being a legal resident of this country, marks her body as outside of the realm of public consideration. Such statements highlight the subaltern position of undocumented immigrants and their awareness about this subaltern subjectivity (Spivak, 1988). Serina also indicates that her subaltern position ultimately results in a type of paranoia, whereby she constantly fears for her own well-being.

Research participants pointed to how policy language validates the stigmas that accompanies being undocumented, which in turn sustains fear-inducing and alienating structures that limit the ways in which individuals in these groups can access resources and living conditions available to the nation's citizens. Several participants discussed the negative impact Trump's executive order for the protection of the interior of the U.S. had on their daily lives, and affected day-to-day decision making for members of this group. Nancy has lived and worked in Miami since she moved to the U.S. 13 years ago, and she recalls the deep sadness and fear she felt when Trump announced his plans. She said, "If Mr. Trump stops saying what he is saying that will help, that alone is killing people." She makes the point that Trump's rhetoric is just as damaging to undocumented immigrants as the policies that he puts forth. According to her, Trump's continuous tweets and speeches about this group are as influential to this group as the policies he writes into law.

The negative representation of undocumented immigrants in policies and political rhetoric sustains fear in the daily lives of these individuals. Shelly sees Trump's rhetoric and policies as a critical barrier to undocumented immigrants' leading meaningful lives. She said,

> That policy strikes fears into all immigrants' hearts, undocumented or not, I have a co-worker, and I didn't even know that they could do this, she told me that when she showed up to work there were people there asking them for paperwork, showing that they were citizens or green card holders, so people would show up to your actual job and ask for your paperwork. Her husband was a citizen, so he had paperwork, but for other people they didn't show up to work. They called their friends and family to tell them not to show up to work, so before that Trump Ice agreement there was still fear, but I want to say the threat has become very real, the policy that Trump has put into place it is not a matter of if, but a matter of when, they are going to come.

The increased fears that undocumented immigrants experienced since President Trump took office only added to this group's inability to access any sort of medical services. Shelly's comments reinforce the fear that steams from such dominant discourses, and the way immigrants are forced to adjust their lives in order to survive.

Fear as Health Disparity

Along with the fear of deportation that undocumented immigrants face, they must also operate in fraught spaces knowing they have no means of legal protection. Hiding in public spaces or avoiding them all together is one of the only avenues left available to undocumented immigrants. Many undocumented immigrants interpret their well-being as connected to their ability to remain in this country. Thus, avoiding health institutions is one way for this group to manage their well-being, while simultaneously learning to manage their own health in order to balance the equation.

When it comes to health needs, most undocumented immigrants that were interviewed spoke about avoiding medical services altogether, either because of cost, or because of the mistrust in the medical system, or the need to prioritize work, or due to a combination of these factors. What was clear among this group was that they constantly avoided medical systems due to a multitude of fears that are a result of policies that frame them as deviants. Participants not only described an ultimate fear of deportation, but other more immediate fears that stem from their lack of access. They were afraid of missing work to visit the doctors because they could lose their jobs for requesting time off. In addition, they were fearful of going to seek health service and not having enough to cover the cost without insurance. Additionally, there was the fear of being questioned about their accent, fear of not having requested documentation, fear that their medical information could later be used to track them down, and fear that they would need prescriptions or a second visit that they could not afford. Even such things as taking public transportation to go visit a doctor operated as a fear that creates health disparities for this group.

Nancy explained that she knew someone "diabetic and the doctor said they must try not to work too hard, to take time off, how is he supposed to do that, how does he pay his rent?" Evident in Nancy's narrative is a structural double-bind. As Nancy argues, to maintain his health, her friend needs to take time off work, but he cannot afford not to work if he wants to take care of his health. Being "kicked out on the street" is a constant worry, Nancy noted, unlike the "supportive" community back "home," who are more loving, caring and are willing to look out for their neighbors.

For a few of the research participants like Nancy and Troy, the cost of accessing healthcare is intertwined with the precarity of their job situations. With their "illegal" label, undocumented immigrants, according to both Nancy and Troy, find it imperative to keep the jobs they have, because getting new jobs is close to impossible due to their inability to produce required identification documents. Troy said,

> When you are illegal here, you have to find a way to have a roof over your head, and for you to have a roof over your head, you have to work hard. You have to wake up early, come home late at night, the money is not enough, and you know if you miss one day of work you could lose the job, and you miss one month's rent and you are out on

your own, so, if you feel sick, or if you are not at your best, you still have to work. Because I see people who are out there going to work sick as a dog, and you have to keep going because you will lose that job, and you don't know if you will get another one, so that ends up being a lot of stress. You don't get time to just relax or to recoup.

In addition to direct and indirect cost-related structural barriers they face, several research participants said that visiting medical facilities was not their first choice when they became ill. The fear of being questioned in those spaces made it difficult to think of accessing such facilities as a first option. It is only when undocumented immigrants face major health crisis that they feel compelled to seek out medical treatment. In such cases, their lack of trust in the medical system leads to seemingly deceitful ways of interacting with the system. Pat said,

> Sometimes you might use some else's identification to go to the doctors, sometimes you have to get crafty. Just to go see a doctor, sometimes when you are illegal you have to be like let me do something illegal because I don't have any other choice and I don't want to die.

For this group to be able to survive in a space that is structured with dominant anti-immigrant discourse they must find creative and strategic ways to manage their health and well-being, similar to what Pat describes. This creates additional stress for this group because their aim is to avoid detection, but in extreme cases they must circumvent the system in order to access the care they need, which sometimes makes them more vulnerable.

Several participants mentioned they have to make difficult choices on whether to break the rules to support their health or suffer the consequences of not receiving treatment. Maxine mentioned that "the medical service is more advanced in the U.S., so attempting to return home for treatment would be a waste of time." For Troy and Ricardo, finding a way around their limitations was the only real option as self-deportation was never an option in their mind. As I discuss in the next section, group solidarity and ideas of community are valuable resources for undocumented immigrants looking to access medical service.

Wellness, Solidarity, and Resistance

Troy and Maxine stated that undocumented immigrants in the U.S. need more collective voice, more representation.

> Those of us who are here, who have lived under these statuses, who understand the problems, we are going to have to let our voices be heard for those who cannot be heard, by protest or going out to vote for the right people.

Troy explained. Until such shift in representation and policies have occurred, undocumented immigrants are left to survive on their own despite the odds being stacked against them. For survival, being healthy and having access to healthcare are essential. Research participants mentioned the multitude of ways they negotiate health in terms of the solidarity they experienced with other undocumented immigrants. In this instance, solidarity refers to the support undocumented immigrants receive from others who have shared similar experiences. Participants indicated that most of their health needs are met due to the information received from others who have shared similar struggles. The theme of solidarity was common among all undocumented immigrants that were interviewed, whereby they attributed their ability to survive in this country to the material, psychological, and emotional support they received from their community.

For immigrants like Nancy and Beverly, they were willing to migrate to the U.S. because they knew they had a support system to help them navigate their new location. Karen mentions that it is only with the knowledge offered by fellow group members who understood her situation that she could survive. They suggest that undocumented immigrants who are new to this country must learn to navigate the system without being detected, and community is critical in this regard. Beverly said,

> You have to have someone. You can't just jump and come to the states. You have to have someone to help give you a push start, you have to have someone who is aware...someone to at least let you stay with them for a few weeks or a month, just to get you started you know. But just to come here with no community, you won't survive.

Pat sees these networks of solidarity as "silent networks," as havens for undocumented immigrants that help them figure out how to survive in this new cultural environment. Pat stated,

> Yes, they help you out because they know like, you don't have a choice, you especially, when it comes to the home health aide jobs. Like, you get one quick, and you stay there for a week and you can make some money, some cash of course, so family, community, they help a lot.

For undocumented immigrants such as Pat, being able to work and provide for herself and family is only possible through networking with individuals who have shared similar experiences.

According to Shelly, when it comes to seeking out medical services the first, and at times, the only option undocumented immigrants have is to turn to their local networks for answers. She said, "My friends were important, you know, they tell you what not to do, give you directions. They will say this is the bank you can go to open and account where they don't ask for much information you know." Shelly added that members of her community work the system to get healthcare, particularly when it comes to potential medical emergencies, knowing where to go, but more importantly knowing where to avoid. Having key information of this sort is valuable to undocumented immigrants' ability to survive as agents in this unwelcome environment.

Many undocumented immigrants mistrust the systems around them. The health system is not different, as Nancy recalled being warned by friends to not give out her information to hospitals because that information could later be used to locate her. She explained:

> There is too much questioning at the hospital, they are asking for all sort of things, calling for your ID...I don't want to deal with any of that, more than anything, you don't want your information to go into the system, once it hits that computer, they could do anything with it, you never know when your information could come back to hurt you.

Distrust in the medical system is a major health disparity for undocumented immigrants living in the U.S. To navigate this structural limitations, undocumented immigrants I interviewed rely on community networks in order to survive. These networks provide the communicative resources needed to challenge the dominant structures that surround them. For Pat, knowing which doctors were immigrant-friendly and which doctors were not was valuable information that, she said, allowed her to maintain good health without being detected.

Most of the undocumented immigrants that were interviewed spoke about how their network constantly helped them find creative ways to navigate the limitations of the structures around them. Troy highlights this point when he said,

> I mean you have situations where like it is either mom, or mom and the children back at home and you really need the money to help them, or they are here with you and you do not have a way to survive, so you turn to whatever you need to do to survive and that is something that the Trump administration doesn't understand. People help people survive.

In situations such as those that Ricardo and Troy face, one strategy is to fall back on the collective. According to Troy and Beverly, immigrants can survive in this country because of the close-knit communities that they participate in. Migrating is a challenging process that involves making sacrifices to be able to gain economic sustainability. One sacrifice these immigrants made when they moved from a less developed country to a global economic powerhouse like the U.S. was to forego the relatively accessible healthcare they received in their native countries.

Communication Strategies

Trump's executive order helped to reify the uneven power structures that undocumented immigrants in the U.S. face discursively and materially. When considering that most health messages produced in the U.S. are geared towards citizens with adequate access to the healthcare system, it becomes important to ask how dominant forms of communication affect those who lack similar access (Hacker, Anies, Folb, & Zallman, 2015). While immigration-unfriendly policies might not directly speak to the health system, they nevertheless generate and circulate anti-immigrant discourses that reinforce structural inequalities and individual fears by framing undocumented immigrants as unworthy of public services.

In this chapter, former President Donald Trump's executive order was chosen as a focal point to highlight the role of policy as a barrier for undocumented immigrants because all 16 participants in this research study talked about the role of the former President in marginalizing them and curtailing their access to health. It was not in the initial interview questions to discuss the former President's executive order, but after completing the first few interviews it was clear that his discourse was important to understanding how this group negotiated access to health.

Critical to this endeavor is understanding how these migrants make sense of/communicate about health. However, there is not much scholarship that speaks to this issue. In fact, a search of the Communication Abstracts database, using "undocumented immigrants" as key words, does not yield any articles that address health issues among illegal/undocumented immigrants directly, let alone present narratives from undocumented immigrants on how they navigate health and well-being. This chapter serves as an entry point into this critical topic at a time when the U.S. is rife with rhetoric that seeks to erect walls, demonize, and persecute undocumented immigrants. Through interviews with undocumented immigrants in South Florida, we tried to document how this community communicates about health amid structures that limit access to mainstream health platforms. Based on our interpretation of the interview data, here are a few action steps we'd like to offer even as we want to note that action steps, particularly when such initiatives affect lives of those at the margins of our society, are always dynamic, contextual and require intense listening of life stories that exist at the margins.

First, we argue that the research participants, all of who have been undocumented immigrants, actively forge meanings of health and survival through an acknowledgment and performance of their subaltern cultural positions in engagements with structural restrictions that their cultural positioning brings. This argument aligns with the culture-structure-agency axes of the CCA, which we adopted as a theoretical backdrop of this chapter. Hence, it is critically important that any health promotion initiative recognize that individuals at the margins of our society can and do indeed communicate about their health needs and strategies to navigate health systems within the constraints they face. This recognition should replace the impetus to impose on those at the margins what health experts *think* are needs and strategies of the margins.

Second, the restrictions that accompany being an undocumented immigrant create various structural challenges for individuals who must navigate such limitations in creative ways. Situated in the narrative of the research participants is a powerful sense of survival that is sustained by the need for individuals to support someone other than themselves. Troy's story highlights the way undocumented immigrants see solidarity as a necessity for their survival. Due to the need to support others in their community, finding a way around the restrictions of the system is vital for this group. Hence, policy makers might want to adopt a more ground-up collaborative approach to policy making.

The importance of community and solidarity in the lives of our research participants points to the likelihood that health promotion/ policy initiatives must involve and target the community and essentially create pathways for listening to the community in ways that enable community narratives to dictate health problems and possible solutions that are important to the community. Thus, policies such as Trump's executive order for the protection of the interior of the U.S., limits the movement of undocumented immigrants and only induces fear. Survival and solidarity, on the other hand, become critical to living a healthy and meaningful life in limiting circumstances for our research participants.

Notes

1 The term 'undocumented immigrant' refers to foreign nationals residing in the U.S. without legal immigration status. It includes persons who entered the U.S. without inspection and proper permission from the U.S. government, and those who entered with a legal visa that is no longer valid (Briggs, 2009).

2 Executive Order 13768 titled Enhancing Public Safety in the Interior of the United States. "Section 5 of the order prioritizes removal of aliens who have been convicted of any criminal offense; have been charged with any criminal offense, where such charge has not been resolved; have committed acts that constitute a chargeable criminal offense; have engaged in fraud or willful misrepresentation in connection with any official matter or application before a governmental agency; have abused any program related to receipt of public benefits; are subject to a final order of removal, but who have not complied with their legal obligation to depart the United States; or in the judgment of an immigration officer, otherwise pose a risk to public safety or national security" (Tal & Shoichet, 2017).

Recommended Readings

Derose, K. P., Escarce, J. J., & Lurie, N. (2007). Immigrants and Health Care: Sources of Vulnerability. *Health Affairs*, 26(5), 1258–1268.

Edwards, J. (2014). Undocumented Immigrants and Access to Health Care: Making a Case for Policy Reform. *Policy, Politics, & Nursing Practice* 15(1–2), 5–14.

Newton, L. (2009). *Illegal, Alien, or Immigrant: The Politics of Immigration Reform.* New York: New York University Press.

Passel, J. S., & Cohn, D. (2009). *A Portrait of Unauthorized Immigrants in the United States.* Washington, DC: Pew Hispanic Center.

References

Basu, A., & Dutta, M. J. (2009). Sex Workers and HIV/AIDS: Analyzing Participatory Culture-Centered Health Communication Strategies. *Human Communication Research*, 35(1), 86–114. doi:10.1111/j.1468–2958.2008.01339.x

Biswas, D., Toebes, B., Hjern, A., Ascher, H., & Norredam, M. (2012). Access to Health Care for Undocumented Migrants from a Human Rights Perspective: A Comparative Study of Denmark, Sweden, and The Netherlands. *Health Human Rights,*. 2012 Dec 15;14(2): 49–60.

Bloemraad, I., Korteweg, A., & Yurdakul, G. (2008). Citizenship and Immigration: Multiculturalism, Assimilation, and Challenges to the Nation-State. *Annual Review of Sociology*, 34(1), 153–179. doi:10.1146/annurev.soc.34.040507.134608

Briggs, V. M. (2009). The State of U.S. Immigration Policy: The Quandary of Economic Methodology and the Relevance of Economic Research to Know. *Journal of Law, Economics and Policy*, 5(1): 177–193.

Capps, R., Castañeda, R. M., Chaudry, A., & Santos, R. (2007). *Paying the Price: The Impact of Immigration Raids on America's Children.* Washington, DC: National Council of La Raza.

Cheong, P. (2007). Health Communication Resources for Uninsured and Insured Hispanics. *Health Communication*, 21(2), 153–163. doi:10.1080/10410230701307188

Dutta, M. J. (2008). *Communicating Health: A Culture-Centered Approach.* London, England: Polity Press.

Dutta, M. J. (2010).The Critical Cultural Turn in Health Communication: Reflexivity, Solidarity, and Praxis. *Health Communication*, 25, 534–539.

Dutta, M. J. & Zoller H. M. (2008). Theoretical foundations: Interpretive, critical, and cultural approaches to health communication. In H. M. Zoller & M. J. Dutta (Eds.), *Emerging Perspectives in Health Communication* (pp. 1–18). New York: Routledge.

Edwards, J. (2014). Undocumented Immigrants and Access to Health Care: Making a Case for Policy Reform. *Policy, Politics, & Nursing Practice*, 15(1–2), 5–14.

Hacker, K., Anies, M. E., Folb, B., & Zallman, L. (2015). Barriers to Health Care for Undocumented Immigrants: A Literature Review. *Risk Management and Healthcare Policy*, 175. doi:10.2147/rmhp.s70173

Karp, R. J., Rhee, D., Feldman, D., & Bouchkouj, N. (2007). Outreach to Immigrant Communities: Teaching Pediatric Residents about Access to Health Care. *Journal of Health Care for the Poor and Underserved*, 18(3), 510–515. doi:10.1353/hpu.2007.0060

Kullgren, J. T. (2003). Restrictions on Undocumented Immigrants' Access to Health Services: The Public Health Implications of Welfare Reform. *American Journal of Public Health*, 93(10), 1630–1633.

Lee, Y., Ottati, V., & Hussain, I. (2001). Attitudes Toward "Illegal" Immigration into the United States: California Proposition 187. *Hispanic Journal of Behavioral Sciences*, 23(4), 430–443. doi:10.1177/0739986301234005

Lupton, D. (1994). Toward the Development of Critical Health Communication Praxis. *Health Communication*, 6, 55–67. doi: 10.1207/s15327027hc0601_4

Newton, L. (2009). *Illegal, Alien, or Immigrant: The Politics of Immigration Reform*. New York: New York University Press.

Passel, J. S. (2005). The Size and Characteristics of the Unauthorized Migrant Population in the U.S.: Estimates Based on the March 2005 Current Population Survey. Pew Hispanic Research Reports, Washington, DC. http://pewhispanic.org/reports/report.php?ReportID=61

Passel, J. S., & Cohn, D. (2009). *A Portrait of Unauthorized Immigrants in the United States*. Washington, DC: Pew Hispanic Center.

Spivak, G. C. (1988). *Can the Subaltern Speak?* Basingstoke: Macmillan.

U.S. Bureau of the Census. (2008). *Native and Foreign-Born Populations by Selected Characteristics: 2007*. Washington, DC: United States Department of Commerce.

U.S. Census Bureau. (2007). Educational Attainment in the United States: 2007. Retrieved from http://blueprod.ssd.census.gov/prod/2009pubs/p20-560.pdf

5 Language Barriers as a Social Phenomenon

Distinctive Impacts on Health Communication in Japan and the United States

Sachiko Terui and Elaine Hsieh

Papina, from the Philippines, was involved in a car accident soon after she came to Japan. Her Japanese proficiency at the time was near-novice, limiting her to brief greetings. The other driver fled. No one was around to call for an ambulance or the police. Experiencing great pain and shock, Papina drove to a hospital nearby for emergency treatment. To her surprise, she was turned away. She was told to come back the next day. Papina believed that she was sent back home because she did not come in with an ambulance.

Cherri, from China, is a doctoral student at a Japanese university. Cherri writes research manuscripts and presents conference papers in Japanese. When she got a fever, she went to a hospital to obtain antibiotics. Cherri's doctor prescribed painkillers instead. Although Cherri had language proficiency in communicating her perspectives and needs, she decided not to say anything because she didn't know how to express her disagreement politely without offending her doctor. Instead, Cherri visited another hospital, hoping the physician would offer her preferred medication.

Language barriers faced by immigrants and refugees have been widely recognized as a social determinant of health. Nevertheless, the literature has predominately focused on the impacts of language barriers on provider-patient interactions. Papina's and Cherri's cases demonstrate that language barriers can influence patients' health and health communication in all stages of care (Terui, 2017). This chapter examines how individuals' experiences of language barriers are constructed and limited by their host society's sociopolitical and sociocultural contexts. Our conceptualization of language barriers extends the Model of Bilingual Health Communication (Hsieh, 2016) and echoes with culture-centered approach (Dutta, 2008) and Integral Fusion (Hsieh & Kramer, 2021).

DOI: 10.4324/9781003230243-5

Reconceptualizing Language Barriers as Localized, Situated Experiences

In the *Model of Bilingual Health Communication*, Hsieh (2016) conceptualized bilingual healthcare as a socially constructed, goal-driven communicative activity that requires multi-party coordination on the meanings and processes of healthcare delivery. In addition, language-discordant patients' experiences are situated in the larger society, shaped by the corresponding normative expectations of the sociocultural and sociopolitical environments (Hsieh, 2018). As such, system-level influences can impact all aspects of care, resulting in diverging experiences, meanings, and outcomes. To truly appreciate language barriers, Hsieh (2016) urged researchers to "examine the impacts of these system-level influences in enhancing/compromising quality care" and "explore the system-level structures that best promote successful bilingual health care" (p. 274). In this chapter, we aim to explore the various system-level influences that shape language-discordant individuals' experiences of health and illness in Japan and the United States.

Our approach to our participants' experiences is grounded in culture-centered approaches (Dutta, 2008). *A culture-centered approach* invites marginalized communities to engage in dialogues that challenge existing social structure/order, address historically situated social injustice, and collaborate and co-create structures and knowledge with the larger society (Dutta, 2018). Dutta (2007) conceptualized culture as "a complex and dynamic web of meanings that is continuously in flux, as it interacts with the structural processes that surround the culture" (pp. 310–311). Dutta's focus on the structural processes echoes with our interests to examine "the organization of social systems, the patterns of distribution of resources, and the patterns of control of these resources that are inherent in the production and reinforcement of social inequities" (p. 319). In addition, because a culture-centered approach recognizes the potential bias of the larger society and legitimizes the perspectives of the marginalized, such an approach is particularly valuable to examine how language-discordant individuals experience disparities and alienation.

Finally, *Integral Fusion*, a type of cultural consciousness proposed by Hsieh and Kramer (2021), guides our understanding and analysis of our participants' experiences. Integral Fusion is a result of intercultural interactions. As individuals travel between and across different cultures, they develop cultural perspectives that enrich their understanding of their realities. In addition, their experiences are situated in the larger society, resulting in pan-evolutionary effects that change both the cultural sojourners and the host society (Hsieh & Kramer, 2021). In a pluralistic society, its cultural members constantly and continuously engage in dynamic interactions, through which individuals negotiate, resist, and collaborate to reach mutually agreeable solutions (Terui & Hsieh, 2020). Cultural members' interactions are influenced by and actively shape the evolving, shifting political, economic, and dialogic forces within the larger society. In short, we view culture as a living process through which cultural participants and their host society continuously shape and are shaped by each other's presence and experiences.

The voice of marginalized populations, situated in their cultural perspectives and contexts, provides invaluable insight into how they construct meanings in health and illness, understand health behaviors, and identify possible solutions. By examining immigrants' and refugees' experiences of language barriers as localized, situated experiences, we aim to explore how such experiences can be shaped and constrained by the host society's larger sociopolitical and sociocultural contexts.

Language Barriers as a Social Phenomenon

The literature on language barriers has provided opportunities to address health disparities experienced by immigrants and refugees. Within the literature, an overwhelming number of studies centered on provider-patient interactions. Few studies have theorized language barriers in health contexts. A lack of theoretical framework reflects a common misconception – assuming language barriers are practical, technical problems in healthcare settings, rather than communicative challenges involving the intersections of medicine, culture, language, and one's lived environments.

For example, in Segalowitz and Kehayia's (2011) extensive review of language barriers in healthcare, language barriers are defined as "language-based obstacles to successful communication *between a patient and a health care provider* that have *consequences* for health care delivery" (emphasis added; p. 482). They emphasized the importance of examining language barriers in healthcare because of "its *universality* and the very high stakes that may be involved in miscommunication" (emphasis added; p. 486). We agree that language barriers in healthcare have high stakes. Their definition and conceptualization, however, failed to capture the complex, multidimensional, and nuanced nature of language barriers in healthcare in three ways.

First, it is important that we expand the investigation of language barriers in health contexts beyond provider-patient interactions. Although language barriers may be most salient and observable in medical encounters, they also impact individuals' access to care and health maintenance in everyday life (e.g., obtaining health information, navigating healthcare systems, and maintaining treatment adherence; Terui, 2017). By looking beyond medical encounters, researchers can identify a wide range of intervention points and solutions that address the impacts of language barriers on the access to, process of, and outcomes of care.

Second, individuals' experiences of language barriers vary in intensity and are often shaped by their levels of language proficiency and sociolinguistic skill. By focusing their investigation of language barriers during medical encounters, researchers inadvertently limited their attention to the negative consequences of clinical care (Suarez et al., 2021). However, the impacts of language barriers are not limited to clinical consequences. For example, language barriers may be intentional discrimination and/or structural barrier utilized by a host society that aims to alienate cultural Others. Recognizing such hostile attitudes, immigrants and refugees may avoid preventive care, delay help-seeking behaviors, and rely on interpersonal networks for illness management (Hsieh & Kramer, 2021).

In addition, the presence of language barriers should not be conceptualized as a dichotomous, either/or phenomenon limited to "foreigners." For example, a host society or health facility may provide language access (e.g., interpreters and translated materials) for certain groups of language-discordant patients (e.g., deaf patients using American Sign Language), but not others (e.g., Spanish-speaking migrant workers). English-speaking foreign patients in Taiwan may be less likely to experience language barriers than local elderlies who speak only Taiwanese because all physicians learn medicine through English textbooks and use English for patient record-keeping, but not all physicians can speak Taiwanese (i.e., Mandarin is the official language in Taiwan; Hsieh, 2018).

Finally, solutions to language barriers cannot be one-size-fits-all. Segalowitz and Kehayia's (2011) assumed that language barriers in healthcare can be addressed through universal solutions. While language-discordant individuals may share universal experiences, they also face unique challenges and barriers due to cultural particulars within a host society. Different host societies often entail distinct sociocultural and sociopolitical environments. These environments and their cultural particulars hold diverging forces in shaping (a) the meanings of health and illness, (b) the normative expectations of healthcare behaviors, and (c) the social resources that are available to cultural Others (e.g., immigrants and refugees).

Hsieh (2018) argued that (a) language discordance is a social phenomenon that may entail diverging meanings and experiences in different countries, (b) language-discordant patients may not share similar experiences even if they are in the same country, and (c) disparities in language concordance may be confounded with other disparities and cultural particulars that are unique to a host society. For example, in the United States, language-discordant care generally means that the patient has limited English proficiency (rather than the provider is using his second language); in contrast, in Japan, language-discordant care may mean that both patients and their physicians communicate in their second language (e.g., English; Terui, 2017). In addition, depending on the patients' ethnicity and/or country of origin, language-discordant patients may experience preferential treatment (e.g., an English-speaking, white patient from France) or potential discrimination (e.g., a Bantu-speaking, black patient from Zimbabwe) in a host society even though both would be considered to receive language-discordant care (Hsieh, 2018; Terui, 2017). In short, it is important to recognize that language barriers in health contexts are more multidimensional than the literature depicted.

In summary, we argue that language barriers are complex, multidimensional, and nuanced social phenomena. Individuals' experiences of language barriers are influenced by the culture, policies, and lived environments in the corresponding host society.

Health Policies and Access to Care for Immigrants and Refugees

How immigrants and refugees experience their health and language barriers in healthcare largely depends on the culture of the host society, its approaches to healthcare, and the availability of social resources (Hsieh, 2018). To further delineate host societies and local authorities' willingness to make accommodations for immigrants and refugees, we will first examine policies related to language access in healthcare in Japan and in the United States. Our analysis centered on social policies and legal regulations related to providing culturally and linguistically appropriate care in these two countries.

Health Policies and Language Access in Japan

Under the Japanese social security system, immigrants and refugees with valid documentation who stay in Japan more than 90 days are eligible to have national health insurance (国民健康保険 Kokumin kenko hoken; Okubo, 2004). This national health insurance provides equal quality of medical treatment and access to healthcare to every insurance holder. However, when it comes to social resources, specifically language services, the Japanese state of being a jus sanguinis[1] reinforces the tendency to exclude immigrants and refugees without Japanese blood (Sato, 2009). The Japanese government sets no legislative guidelines for providing language services to immigrants and refugees, except for Japanese returnees from China (Iida, 2010). Those with Japanese blood are entitled to receive government support to have access to healthcare interpreters (Iida, 2010, 2011). Immigrants and refugees without Japanese blood primarily rely on services provided by local governments, non-profit organizations, and medical institutions (e.g., multilingual websites, volunteer interpreters, and accessibility technologies; Nakamura, 2012).

Health Policies and Language Access in the United States

Unlike Japan, immigrants' and refugees' children are US citizens as long as they were born in the United States and its territories. The US government offers Medicaid and Medicare for US citizens and permanent residents who meet specific qualifications. Medicare is a government health insurance program available for ones who (a) are 65 or older, (b) are younger than age 65 with specific types of disabilities and/or are with end-stage renal disease (Centers for Medicare & Medicaid Services, 2021a). Medicaid is a needs-based program funded by both federal and state governments. One must meet income-based eligibility to receive the service (Centers for Medicare & Medicaid Services, 2021b). Individuals who do not meet these criteria select their own health providers based on quality and cost either by themselves or through employer-based health programs (De Gagne et al., 2014). Choosing health insurance can present additional obstacles to maintaining good health for immigrant populations who are not familiar with the US social and healthcare systems (De Gagne et al., 2014).

With the continual increases not only in the number of immigrants and refugees, but also in the diversity of these groups, the Office of Minority Health at the U.S. Department of Health and Human Services published the National Standards for Culturally and Linguistically Appropriate Services in Health and Health Care (CLAS Standards). The CLAS Standards require healthcare institutions receiving government funding to provide linguistically and culturally appropriate healthcare (Barksdale et al., 2017). Unfortunately, such a policy does not ensure successful mitigation of adverse effects caused by language barriers because not all medical providers are knowledgeable about laws and policies and how to implement them in their institutions (Barksdale et al., 2017). In fact, several studies suggest that legislation and policies have limited impacts on healthcare providers' use of language-related services (Ginde et al., 2010).

Method

Data used in this chapter were collected by the first author through semi-structured, in-depth interviews with language-discordant immigrants and refugees living in Japan (N = 30) and the United States (N = 30). Participants recruited in Japan are from 13 countries, and the participants recruited in the United States are from ten countries. Both English and Japanese languages were used for data collection. More than 50 hours of interview data were transcribed verbatim.

The data gathered using Japanese was first analyzed in Japanese before translating them into English. This procedure allowed us to preserve the cultural contexts, ensuring minimal distortions and lost meanings in the translation processes (Squires, 2009). Using narrative approach (Fisher, 1987), we explored the ways these participants understand their experiences of facing language barriers in managing health. We identified major issues salient to our language-discordant participants through applied thematic analysis (Guest et al., 2011), highlighting their experiences in accessing healthcare and related processes and the sociopolitical and sociocultural elements of their lived environments.

Challenges and Recommendations

Revisiting Papina's Case

Language barriers compromise patients' familiarities and accessibilities with the healthcare systems in their local communities. Many participants shared their concerns about their language and interpersonal skills in communicating with medical providers. Such concerns can arise from lack of proficiency and uncertainties about sociocultural norms. However, they also noted that these concerns do not always prevent them from seeking medical treatments because they know the locations of the hospitals and clinics and because they believe that they can receive treatment as long as they get to a healthcare facility. Such attitudes are shared by immigrants and refugees in both Japan and the United States.

However, when it comes to an emergency, unexpected waiting time could be troublesome and life-threatening, and knowing the locations of healthcare facilities is not adequate to promptly utilize resources in Japan. Immigrants and refugees in Japan experienced language barriers in accessing emergency care, particularly with the ways to use ambulances. Papina explained,

> After I came to Japan, I had a car accident. I drove to the hospital by myself. There is no one who could call 119 and the police for me. The other driver fled, and I was alone... [When I arrived at the hospital,] they said, "Not today. Come back tomorrow morning. Not tonight. You are okay today." They said it's because I didn't come in an ambulance.

Papina did not feel confident to call 119, a local telephone number for emergency and an equivalent to 911 in the United States. Thus, she drove to the hospital by herself, believing that she would be able to see a doctor once she got there. Many participants said that they would have made the same decision as Papina, visiting an emergency care unit by themselves without using an ambulance. Remembering the time when she accompanied a friend to a hospital in an ambulance, Ida explained, "I was surprised. The Japanese ambulance came so quickly! In my country [Indonesia], it's faster to go to hospitals by ourselves compared to calling an ambulance. And we'd have to pay for it."

Calling an ambulance requires individuals to articulate the specific nature and the exact location of the emergency, which may demand the kind of linguistic skills (e.g., proficiency, accuracy, and clarity) that language-discordant individuals may not have – particularly in an emergency situation that involves heightened emotions and compromised cognitive abilities. This problem is reduced when the incident happens at or near the place they live. Individuals typically know their address and can articulate it without much difficulty. However, when the need for an ambulance occurs outside the individual's familiar areas (e.g., the cases of traffic accidents), it is difficult to identify the exact location. This problem is exacerbated in Japan because only major Japanese highways have names – neighborhood streets do not. Articulating the specific location takes more time and is more nuanced. Thus, language-discordant individuals must possess a higher level of communicative skills to convey their situations and needs. They also face a higher risk of delayed care (e.g., ambulance misdirected to the wrong place) as a result of miscommunication. Together, such concerns can reduce a person's self-efficacy in seeking emergency care through paramedics.

Revisiting Cherri's Case

Language-discordant individuals learn appropriate and desirable behaviors in their host societies through daily interactions and observations. Having learned what could be perceived as culturally appropriate ways, these cultural sojourners work to perform these identities in medical encounters, aiming for desirable identities, relationships, and health outcomes. Nevertheless, they face unique challenges that prevent them from asserting desirable identities due to language barriers.

Many immigrants and refugees in Japan are aware that Japanese society places high value on politeness, including the belief that politeness and agreeableness are key components to successful interaction (Lebra, 2004). In provider-patient interactions, politeness and agreeableness play more important roles, especially in light of the power differences present in provider-patient dyads. Medical providers have more power based on the amount of information they hold about medical treatment and their high social status in Japan. When disagreements occur in provider-patient interactions, patients face difficulties in communicating their thoughts and preferences in an effective manner. Cherri shared her narrative.

When I was in China, I used Kampo (漢方: Chinese traditional medicine). I have a pretty good idea of which part of my body suffers and what I need to heal. I went to a hospital when I got a fever. Although I thought I needed a particular medicine to draw out the irritation, I was prescribed a painkiller. I couldn't point it out. Isn't it awkward if I explain to the doctor how the human body works? I would say things if it were in China. The Chinese doctor would understand what I am saying without that much effort. Japanese is less direct than Chinese. I try not to say a lot because I don't know the better ways to communicate my concerns... in the Japanese way.

Cherri was in a bind. She recognized that she did not have the linguistic and interpersonal skills needed to discuss her preferred treatment without implying that she is more knowledgeable about Kampo and other medicine than her doctor, a serious face threat to physicians in Japanese culture. As a result, she decided to forego her agenda and visited a different clinic hoping that the next provider would offer her what she wanted.

Other participants recruited in Japan shared similar experiences. During the interviews, the first author found that they have high language proficiency in Japanese, allowing them to communicate their concerns in detail. However, their language proficiency is not high enough to communicate nuanced meanings without being direct or blunt. If they have had language skills similar to those of native Japanese speakers, they would have been better able to express their concerns without offending medical providers. Daily interactions taught them that culturally inappropriate interactions may contribute to social sanctions (e.g., less friendly interactions). They decided not to speak up about their concerns or disagreements to avoid potentially negative consequences (e.g., unfavorable treatment). In short, language-discordant patients in Japan may face prolonged time to receive treatment and increased financial burdens due to the sociocultural and sociopolitical contexts.

Universalities and Cultural Particulars of System-Level Forces

The narratives collected in Japan and the United States show both cross-environmental and environment-specific influences on language barriers. Participants in both countries indicated an awareness of the impacts of their language barriers both inside and outside provider-patient interaction. Charmaz (1991) described that individuals' experiences of chronic illness are not static but often fluctuate between high and low points as they adapt to illness conditions and manage activities in everyday life. Our participants' experiences with language barriers echo with such an understanding. When they feel ill, their language proficiency decreases due to their reduced cognitive abilities for everyday tasks. Participants recruited in Japan and the United States both mentioned that when they are sick, their interlocutors (e.g., friends and physicians) can face greater language barriers when communicating with them. For our participants in Japan and the United States, their experiences with the oscillating struggles with language barriers and the perceived burdens placed on social interactions with native-speaking others are fundamentally similar. From this perspective, the sociocultural and sociopolitical environments do not significantly influence language barriers, affirming the concept of universality in language barriers depicted in Segalowitz and Kehayia (2011). Nonetheless, such a concept is not applicable in a number of situations.

As demonstrated in Papina's case, some narratives shared by participants recruited in Japan highlighted that the lack of knowledge about local procedures accentuates the adverse influences of language barriers, positing a critical challenge to accessing healthcare, especially in an emergency. Similar to the notion that language-discordant patients tend to be unaware of environment-specific diseases, attributed by some to a lack of social interaction with local individuals (Ndiaye et al., 2011), language barriers tend to require additional effort to learn local procedures needed to utilize resources (Wakimoto et al., 2013). Frequently, language-discordant patients do not recognize the need for such information until encountering problematic situations or outcomes (e.g., an emergency; Wakimoto et al., 2013).

Participants in both countries shared the experiences of obtaining information and perceptions about healthcare through their social networks. Participants indicated that interpersonal interaction and interpersonal relationship management largely affect access to healthcare. In particular, language barriers (a) contribute to developing distorted knowledge and (mis)understandings of healthcare in the host society, and (b) impose additional obstacles in managing interpersonal relationships within an individual's limited social network. The predominant difference in the impact of these distortions and misunderstandings of healthcare systems in the United States and Japan is whether or not these language-discordant individuals can dispel distortion and misunderstandings by obtaining firsthand experiences through using the healthcare system in their host societies. Relatively manageable healthcare cost in Japan presents fewer obstacles to obtaining firsthand experiences than healthcare costs in the United States. Having the correct information about the local healthcare system is critical for gaining timely and effective access to healthcare.

The accessibility to healthcare interpreters in the local environments also influences language-discordant patients' access to healthcare. Lukes and Miller (2002) noted that immigrant and refugee populations tend to view a lack of visible symptoms or noticeable discomfort as less crucial in seeking healthcare, thereby placing little weight on preventive care. Some of our language-discordant participants indicated that symptoms are not critical enough to place burdens on other people. As a result, they prioritized harmony in interpersonal relationships and/or avoided trouble or inconvenience to others. Such concerns may be particularly heightened for immigrants and refugees as they are motivated to conserve resources within their limited support networks in case of future needs. Most of the participants recruited in Japan did not have easy access to healthcare interpreters, and they typically bring their family members and friends as an interpreter. Even when language-discordant patients want to visit hospitals/clinics, these participants in Japan sometimes have to wait for their friends' or family members' availability to schedule an appointment for medical treatment. Relationship and identity management can be costly, particularly when individuals have close and limited social networks, as is often the case with immigrants and refugees in general and recent immigrants in particular.

Our findings also support previous studies which demonstrated that language barriers produce less effective provider-patient communication due in large part to the patients' lack of linguistic abilities in expressing their concerns, symptoms, and preferences for treatment, as well as their proficiency in understanding the information given by their medical providers (Flores, 2006). We argue that such difficulties in provider-patient interaction do not always reflect language-discordant patients' lack of language proficiencies. Individuals with high levels of language proficiency still encounter substantial miscommunication in sharing information that is less accurate than it may appear. Some participants recruited in both countries reported that they *think* they know how to express their symptoms, but they also wonder whether or not the words they use are accurate. These participants noted that there are many words and expressions they heard in daily conversations, and they used these words and expressions in the interactions with their providers, believing that they knew the meanings. However, they later wondered how accurately they explained their perspectives and symptoms. When medical providers observe language-discordant patients speaking fluently and their explanations make sense to the medical providers, the medical providers may not recognize possible misunderstandings (Hsieh, 2016). Being able to say specific words, even with excellent pronunciation, does not always mean that individuals understand the nuanced meanings the words carry (Maddux, 2002). To express a person's symptoms and provide information about how one feels in culturally appropriate and understandable ways, individuals must be able to do more than just naming the symptoms (Holland & Quinn, 1987).

Similarly, having a high degree of language proficiency does not always lead to better care. When healthcare providers perceive their patients have a high degree of language proficiency, they may formulate inaccurate assumptions about the patients. Some participants recruited in the United States shared that local individuals in the United States may not recognize language-discordant patients' lack of familiarity with local norms. Healthcare providers often overestimated patients' knowledge and understanding of procedures and treatment due to their high level of language proficiency. Participants who have lived in multicultural, multilingual communities (e.g., Miami and New York City) often raised such concerns. In other words, large, multilingual, and multicultural communities may hold differing expectations and assumptions for language-discordant patients when compared to smaller, less diverse communities. This particular challenge is mentioned only by participants recruited in the United States, underscoring the notion that each environment, even within the same country, contributes to differing influences of language barriers on experiences of health management, as well as the quality of provider-patient interaction.

Furthermore, the Japanese environment provides unique advantages and challenges for language-discordant individuals whose native language is English. A few participants recruited in Japan were native speakers of English. Their narratives reflect the influences of language hegemony and language hierarchy. Their narratives illustrate that, to a certain degree, language-discordant patients expect their medical providers to be able to communicate in English. Such an expectation was not shared among other participants in Japan nor those recruited in the United States: None of them blamed the medical providers' language skills in patients' native language (i.e., Chinese and Spanish, etc.) as being the cause of miscommunication. Such a hegemonic power of the English language creates unique interactional dynamics in provider-patient dyads.

Finally, narratives support the idea that language barriers do not always function negatively in healthcare settings. Previous literature has depicted language barriers as obstacles in provider-patient communication (Street, 1992). However, we argue that language barriers do not always provoke weak and inferior patient roles. Individuals with language barriers sometimes strategically use their non-native status as a resource useful in meeting healthcare goals (Terui, 2012). For example, when teased about his uncertainties/anxieties (and needs for social support), the participant in the United States embraced the powerless identity. It allowed him to play an active and engaged patient role without worrying too much about being seen as annoying. By reframing the nature of language barriers, it is possible for patients to be more comfortable when engaged in language-discordant provider-patient interactions. As strategic actors, individuals actively negotiate and shape contexts to further their goals (Goodwin & Duranti, 1992). As they co-evolve with the deep cultural and social norms and contexts in host societies, language-discordant individuals also actively and strategically re-arrange and negotiate their tasks, identities, and relationships within the immediate, interactional, localized contexts.

In conclusion, language proficiency alone does not overcome the adverse effects of language barriers. Language-discordant patients understand their language barriers in the context of their surrounding sociocultural and sociopolitical environments. The sociocultural and sociopolitical environments place both shared and unique challenges for language-discordant patients to navigate their management of health and illness. It is necessary to consider the fluctuating, multidimensional nature of language barriers when developing interventions to deepen understanding and ultimately to improve health among language-discordant patients.

Note

1 Jus sanguinis is a principle of nationality law by which citizenship is determined or acquired by the nationality or ethnicity of one or both parents.

Recommended Readings

Hsieh, E., & Kramer, E. M. (2021). *Rethinking culture in health communication: Social interactions as intercultural encounters.* Wiley.

Jacobs, E. A., & Diamond, L. C. (Eds.). (2017). *Providing health care in the context of language barriers: International perspectives.* Multilingual Matters.

Peled, Y. (2018). Language barriers and epistemic injustice in healthcare settings. *Bioethics, 32*(6), 360–367.

Schouten, B. C., Cox, A., Duran, G., Kerremans, K., Banning, L. K., Lahdidioui, A., van den Muijsenbergh, M., Schinkel, S., Sungur, H., Suurmond, J., Zendedel, R., & Krystallidou, D. (2020). Mitigating language and cultural barriers in healthcare communication: Toward a holistic approach. *Patient Education and Counseling, 103*(12), 2604–2608.

Terui, S. (2017). Conceptualizing the pathways and processes between language barriers and health disparities: Review, synthesis, and extension. *Journal of Immigrant and Minority Health, 19*(1), 215–224.

References

Barksdale, C. L., Rodick, W. H., Hopson, R., Kenyon, J., Green, K., & Jacobs, C. G. (2017). Literature review of the National CLAS Standards: Policy and practical implications in reducing health disparities. *Journal of Racial and Ethnic Health Disparities, 4*(4), 632–647. https://doi.org/10.1007/s40615-016-0267-3

Centers for Medicare & Medicaid Services. (2021a, April 12). *Medicare program: General information.* https://www.cms.gov/Medicare/Medicare-General-Information/MedicareGenInfo

Centers for Medicare & Medicaid Services. (2021b, April 12). *Medicate managed care eligibility and enrollment.* https://www.cms.gov/medicare/eligibility-and-enrollment/medicaremangcareeligenrol

Charmaz, K. (1991). *Good days, bad days: The self in chronic illness and time.* Rutgers University Press.

De Gagne, J. C., Oh, J., So, A., & Kim, S.-S. (2014). The healthcare experiences of Koreans living in North Carolina: A mixed methods study. *Health & Social Care in the Community, 22*(4), 417–428. https://doi.org/10.1111/hsc.12098

Dutta, M. J. (2007). Communicating about culture and health: Theorizing culture-centered and cultural sensitivity approaches. *Communication Theory, 17*(3), 304–328.

Dutta, M. J. (2008). *Communicating health: A culture-centered approach.* Polity Press.

Dutta, M. J. (2018). Culture-centered approach in addressing health disparities: Communication infrastructures for subaltern voices. *Communication Methods and Measures, 12*(4), 239–259. https://doi.org/10.1080/19312458.2018.1453057

Fisher, W. R. (1987). *Human communication as narration: Toward a philosophy of reason, value, and action.* University of South Carolina Press.

Flores, G. (2006). Language barriers to health care in the United States. *New England Journal of Medicine, 355*(3), 229–231. https://doi.org/doi:10.1056/NEJMp058316

Ginde, A. A., Sullivan, A. F., Corel, B., Caceres, J. A., & Camargo, C. A., Jr. (2010). Reevaluation of the effect of mandatory interpreter legislation on use of professional interpreters for ED patients with language barriers. *Patient Education and Counseling, 81*(2), 204–206.

Goodwin, C., & Duranti, A. (1992). Rethinking context: An introduction. In A. Duranti & C. Goodwin (Eds.), *Rethinking context: Language as an interactive phenomenon* (pp. 1–42). Cambridge University Press.

Guest, G., MacQueen, K. M., & Namey, E. E. (2011). *Applied thematic analysis.* Sage.

Holland, D., & Quinn, N. (1987). Culture and cognition. In N. Quinn & D. Holland (Eds.), *Cultural models in language and thought* (pp. 3–40). Cambridge University Press.

Hsieh, E. (2016). *Bilingual health communication: Working with interpreters in cross-cultural care.* Routledge.

Hsieh, E. (2018). Reconceptualizing language discordance: Meanings and experiences of language barriers in the U.S. and Taiwan. *Journal of Immigrant and Minority Health, 20*(1), 1–4. https://doi.org/10.1007/s10903-017-0556-x

Hsieh, E., & Kramer, E. M. (2021). *Rethinking culture in health communication: Social interactions as intercultural encounters.* Wiley.

Iida, N. (2010). Zainichi gaikokujin wo taisyou toshita gengohosyou wo kangaeru: Komunitei tsuuyaku no genjyou to kadai kara [The present condition and problems of community interpreters involved in the support system for returnees from China: A study of interpreter roles]. *Ritsumeikan Ningenkagaku Kenkyuu, 21*, 75–88.

Iida, N. (2011). Zaijyuu gaikokujin oyobi iryou kankou mokuteki no hounichi gaikokujin ni taisuru iryoutuuyaku no genjyou to kadai [The present condition and problems of medical interpreters for the foreigners living in Japan and visiting Japan]. *Ritsumeikan Ningenkagaku Kenkyuu, 23*, 47–57.

Lebra, T. S. (2004). *The Japanese self in cultural logic.* University of Hawai'i Press.

Lukes, S. M., & Miller, F. Y. (2002). Oral health issues among migrant farmworkers. *Journal of Dental Hygiene, 76*(2), 134–140.

Maddux, J. E. (2002). Stopping the "madness": Positive psychology and deconstructing the illness ideology and the DSM. In C. R. Snyder & S. J. Lopez (Eds.), *The Oxford handbook of positive psychology* (pp. 13–25). Oxford University Press.

Nakamura, Y. (2012). Iryou tuuyakushi: Komunikeeshon wo shien suru senmonshoku [Medical interpreters: Experts to assist patient-physician communication]. *Jichitai Kokusaika Foramu, 276*, 2–4.

Ndiaye, K., Krieger, J. L., Warren, J. R., & Hecht, M. L. (2011). Communication and health disparity. In T. L. Thompson, R. Parrott, & J. F. Nussbaum (Eds.), *The Routledge handbook of health communication* (2nd ed., pp. 469–481). Routledge.

Okubo, T. (2004). Kokumin kenkou hoken seido to cyouka taizai gaikokujin [National health insurance and over-stayed foreigners in Japan]. *Shakai Kenronsyuu, 4*, 141–153.

Sato, B. (2009). *Zainichi "gaikokujin" dokuhon: Boodaares shakai no kisochishiki* [Reading about "foreigners" living in Japan: Fundamental knowledge about borderless society] (3rd ed.). Ryokuou Shuppan.

Segalowitz, N., & Kehayia, E. (2011). Exploring the determinants of language barriers in health care (LBHC): Toward a research agenda for the language sciences. *Canadian Modern Language Review, 67*(4), 480–507. https://doi.org/10.3138/cmlr.67.4.480

Squires, A. (2009). Methodological challenges in cross-language qualitative research: A research review. *International Journal of Nursing Studies, 46*(2), 277–287. https://doi.org/10.1016/j.ijnurstu.2008.08.006

Street, R. L., Jr. (1992). Analyzing communication in medical consultations: Do behavioral measures correspond to patients' perceptions? *Medical Care, 30*(11), 976–988.

Suarez, N. R. E., Urtecho, M., Nyquist, C. A., Jaramillo, C., Yeow, M.-E., Thorsteinsdottir, B., Wilson, M. E., & Barwise, A. K. (2021). Consequences of suboptimal communication for patients with limited English proficiency in the intensive care unit and suggestions for a way forward: A qualitative study of healthcare team perceptions. *Journal of Critical Care, 61*, 247–251. https://doi.org/10.1016/j.jcrc.2020.10.012

Terui, S. (2012). Second language learners' coping strategy in conversations with native speakers. *Journal of International Students, 2*(2), 168–183.

Terui, S. (2017). Conceptualizing the pathways and processes between language barriers and health disparities: Review, synthesis, and extension. *Journal of Immigrant and Minority Health, 19*(1), 215–224. https://doi.org/10.1007/s10903-015-0322-x

Terui, S., & Hsieh, E. (2020). Managing communicative challenges and interactional dilemma: Native speakers' responses to non-native speakers' lack of understanding. *Discourse Processes, 57*(1), 48–65. https://doi.org/10.1080/0163853X.2019.1624333

Wakimoto, T., Chisaki, M., & Uchida, K. (2013). Iryoo tsuuyakushi kara mita gaikokujin shinryou no arikata. [Medical interpreters' perspectives on treatments provided to foreign individuals]. *Shounika Shinryou, 76*(6), 971–975.

6 Mapping Young Female Refugees' Personal Communication System for Health Promotion

A Pilot Project in the United States

Hua Wang

Globally, every two seconds someone is forcibly displaced from their home; by June 2019, forced migration had uprooted an unprecedented 71 million people due to natural and manmade disasters; among them, 26 million were refugees who had to flee their countries because of persecution, war, or conflict (UNHCR, 2019). Refugees suffer from the lack of basic necessities and access to lucid information and health services (Cheng et al., 2018). Young female refugees are particularly vulnerable to sexual violence, sexually transmitted infections, unwanted pregnancies, unsafe abortions, as well as maternal morbidity and mortality (Cheng et al., 2018). This chapter provides insights from a pilot project called RYMBI, which aimed at developing an educational program to promote sexual and reproductive health among young female refugees in Clarkston, Georgia in the United States (Wang, 2018).

The project name RYMBI was used to represent our human-centered approach in the collaborative process of intervention design to honor the symbiotic relationships built in various refugee-serving support and learning networks. Our institutional partners included: Advocates for Youth (a nonprofit organization advocating honest sexuality education and young people's reproductive rights), the International Rescue Committee (IRC) in Atlanta (a flagship refugee resettlement agency in the United States and globally), and the Oakhurst Medical Centers (a refugee-serving health service providing organization in Georgia). Located on the outskirts of Atlanta, Clarkston has been designated as a refugee resettlement site since the 1980s. In 30 years, the city went from being 90% white to 82% non-white. Today, it is home to people from more than 40 countries, many of whom are refugees. The United States refugee resettlement policy prioritizes population groups that are the most vulnerable but have the best prospects for long-term integration, such as women and children. According to a report by the Migration Policy Institute, over half of the refugees from top resettlement origin countries

DOI: 10.4324/9781003230243-6

such as the Democratic Republic of the Congo and Burma were women and children (Blizzard & Batalova, 2019).

RYMBI focused on young adult female refugees because young adults have the greatest potential to bring about positive change in the refugee communities. Compared to other age groups, they are more likely to be adaptable in a new environment; receiving education in English language; and helping their parents, siblings, and peers to fulfill their needs during the resettlement process. They can serve as opinion leaders because they are active members of the community and have the qualities and skills to obtain, translate, and disseminate new information among those who already rely on them routinely and trust them deeply. Understanding how they are connected with the rest of the world can shed light on not only the complex challenges but also intriguing opportunities for innovative and effective health intervention design. The RYMBI project adopted a human-centered design thinking process with insights obtained through a simulated in-take experience with a refugee resettlement case manager, participant observations at the cultural orientation for newly arrived refugees, interviews with 22 young refugees and 16 refugee-serving experts, and secondary research on current literature and refugee databases (Wang, 2018).

This chapter focuses on the conceptual frameworks of a personal communication system and networked individualism. It also describes a mapping method used for intervention design so we can meet the intended audiences where they already are and work closely with them to create innovative and effective health programs. I begin with a brief literature review that highlights decades of research on social networks and health, the role of technologies in personal networks and well-being, and how understanding the social context of an individual's everyday life can better inform health intervention design. I then use the RYMBI project to illustrate how mapping a personal communication system can be accomplished. I conclude this chapter by discussing the lessons that our team has learned and their important implications for future endeavors.

Literature Review

Social Networks and Health

A social network is made of a set of social actors and their interconnected relationships (Perkins et al., 2015). We human beings are fundamentally social beings as biologically wired during the evolutionary process. Each of us is deeply embedded in complex webs of connections in the world. These social connections and interactions are at the core of our everyday life and become ever more important in the times of need. There are two approaches to studying social networks: The sociocentric approach takes a bird's eye view to examine all actors and their interconnectedness within a network, be it in an organization or a neighborhood. The egocentric approach takes on the perspective from one central actor as the ego and evaluates other actors as alters in the ego's personal network and their relationships (Perkins et al., 2015).

Decades of research has shown that the people with whom we are associated and spend time together are closely related to our own health and well-being, from the emotions we feel and the person we vote for to the diseases we contract and how long we live (e.g., Berkmann, 1984; Christakis & Fowler, 2009, 2013; Valente, 2010). For example, the risk of mortality for individuals with a meager network is doubled whereas those with a robust network benefit from their social capital with more emotional stability, psychological resilience, instrumental support, and better quality of life (Berkmann, 1984; Ikeda & Kawachi, 2010; Sluki, 2010). Social networks are critical for designing and evaluating effective interventions to change health behaviors and outcomes (Hunter et al., 2019; Latkin & Knowlton, 2015; Valente, 2012), especially among vulnerable and marginalized population groups (e.g., Perkins et al., 2015) and sensitive issues such as sexual and reproductive health (Hunter et al., 2019). Engaging young refugees to leverage knowledge from a

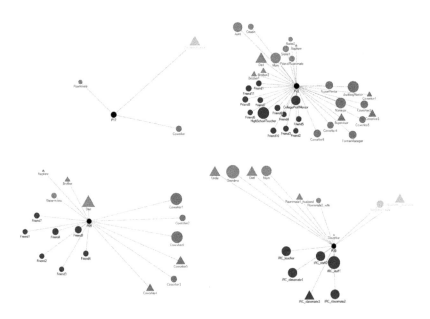

Figure 6.1 Examples of young female refugees' personal network visualization.
Note: The network graphs were created using NodeXL. Node shape indicates sex: disk = female, solid triangle = male; node size indicates age: the larger the older; node color indicates relationship: red = family/household, orange = neighbor, blue = school/education, green = work, black = participant; the distance from the participant to each alter indicates the closeness.

network perspective proved to be fruitful in RYMBI. However, one major challenge is to address the role of emerging technologies in the dynamic between social networks and health (Valente & Pitts, 2017).

Networked Individualism

Scholars have long debated about how new information and communication technologies (ICTs) affect social cohesion and isolation in a society (Hampton & Wellman, 2018), although most would agree that they often serve as a double-edged sword. Regardless of a utopian or a dystopian view one holds in this debate, an undeniable trend is that the rapid diffusion of new ICTs such as mobile phones, personal computers, and social networking platforms has had a profound impact on the ways we organize and maintain our relationships (Boase & Wellman, 2006). In the early days of this digital revolution, Wellman (2001) proposed the concept of *networked individualism* and argued that we are shifting the forms of our social interactions from "door-to-door" in the agrarian society and "place-to-place" in the industrial society to become "person-to-person" in the contemporary network society. With ample empirical evidence, Rainie and Wellman (2012) explicated that networked individualism is the new social operating system: People are increasingly connected as networked individuals, with their social life centered around themselves and interwoven with mediated communication networks.

Networked individualism appreciates the social affordances of ICTs and supports the agency of an individual. For example, Wellman and colleagues (2003) articulated key characteristics of the internet that could enable users to overcome geographic barriers and stay connected 24/7 and personalize their communication with different people and social groups for different purposes. National surveys have shown that when Americans spent more time on the internet, they actually developed larger and more active networks both online and offline (Boase et al., 2006; Wang & Wellman, 2010). Recent in-depth interviews with older adults have also suggested that people do leverage new ICTs for social engagement and support (Wang et al., 2018). Essentially, all newly arrived refugees in the United States are provided a mobile phone with base plans. They heavily depend on these digital devices to stay connected with their loved ones while adapting to the American culture.

Personal Communication System

What prompted the investigation and subsequent conceptualization of personal communication system was the concern about declining social connectivity in the United States. McPherson, Smith-Lovin, and Brashears (2006) analyzed data from the General Social Survey in 1985 and 2004 about adult Americans' core discussion network (i.e., people with whom they discussed important matters with). They found that over two decades their average network size decreased by almost a third (one confidant), from 2.94 to 2.08 and the number of people who reported not having any one to confide with nearly tripled. However, their data did not include any information about the respondents' use of ICTs.

Using the framework of networked individualism and acknowledging that social networks were increasingly individual-centered and personal (Wellman, 2001, 2007), Boase (2008) introduced the concept of personal communication system based on his analysis of a nationally representative survey of 2,200 adult Americans. The results regarding personal network size showed a mean of 51 alters and a median of 35 alters, due to a positive skew; the results regarding personal network composition showed an average of 30% as friends, 22% as immediate kin, 20% as extended kin, 18% as coworkers, and 10% as neighbors (Boase, 2008; Boase et al., 2006). More importantly, Boase (2008) discovered that (1) virtually all respondents drew upon a variety of communication channels, including in-person contact and ICTs, as an active system to manage their social activities and fulfill their personal needs; and (2) those who were heavy communicators had larger and more diverse networks than light communicators. Therefore, personal communication system is an apt conceptual approach for working with young refugees because they rely on maintaining and expanding their personal networks to build a better life in the United States. This is especially important for women and girls who are typically deprived of rights or autonomy of owning or accessing ICTs in most of the countries where refugees came from. Three research questions were central to the mapping of these young female refugees' personal communication systems:

RQ1:   What were the characteristics of their personal networks?
RQ2:   What were the communication channels they used to stay connected?
RQ3:   What functions of the ICTs could they benefit from?

In essence, these research inquiries were centered around three fundamental aspects of an individual's personal communication system: who, how, and what. Specifically, RQ1 asked who were the alters in these young female refugees' personal networks; RQ2 asked how they communicated with them; and RQ3 asked what type of information they shared.

Methods

Participants

As part of the RYMI project, data were collected through semi-structured interviews with 22 IRC clients in February 2018, including 17 young adult female refugees who are the focus in this chapter: They aged

Table 6.1 Participants' demographic characteristics

Project ID	Sex	Age	Nationality	Marital Status	Parental Status	Legal Status	Country of Birth	Age Left Home	Years in the USA
P01	F	20	Congolese	Single	No	Refugee	DRC*	9	8
P03	F	22	Congolese	Single	No	Refugee	DRC	15	5
P04	F	19	Congolese	Single	No	Refugee	Tanzania	14	5
P05	F	19	Congolese	Single	No	Refugee	DRC	7	2
P06	F	19	Congolese	Single	No	Refugee	DRC	NA	2
P08	F	20	Sudanese	Single	No	Refugee	Sudan	5	7
P09	F	20	Burmese	Single	No	Refugee	Thailand	12	9
P11	F	22	Burundian	Single	No	Refugee	Tanzania	11	11
P12	F	21	Syrian	Single	No	Refugee	Syria	14	2
P14	F	23	Central African	Single	Yes	Refugee	CAR**	10	7
P15	F	22	Burmese	Single	No	Refugee	Burma	7	8
P17	F	25	Somalian	Single	No	Refugee	Somalia	19	2
P18	F	19	Burmese	Single	No	Refugee	Thailand	11	9
P19	F	22	Congolese	Married	Yes	Refugee	DRC	3	1
P20	F	20	Burmese	Single	Yes	Refugee	Burma	17	1
P21	F	25	Burmese	Married	Yes	Refugee	Burma	12	8
P22	F	23	Burmese	Single	No	Refugee	Thailand	12	11
P02	M	21	Congolese	Single	No	Refugee	DRC	1	6
P07	M	23	Congolese	Single	No	Refugee	DRC	20	2
P10	M	18	Congolese	Single	No	Refugee	DRC	11	2
P13	F	24	Afghan	Married	Yes	*Immigrant*	Afghanistan	22	2
P16	F	23	Nigerian	Engaged	No	*Immigrant*	Niger	20	4

Note: P02, P07, and P10 were male refugees; P13 and P16 were legal immigrants. They were included for comparisons with the main group of female refugees.
*DRC denotes the Democratic Republic of the Congo.
**CAR denotes the Central African Republic.

19–25 (M = 21.24, SD = 1.98, *Median* = 21, *Mode* = 20); came from different cultural backgrounds; 12% were married; 24% had children; three young male refugees and two female legal immigrants were included for comparisons with the main group of young female refugees (see Table 1).

Their journey of forced migration started at a young age: 88% were forced to leave their home before they were 16; 29% were born in a refugee camp outside of their home country; 69% had a lengthy stay in other countries before being admitted by the United States; and for all participants, their first and final resettlement destination in the United States was Clarkston. They had lived in Clarkston at various lengths, ranging from 1 to 11 years (M = 5.76, SD = 3.51, *Median* = 7, *Mode* = 2); 24% were taking English language classes, 18% were attending high school, 41% were going to college, and 18% graduated from college; 53% had either a part-time or a full-time job.

Procedure

With the Institutional Review Board's approval, participants were recruited through the IRC's network in Clarkston. Essential services such as transportation and childcare were provided for free, and each participant also received a $25 gift card. Most interviews lasted about an hour and were completed in English. Four participants needed help from an interpreter, so the interviews took up to 2.5 hours. To ensure participants' anonymity and privacy, they were each assigned a unique project ID and no audio or video recordings were used. The questions were divided into four sections: (1) their journey to the United States, (2) their activities on a typical school/work day and a typical day off, (3) their personal social networks and how they kept in contact with people important to them, and (4) their challenges and aspirations. Information was recorded through handwritten notes and entered into an Excel spreadsheet.

All questions were intended to gather contextual information about participants' experiences as being resettled in the United States and to identify barriers and opportunities for designing effective health education interventions. In particular, their answers to the second and third sections of the interview were most relevant to the research questions in this article. The second section used a modified time-diary method to help participants recall their major daily activities and any involvement of social interactions and ICT use (c.f., Adam et al., 2007; Nie & Hillybus, 2002; Robinson, 1999; Stepanikova et al., 2010). Each participant was first asked to recall what they did during a typical school/work day recently, starting from the time they woke up till the time they went to sleep. If the activity involved anyone else or the use of any ICT, it was noted on the data collection instrument. Then the procedure was repeated but focusing on a typical day off school/work.

The third section of the interview used a modified personal network mapping method to help participants identify people they were in regular contact with and people who were important to them (c.f., Hogan et al., 2007; McCarty et al., 2007; Sluki, 2010). They were shown the mapping tool with the word "ME" handwritten in front of them at the center of a 2 × 2 grid, indicating four groups of social ties: family/household, neighborhood, work, and school. Following the conventional "name generator" procedure in social network analysis, participants were then asked to list all the people who lived in their household along with basic information such as the nature of their relationship and two demographic variables: sex and age. This procedure was repeated for people they interacted with regularly in their neighborhood, at work, and at school or any educational setting. After that, participants were further probed to recall anyone important that they stayed in contact beyond the local community. This gave them a chance to include family and close friends at a distance.

Data Analysis

The data analyses were primarily qualitative and supplemented with quantitative measures wherever numeric values could be derived from the participants' answers. First, to take advantage of the rich information from the in-depth interviews, an iterative process was adopted for a thematic analysis with inductive reasoning based on the grounded theory (Braun & Clarke, 2006; Corbin & Strauss, 2014). The topic themes were directly connected to the three research questions regarding participants' personal relationships, social activities, and ICT use. Second, each participant's personal network size was calculated based the number of alters they disclosed, their network composition was determined by the nature of their relationships with the alters, the most influential alters were self-identified, both mediated and non-mediated communication channels were tallied. Descriptive and inferential statistics were analyzed using SPSS v26. The personal network graphs were created in NodeXL.

Results

Characteristics of Young Female Refugees' Personal Networks

Results regarding RQ1 showed that participants' personal network size ranged from 3 to 34 ($M = 15.35$, $SD = 6.59$). This means, a young female refugee participant had, on average, about 15 alters in their networks. A closer investigation of the data suggested that the participant with the smallest network (P17) lost both of her parents during the Somali civil war and fled home at the age of 19, went through the refugee camp in Kenya, and arrived in the United States alone in 2016. She was socially isolated as her entire world only included three other people: a roommate to split the rent, a coworker to share the ride to a chicken factory, and a driving instructor (see Figure 6.1). On the other hand, the participant with the largest network (P15) had a much busier life. At age 7, she fled Burma and stayed in the refugee camp in Thailand until her family was accepted by the United States. After having lived in Clarkston for eight years and now attending college, she had a full house with three generations of family members, plus newly arrived refugee relatives and a good friend who shared a room with her; lots of friends she met through the refugee camp, high school, and college; many people she kept close contact with through her part-time job and volunteer work (see Figure 6.1). However, participants' network size and the number of years they had lived in Clarkston were not significantly correlated ($r = .35$, $p = .17$).

Results regarding RQ1 showed that participants' personal network composition were: 19–69% family/household ties ($M = 37$, $SD = .13$), 8–75% through school ($M = 36$, $SD = .16$), 7–36% through work ($M = 24$, $SD = .11$), 9–33% neighbors ($M = 19$, $SD = .09$), and 6–50% family and friends outside of the United States ($M = 22$, $SD = .16$). On average, 24–86% were family near and far combined ($M = 47$, $SD = .17$). One participant (P21) had only two types of ties (local family and work); one participant (P06) had all five types of ties. All the other participants had three or four types of ties. For example, one participant (P09) lived in an apartment with her dad, older brother, sister-in-law, and one-year-old nephew; made seven friends through high school and college; and had six regular contacts through her part-time job as a tutor at a community center (see Figure 6.1). Another participant (P20), a single mother and a survivor of domestic violence, managed to care for her two-year-old daughter by sharing an apartment with a married couple but regularly called her parents in a refugee camp in Bangladesh and her grandmother and uncle back in Burma; met another couple in the same apartment complex who helped her with transportation sometimes; and relied heavily on her six connections at the IRC resettlement staff, English language instructor, and classmates (see Figure 6.1).

Of all the people participants had in their social networks, they were asked to identify the most influential alters. Results showed that parents (mother, father, or both) were most frequently mentioned ($n = 14$); followed by friends (mostly female friends plus two male friends, $n = 10$); mentors (such as a teacher, professor, and coach; $n = 5$); siblings, boyfriends, and refugee resettlement staff each received two mentions; and one participant also mentioned a coworker.

Popular Communication Channels among Young Female Refugees

Analysis of the time-diary data showed that 15 out of the 17 young female refugee participants reported spending considerable time helping with house chores (e.g., cooking and cleaning; n = 15) and seven also mentioned caregiving (e.g., babysitting, helping their parents and refugee friends). Regarding RQ2 about the use of various communication channels, social media were mentioned 41 times (YouTube = 11, Facebook = 10, SMS = 6, Snapchat = 6, WhatsApp = 3, Instagram = 3, LinkedIn = 1, Viber = 1), face-to-face was mentioned 16 times (quality time with friends = 10, quality time with family = 6), watching television was mentioned seven times, and email was mentioned three times.

One participant (P17) was the only person who did not use any ICTs at all. She disclosed that her daily routine was to wake up at 3 am and ride on the bus and in a car with another woman in the neighborhood to work from 4 am to 1 pm at a poultry factory. She went to take English and driving lessons after work and no time or money for anything else. However, it was also worth noting that all participants had a smartphone and a great majority of mediated activities took place through their mobile phone rather than a networked computer or laptop. As one participant (P06) well put, "chatting with friends whenever and wherever she wanted made her so happy and with their constant support she felt that no one could stop her from doing what she truly wanted."

ICT Use by Young Female Refugees

Results regarding RQ3 revealed that participants adopted ICTs for a variety of reasons. The first major reason was to stay in touch with family and close friends, near and far, on a regular basis. Facebook messenger, SMS, Snapchat, WhatsApp, Instagram, and Viber, whichever helped them to reach and stay connected with those important people in their lives regardless of their geographic locations. The second major reason was to learn English by watching news and subtitled drama on television or short videos on YouTube. The third major reason was to use arts in the media for inspiration and enjoyment. For example, many participants said they used YouTube to listen to music and watch movies that helped them maintain a deep connection with their home culture and faith. Others simply watch funny videos to get a laugh and release their stress.

One participant (P12) said that she loved going to school back home in Syria with the three boys in her neighborhood, but her family had to flee when violence worsened and all three boys were kidnapped, tortured, and murdered. At the age of 14, she arrived in Jordan along with her family. Although they experienced heavy discrimination as refugees, her hard work at school earned her a Jordanian scholarship for university education. However, she gave up the scholarship when her family was admitted by the United Stated and moved to Clarkston in hope for a better future with public safety, job security, and higher education. Although she was accompanied by a professional inter-preter for the interview and kept apologizing to me for her English, I was so impressed that within 2.5 years she was able to understand and answer most of my questions without any help. She told me that even though she was only taking an English language class across the street for two hours each week, she learned English mostly by typing in Arabic on YouTube "the most popular sentence in English" and watch the videos repeatedly in both Arabic and English to practice. She also shared that social media helped her tremendously because she could talk to three of her high school best friends in Jordan through WhatsApp and Facebook Messenger, especially when she was feeling sad and depressed.

Research Findings & Implications

This chapter provides critical details about a pilot project that adopted a personal communication system approach to map out young female ref-ugees' personal networks and the way in which they stayed connected, both in person and through ICTs. Results of qualitative and quantitative analyses suggested the following major findings in response to the three research questions. First, all participants had someone that they were in regular contact with. The smallest network size was three, the largest network size was 34, and the average network size was 15. Compared with results of national surveys of adult Americans with a mean of 51 and a median of 35, the personal network size of young female refugees in this project was overall rather limiting. Their personal network com-position was predominantly family and close friends, both near and far, on average nearly half of the network ties and all the way up to 86%. Their social connections became more diverse through people they met in their neighborhood (often immigrant families or former refugees), at school or in English language classes (other foreign students, high school teachers or college professors), and through full-time or part-time jobs (friendly superiors, mentors, and coworkers).

Second, all participants with one exception adopted a variety of com-munication channels to purposefully manage their daily activities and stay meaningfully engaged with people in their social networks. These communication channels, as predicted, included both face-to-face and ICTs, especially popular social media platforms and applications such as YouTube, Facebook, Snapchat, WhatsApp, and Instagram. And most mediated activities took place on smartphones.

Third, ICTs complemented in-person quality time and facilitated social support, language learning, job hunting, religious practice, and media entertainment. The use of both synchronous and asynchronous apps like Facebook messenger, Snapchat, WhatsApp, and Viber allowed young female refugees to stay in touch with family and close friends despite the challenge with geographic distance and time difference. You-Tube videos were indispensable as the music and movies from their home countries helped them remain culturally rooted, educational videos and subtitled films taught them English, and humorous content brightened their day and lifted up their spirit.

Recommended Strategies

By using a personal communication system approach, the RYMBI project offers insights into young female refugees' everyday life and how they navigated complex social systems. A connected life affords the opportunity for a healthier life. Understanding how specific communication channels are used for certain purposes can inform health intervention design, meeting the intended audience where they already are, and facilitate effective program implementation and evaluation. Forced migration can have a disruptive impact on people's social networks, health, and well-being (Sluki, 2008). However, we can leverage the communicative affordances of mobile technologies and social media (Abujarour et al., 2016; Bucher & Helmond, 2018; Schrock, 2015) and develop morally responsible (Birman, 2006; Block et al., 2013) and culturally appropriate intervention programs to promote social inclusion and integration (Andrade & Doolin, 2015; de Jong, 2002).

In addition, six health intervention "design principles" emerged from our fieldwork:

1   Take nothing for granted: Refugees' everyday life is stressful. Even some information may have been given to them, it cannot be assumed that they actually would understand, remember, and follow up with everything.
2   No personal judgments: It helps to build trust if refugees don't feel that they are being judged all the time. Everyone goes through life with ups and downs. We all deserved to be seen and treated the same and as human beings (not just refugees).
3   Meet them where they are: Mapping their everyday schedule, routine activities, and social networks can help us leverage their personal communication systems for health promotion rather than persuading them to do something they are not familiar with.
4   Learning goes both ways: Many of the meetings with the stakeholders suggested that the refugees need to be educated. However, tremendous resilience and wisdom were also demonstrated in their own stories that need to be respected and shared as well.
5   Body, mind, and heart: There are certain communication strategies effective for addressing knowledge and attitudes, but without trust no health campaigns or promotional efforts can last long.

6　Positive, positive, positive: A positive frame for communication campaigns and health education programs will be most beneficial because it amplifies what is already working while minimizing the possibility of re-traumatizing the refugees.

Additional resources include the human-centered design toolkit developed by IDEO (2021) as well as the Digital Health Checklist (Nebeker et al., 2019) for ethical and meaningful engagement with the refugee community throughout a collaborative project.

Recommended Readings

Andrade, A. D., & Doolin, B. (2015). Information and communication technology and the social inclusion of refugees. *MIS Quarterly, 42*, 405–416.

Boase, J. (2008). Personal networks and the personal communication system. *Information, Communication & Society, 11*, 490–508.

Wellman, B. (2001). Physical place and cyber-place: Changing portals and the rise of networked individualism. *International Journal for Urban and Regional Research, 25*, 227–252.

IDEO's Design Kit, https://www.ideo.com/post/design-kit

Nebeker, C., Ellis, R. B., & Torous, J. (2019). Digital Health Checklist for Researchers (DHC_R) at ReCODE Health, https://recode.health/tools/

References

Abujarour, S., Krasmova, H., Wenninger, H., Fedorowicz, J., Olbrich, S., Tan, C.-W., & Urquhart, C. (2016, December). *Leveraging technology for refugee integration: How can we help?* Panel presentations at the 37th International Conference on Information Systems in Dublin.

Adam, E. K., Snell, E. K., & Pendry, P. (2007). Sleep timing and quantity in ecological and family context: A nationally representative time-diary study. *Journal of Family Psychology, 21*, 4–19.

Andrade, A. D., & Doolin, B. (2015). Information and communication technology and the social inclusion of refugees. *MIS Quarterly, 42*, 405–416.

Berkmann, L. F. (1984). Assessing the physical effects of social networks and social support. *Annual Review of Public Health, 5*, 413–432.

Birman, D. (2006). Ethical issues in research with immigrants and refugees. In J. E. Trimble & C. B. Fisher (Eds.), *The handbook of ethical research with ethnocultural populations & communities* (pp. 155–177). Thousand Oaks, CA: Sage.

Blizzard, B., & Batalova, J. (2019, June). *Refugees and asylees in the United States*. Retrieved from https://www.migrationpolicy.org/article/refugees-and-asylees-united-states

Block, K., Warr, D., Gibbs, L., & Riggs, E. (2013). Addressing ethical and methodological challenges in research with refugee-background young people: Reflections from the field. *Journal of Refugee Studies, 26*(1), 69–87.

Boase, J. (2008). Personal networks and the personal communication system. *Information, Communication & Society, 11*, 490–508.

Boase, J., Horrigan, J. B., Wellman, B., & Rainie, L. (2006). *The strength of Internet ties.* Retrieved from https://www.pewinternet.org/2006/01/25/the-strength-of-internet-ties/

Boase, J., & Wellman, B. (2006). Personal relationships: On and off the internet. In D. Perlman & A. L. Vangelisti (Eds.), *The Cambridge handbook of personal relationships* (pp. 709–723). Oxford: Blackwell.

Braun, V., & Clarke, V. (2006). Using thematic analysis in psychology. *Qualitative Research in Psychology, 3,* 77–101.

Bucher, T., & Helmond, A. (2018). The affordances of social media platforms. In J. Burgess, A. Marwick, & T. Poell (Eds.), *The Sage handbook of social media* (pp. 233–253). New York: Sage.

Cheng, I.-H., Advocat, J., Vasi, S., Enticott, J. C., Willey, S., Wahidi, S., et al. (2018). *A rapid review of evidence-based information, best practices and lessons learned in addressing the health needs of refugees and migrants: Report to the World Health Organization.* Retrieved on March 12, 2019 from https://www.who.int/migrants/publications/partner-contribution_review.pdf

Christakis, N. A., & Fowler, J. H. (2009). *Connected: The surprising power of our social networks and how they shape our lives.* New York: Little Brown and Company.

Christakis, N. A., & Fowler, J. H. (2013). Social contagion theory: Examining dynamic social networks and human behavior. *Statistics in Medicine, 32,* 556–577.

Corbin, J. M., & Strauss, A. (2014). *Basics of qualitative research: Techniques and procedures for developing grounded theory* (4th ed.). Thousand Oaks, CA: Sage.

de Jong, J. T. V. M. (2002). Public mental health, traumatic stress and human rights violations in low-income countries: A culturally appropriate model for times of conflict, disaster and peace. In J. T. V. M. de Jong (Ed.), *Trauma, war, and violence: Public mental health in socio-cultural context* (pp. 1–93). New York: Kluwer/Plenum.

Hampton, K., & Wellman, B. (2018). Lost and saved … again: The moral panic about the loss of community takes hold of social media. *Contemporary Sociology: A Journal of Reviews, 47,* 643–651.

Hunter, R. F., de la Haye, K., Murray, J. M., Badham, J., Valente, T. W., Clarke, M., & Kee, F. (2019). Social network interventions for health behaviours and outcomes: A systematic review and meta-analysis. *PLoS Medicine, 16*(9), e1002890.

Hogan, B., Carrasco, J. A., & Wellman, B. (2007). Visualizing personal networks: Working with participant-aided sociograms. *Field Methods, 19,* 116–144.

IDEO. (2021). Design Kit, https://www.ideo.com/post/design-kit

Ikeda, A., & Kawachi, I. (2010). Social networks and health. In K. E. Freedland, J. R. Jennings, M. M. Llabre, S. B. Manuck, E. J. Susman (Eds.), *Handbook of behavioral medicine: Methods and applications* (pp. 237–261). New York: Springer.

Latkin, C. A., & Knowlton, A. R. (2015). Social network assessments and interventions for health behavior change: A critical review. *Behavioral Medicine, 41,* 90–97.

McCarty, C., Molina, J. L., Aguilar, C., & Rota, L. (2007). A comparison of social network mapping and personal network visualization. *Field Methods*, *19*, 145–162.

McPherson, M., Smith-Lovin, L., & Brashears, M. E. (2006). Social isolation in America: Changes in core discussion networks over two decades. *American Sociological Review*, *71*, 353–375.

Nebeker, C., Ellis, R. B., & Torous, J. (2019). Digital Health Checklist for Researchers (DHC_R) Accessed on July 30, 2021, from ReCODE Health https://recode.health/tools/

Nie, N. H., & Hillygus, D. S. (2002). The impact of internet use on sociability: Time-diary findings. *IT & Society*, *1*, 1–20.

Perkins, J. M., Subramanian, S. V., & Christakis, N. A. (2015). Social networks and health: A systematic review of sociocentric network studies in low- and middle-income countries. *Social Science & Medicine*, *125*, 60–78.

Rainie, L., & Wellman, B. (2012). *Networked: The new social operating system*. Cambridge, MA: MIT Press.

Robinson, J. P. (1999). The time-diary method: Structure and uses. In W. E. Pentland, A. S. Harvey, M. P. Lawton & M. A. McColl (Eds.), *Time use research in the social sciences* (pp. 47–89). New York: Kluwer/Plenum.

Schrock, A. R. (2015). Communicative affordances of mobile media: Portability, availability, locatability, and multimediability. *International Journal of Communication*, *9*, 1229–1246.

Sluki, C. E. (2008). Migration and the disruption of the social network. In M. McGoldrick & K. Hardy (Eds.), *Re-visioning family therapy: Race, culture and gender in clinical practice* (2nd ed., pp. 39–47). New York: Guilford.

Sluki, C. E. (2010). Personal social networks and health: Conceptual and clinical implications for their reciprocal impact. *Family Systems and Health*, *28*, 1–18.

Stepanikova, I., Nie, N. H., & He, X. (2010). Time on the internet at home, loneliness, and life satisfaction: Evidence from panel time-diary data. *Computers in Human Behavior*, *26*, 329–338.

UNHCR. (2019). Figures at a glance. Retrieved on October 15, 2019, from https://www.unhcr.org/en-us/figures-at-a-glance.html

Valente, T. W. (2010). *Social networks and health: Models, methods, and applications*. New York: Oxford University Press.

Valente, T. W. (2012). Network interventions. *Science*, *337*, 49–53.

Valente, T. W., & Pitts, S. R. (2017). An appraisal of social network theory and analysis as applied to public health: Challenges and opportunities. *Annual Review of Public Health*, *38*, 103–118.

Wang, H. (2018). *RYMBI: Using human-centered design to promote sexual and reproductive health among refugees in the United States*. Report submitted to the Advocates for Youth, Washington DC.

Wang, H., & Wellman, B. (2010). Social connectivity in America: Change in adult friendship network size from 2002 to 2007. *American Behavioral Scientist*, *53*, 1148–1169. https://doi.org/10.1177/000276420356247

Wellman, B. (2001). Physical place and cyber-place: Changing portals and the rise of networked individualism. *International Journal for Urban and Regional Research*, *25*, 227–252.

Wellman, B. (2007). The network is personal. *Social Networks*, 29, 349–356.
Wellman, B., Quan-Haase, A., Boase, J., Chen, W., Hampton, K., Díaz, I., & Miyata, K. (2003). The social affordances of the internet for networked individualism. *Journal of Computer-Mediated Communication*, 8(3). https://doi.org/10.1111/j.1083-6101.2003.tb00216.x

7 Communicating COVID-19 Health and Safety Measures to Vulnerable Communities

The Case of Refugees and Migrants in Austria and Germany

Judith Kohlenberger and Maria Gruber

With the onset of the Coronavirus pandemic, the relevance of efficient health communication to socially vulnerable groups, including refugees and migrants, has come to the forefront of public and political concern in Austria and Germany, two countries in the heart of Europe with a traditionally high share of immigrant populations. While their national governments informed their citizens on public curfews and a weeks-long lockdown in spring 2020, information in the languages of (forced) migrants was delayed and incomplete, partly even inaccurate. Consequently, many migrants were induced to avoid or delay treatment, to misinterpret or ignore safety measures, or to experience heightened levels of stress and anxiety. Refugees who arrived in Europe in the wake of the great summer of migration in 2015 experienced re-traumatization, were too scared to leave their homes for days and weeks, and reported racial profiling by the heightened police force intent on checking curfew measures. For fear of identification, undocumented and irregular migrants avoided reporting for testing and quarantining.

This led to heated discussions on social inclusion, health equality, and adequate communication policies for minorities, which has historically proven key in containing the spread of infectious diseases (White, 2020), but also sparked xenophobic responses by the political actors and the resident population. This chapter explores the factors reinforcing in/sufficient access to information on health care and health literacy for migrants and refugees in Germany and Austria. Secondly, we examine the types and effectiveness of COVID-19-related health communication targeted at migrants, with a particular focus on the vulnerable group of recently arrived refugees and asylum seekers.

Migrant and Refugee Health Outcomes in Austria and Germany

Marginalized groups, including ethnic minorities and migrant minorities in most European host countries, are disproportionately affected by health

DOI: 10.4324/9781003230243-7

crises like global pandemics. Data show that refugees and migrants tend to have worse health outcomes than the native population, which is both exacerbated by and affects their weaker social networks and economic performance. This is particularly true for Austria and Germany, where being a migrant or descendant of migrants (the latter being referred to as "persons with a migration background") is frequently connected to a lower socio-economic status. In Austria, 17% of the population have foreign citizenship, while roughly one quarter (2.070.000 persons) qualify as "persons with a migration background" (Statistics Austria, 2020a). In Germany, 13.5% hold foreign citizenship (German Federal Statistics Office, 2019) while again, about 26% (21.246.000 persons) are considered to have a "migration background" (German Federal Statistics Office, 2020).

In both countries, "migrants" are a vastly heterogeneous group, including EU-citizens, persons under humanitarian protection, and labor migrants from mostly Eastern European countries. Indeed, the biggest national group of migrants in Austria are Germans (199.993 of all migrants, in absolute numbers). In public discourse, however, "migrant" and "migration background" are typically used to denote nationals that hold lowly qualified jobs and therefore tend to stem from a lower socio-economic stratum. Above all, these are migrants from Turkey and Ex-Yugoslavia, mostly (descents of) so-called low-skilled "guest workers" actively recruited by the Austrian and German governments in the 1960s and 1970s, as well as recently arrived refugees from Syria, Iraq, Afghanistan, and Chechnya. Due to low educational and social mobility in Austria, economic disadvantages associated with in-migration continue well into the second and third generation of migrants, in particular for women and girls, who display much lower employment rates than native females (Statistics Austria, 2020a).

The fact that migrants and refugees tend to be economically more disadvantaged than the native population is also reflected by their health indicators. For instance, data from the Austrian Health Interview Survey 2019 (ATHIS, 2019)[1] shows that while 51% of native Austrians suffer from obesity, a chronic illness strongly associated with social status and income (see, e.g., Moore & Cunningham, 2012), this is true for 61% of migrants from Turkey and Ex-Yugoslavia. The same holds true for smoking: 19% of the native Austrians and 33% of Turkish and Ex-Yugoslavian migrants smoke regularly (ATHIS, 2019). At the same time, migrants tend to assess themselves as less informed than the general population: Hence, 47% of migrant parents of children with special needs state they did not partake in a certain therapy or treatment due to lack of information. For Austrian parents, this ranges at merely 14%. Furthermore, prevention and early screening programs are more often used by natives than by migrants. Finally, economic hardship and poverty typically involve adverse working conditions, odd working hours, and frequent bouts of unemployment, which may be accompanied by a precarious residence status. All these factors have a negative impact on migrants' mental health. In the case of refugees, their recent experience of conflict, war, and displacement acts as an additional stressor and leads to increased levels of anxiety and depression (Kohlenberger et al., 2019).

These findings are, however, not specific to Austria and Germany: Across Europe, exclusivity-driven policies have fueled a resentful climate that reinforces social inequalities among migrant communities, notably in regard to access, availability, and quality of health services (Maldonado et al., 2020). Globally, research shows that ethnic minorities and marginalized groups tend to have poorer health outcomes and more restricted health access (Braveman et al., 2010). Research for the United States shows that ethnic minorities have always displayed higher rates of disease, more aggressive progression of disease, and higher mortality (Williams, 2012). These differences persist even if factors like education and living conditions are taken into account. In immigrant communities, health outcomes tend to deteriorate over time, so that 20 years after migration, Mexican immigrants have a similar health profile as African-Americans (Kaestner et al., 2009). For Europe, data shows that the risk for people in the lowest income group to suffer from a chronic illness like diabetes or asthma is five times that of people in the highest (ATHIS, 2019; Hurrelmann & Richter, 2019). In the UK, health inequalities have widened, and life expectancy has stalled in recent years (Marmot et al., 2020). Health is a highly unequally distributed resource.

For migrants and refugees in European host countries, unequal health outcomes due to socio-economic status are further exacerbated by implicit bias and discrimination in the health care system. This particularly concerns aspects of communication between doctors and patients. Hence, a study for the Netherlands shows that medical staff is more verbally dominant when treating migrants, while at the same time, consultations are shorter (Meeuwesen et al., 2006). Implicit bias can lead practitioners to take the pain of marginalized groups less seriously, an effect that is even more pronounced for migrant women. For humanitarian migrants in European host countries, studies show that asylum seekers, but also persons already granted protection, may shy away from seeking treatment for fear of being deported. In many cases, this fear is legally unfounded, which should be considered a central concern of health communication (Karl-Trummer et al., 2009). Finally, health communication must include health education, in particular as concerns stigmatization of conditions or the religious interpretation of symptoms (Bermejo et al., 2017). In the origin countries of many migrants in Austria and Germany, including the Middle East and Africa, mental disorders are highly stigmatized, which leads to higher rates of somatization and ailments being read as physical rather than psychological symptoms. This can lead to uninformed choices of medical consultation, restricted health access, and in turn to misdiagnoses and chronification of disorders (Elbert et al., 2017). Language barriers, another vital area of accessible health communication, may further contribute to this effect.

The Adverse Effects of COVID-19 on Migrants and Refugees

During the Coronavirus pandemic, the above outlined, already existing inequalities in terms of health outcomes and health communication for marginalized groups were heavily exacerbated, and slowly gained increased academic and public attention. In the United States, studies showed early on that people of color were twice as often affected by a Coronavirus infection than white people (Ford et al., 2020; Razai et al., 2021). In Europe, recent OECD data suggests similarly increased infection rates for migrants: In states like Portugal, Denmark, Norway, and Sweden, the risk for persons born abroad to contract the novel SARS-CoV-2 virus is almost twice as high as for persons born in the country. Similarly, mortality rates seem to be higher for migrants than natives, partly due to higher rates of pre-existing conditions that can exacerbate a COVID infection (OECD, 2020).

On the one hand, this can be explained by socio-economic conditions: Migrants and ethnic minorities have a higher tendency to work in low-skilled frontline jobs, for instance, as delivery workers, in the health care system, or in supermarkets. In Austria, roughly one-third of workers in non-academic health care (i.e., nurses) have a migration background (Statistics Austria, 2020b). 33% of employees in food production and 30% in construction, two labor market sectors that continued production during national lockdowns, hold foreign citizenship (BMA, 2021). Due to the nature of their jobs, migrants in almost all OECD countries have less opportunity to work from home than the native population, which increased their exposure during epidemic peaks. While almost 35% of workers born in Germany were able to work from home during the pandemic, only 20% of foreign-born workers were able to do so (OECD, 2020). In addition to frontline workers, many persons with a migration background have been working in sectors that were hit particularly hard by the crisis. For example, in Vienna, two- thirds of the now unemployed have a migration background. A high share of them was employed in the hospitality sector (EC, 2021). Cramped living quarters, a higher likelihood for pre-existing conditions, a tendency to live in urban centers, and having to rely on public transport further increase migrants' and refugees' infection risk. For the latter, insufficient possibility to socially distance in refugee camps is another risk factor.

However, personal health behavior and socio-economic circumstances only explain part of the higher infection and mortality rates for migrants and refugees. Existing structural discrimination and racism in the health system and society at large seem to be of high importance as well, which became perceptible in a general lack of targeted, accessible COVID-19 communication. While both Austria and Germany can be considered typical migration societies, with a labor market that heavily depends on foreign workers (see, e.g., Fuchs et al., 2015; Hofer & Weyerstraß, 2016), translations of the central hygiene and safety measures to contain the pandemic were often flawed and provided much later than the original German version. Given the high percentages of foreign-born population and persons with a migration background, this was both counterintuitive and inefficient. Furthermore, the lack of efficient COVID-19 communication allowed for scapegoating migrants and refugees for spreading the virus when visiting extended family in their countries of origin or celebrating large religious festivals (see, e.g., Crossland, 2020; Prugger, 2020). According to a European Commission report (EC, 2021), due to the pandemic, there has been an increase in discrimination and scapegoating, which further endangers integration into society and social cohesion. Migrant communities did not feel addressed by and included in national pandemic measures to the same degree as the native population, and were further alienated by negative media coverage. This is corroborated at the global level: An online WHO survey conducted among 30,000 migrants and refugees from 159 countries found that respondents experienced a worsening situation of discrimination, regardless of their residence or employment status (WHO, 2020a).

In addition, the survey found that "nongovernmental and civil society organizations (NGOs), and other supporting organizations do play a key role regarding dissemination of accessible information on COVID-19 to refugees and migrants" (2020, p. vii), an assessment that certainly holds true for Austria and Germany. With the onset of the pandemic in March 2020, COVID-19 information was distributed by NGOs and within migrant communities in a peer-to-peer manner. In the following, we review some of the most important communication strategies that emerged in the course of 2020 and 2021.

COVID-19 Health Communication Strategies to Migrants and Refugees

At the onset of COVID-19 and the first phase of its pandemic spread, it became clear that there was neither a vaccine nor effective medical treatment against the disease at that time. Thus, public health measures provided the only containment strategy for the highly contagious virus (Maldonado et al., 2020). As an essential part of public health strategies, health communication turned into a necessary and central factor for saving lives. Notably, sophisticated health communication strategies have the potential to assist the population in dealing with uncertainty and fear, and in adhering to and understanding new guidelines on behavior (Finset et al., 2020).

While the universal right to health has long been enshrined in various international treaties and laws (Matlin et al., 2018), considerations on how to improve health communication directed at migrants and necessary health literacy have only recently come to the fore in the German-speaking countries (see, e.g., Quenzel et al., 2016). Sørensen and colleagues (2012, p. 3) define health literacy as "knowledge, motivation, and competencies to access, understand, appraise, and apply health information in order to make judgments and take decisions in everyday life concerning healthcare, disease prevention, and health promotion." Health literacy is linked to empowerment strategies (Schulz & Nakamoto, 2013) and is determined not only by individual skills, but also by clarity or complexity of the information (Parker & Ratzan, 2010). Research on health literacy refers to migrants as "hard to reach groups" (see, e.g., Islertas, 2020); in both Austria and Germany, health literacy and the associated ability to navigate the health system are significantly lower among migrants compared to people without a migration background (Berens et al., 2021; BMGF, 2014; Quenzel et al., 2016).

Empirical studies have shown that migrants utilize their host countries' health care systems differently than the native population (see, e.g., Kohlenberger et al., 2019). In this context, Klein and von dem Knesebeck (2018) defined *acceptable* and *unacceptable inequalities*. While personal or cultural preferences are termed as acceptable reasons for differences, lack of information and access barriers are considered unacceptable inequalities. Studies in Germany and Austria have repeatedly shown too little or no information available on certain medical topics in relevant migrant languages (see, e.g., Bozorgmehr, 2016).

During the first phase of the COVID-19 pandemic, the resident population in Austria and Germany received an unprecedented amount of information in the form of 24/7 news coverage and weekly press conferences by experts and high-ranking politicians. Other communication channels that may prove to be more efficient in reaching migrants and refugees were initially overlooked. Available data from the Corona panel survey conducted by the University of Vienna (see, Kittel et al., 2020) suggest that in the first phase of the pandemic, Austrian residents[2] relied heavily on the national broadcast company ORF for information on hygiene and safety measures to contain the Coronavirus. Following the survey data, 11% of the population could neither be reached by traditional nor social media (Lebernegg et al., 2020). In the case of Germany, a similar survey revealed that in March and April 2020, 66% of the German population relied on public broadcasters, while around 20% did not use these media outlets at all. In addition to the importance of personal contacts as a source of information, mediated, among others, via online messaging services, many also relied on official information provided by governmental authorities or research institutions (Viehmann et al., 2020). However, aiming first and foremost at statistical representativeness, both surveys generally focus on residents of the respective country, whereby the aspect of a possible "migration background" of the respondents was not considered further (Figure 7.1).

Globally, surveys suggest that official news coverage of the country of residence can also serve as a major source of COVID-19 information for migrants and refugees: In a WHO survey, 77% of respondents relied on their host country's news to receive updates on the pandemic. This was followed by social media, a circumstance that can and was positively exploited by NGOs and civil organizations catering to migrants and refugees. Interestingly, more than 40% of respondents turned to news from their country of birth to inform themselves about the pandemic. On the one hand, this must be considered a coherent and intuitive strategy, as home country media are often reverted to when language barriers or lack of trust keep migrants from using media of the receiving country (Piga, 2007; Sauer, 2010). On the other hand, however, a rather large percentage of the migrants informed by foreign media may also give rise to concern, as hygiene and safety measures to contain the virus may differ drastically between home and host country. The effects of obtaining one's COVID-19 information chiefly from one's country of

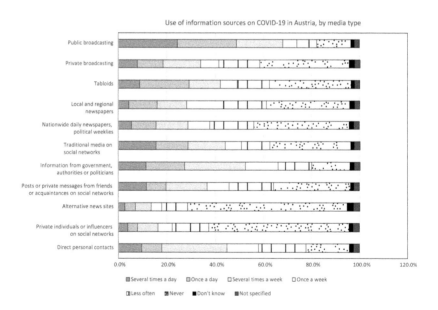

Figure 7.1 Note: Chart based on Data from the Austrian Corona Panel (Wave 4: April 2020), Question 77: "How often have you followed news on the Corona crisis from the following sources?". n = 1528. Source: Kittel et al. (2020).

origin while residing in another part of the world have, so far, not been studied in a comparative or longitudinal manner (Figure 7.2).

Scholarly debate on effectively reaching out to migrants increasingly points to an *inclusive migrant-sensitive* strategy, taking into account which existing services can be specifically provided to migrants and adapted to their needs for better access (Klein & von dem Knesebeck, 2018; Razum & Spallek, 2014). Health communication strategies targeting migrants should not focus on assimilating migrants and lecturing them to deal with the general information tailored to the native population. Instead, information must be developed, provided, and communicated in a way that meets the needs and preferences of the particular group. It must be easily accessible, retrievable, understandable, assessable, and applicable (Berens et al., 2021).

Accordingly, a variety of research on migrants' health literacy, their use of and access to the German and Austrian health care systems consistently highlight the importance of health communication that is tailored to the respective migrant target group (Anzenberger et al., 2015; Quenzel et al., 2016), language-specific (Bermejo et al., 2012) and culturally sensitive (Ganahl et al., 2016). Unsurprisingly, this also resonates in the recommendations that current research on COVID-19 measures direct at policymakers: Different migrant groups must be deliberately considered and addressed explicitly in national but also global COVID-19 outreach campaigns (Biddle et al., 2021; Maldonado et al., 2020). Moreover, according to the World Health Organization (WHO, 2020b) and the International Organization for Migration (IOM, n.d.), such efforts need to be taken timely and without delay.

Furthermore, research has shown that different migrant groups prefer or are used to different information channels and sources. In terms of effective channels for reaching migrants with information on

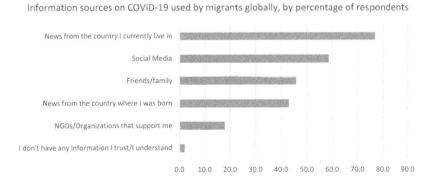

Information sources on COVID-19 used by migrants globally, by percentage of respondents

Figure 7.2 Note. Chart based on WHO Data from a total of 22.649 respondents for each information item; potential overlap of categories "friends/family" and "news from the country where I was born". Source: WHO (2020a).

COVID-19, Maldonado and colleagues (2020) suggest in their review of European public health communication aimed at migrants during the pandemic that there should be an increased collaboration with nongovernmental organizations and migrant community groups at the national level. Furthermore, it is vital to provide COVID-19 help-lines in various migrant languages; in this regard, cooperation with NGOs and community groups is repeatedly recommended (Maldonado et al., 2020). Biddle and colleagues (2021), who analyzed the pandemic response in German refugee shelters, emphasize the high relevance of oral information (through language mediators) to prevent misinformation and panic, but also downplaying.

The significance of oral information and the involvement of NGOs and community groups in health communication has been discussed in Austrian studies even before the pandemic, highlighting the need for *direct communication channels* (Anzenberger et al., 2015) and so-called *migrant-to-migrant health guides* ("MiMi Gesundheitslots*-innen"). This concept relies heavily on engaging with migrant networks and their confidants (Ganahl et al., 2016) and is also supported by international research, which shows that people in emergency situations primarily turn to their own social network, family, and friends (see, e.g., National Academies of Sciences, Engineering, and Medicine, 2017). In addition, European-focused studies have shown that migrant groups can be reached culturally appropriately and effectively with *eHealth* or *mHealth*[3] applications (Fernández-Gutiérrez et al., 2019). For the German context, recent studies (see, e.g., Islertas, 2020; Koschollek et al., 2020) confirm the potential to address specific migrant groups with target group-specific information via new media.

Shortcomings, Gaps, and Best-Practice Examples

Maldonado and colleagues (2020) argued that the efforts of European governments in reaching out to their migrant populations in their COVID-19 communication strategies can and should be improved on several levels. Despite the availability of translated COVID-19 guidance provided by the IOM and WHO in a variety of languages, many European governments have, so far, refrained from referring to these resources on national websites (Maldonado et al., 2020). For Germany, it has been shown that the COVID 19 pandemic presented the host authorities and infection control institutions with a particularly complex challenge, due to the lack of nationwide guidance on refugees in the national pandemic plan (Biddle et al., 2021).

Moreover, there were considerable differences to be observed in the content of migrant-oriented health communication measures, most of which focused on hygiene such as hand washing, face masks, and keeping physical distance. In contrast, information on testing strategies and vaccination awareness was hardly made available in migrant languages (Maldonado et al., 2020). In Austria, the COVID-19 information provided to migrants by the Austrian Integration Fund (ÖIF) in April 2020 was significantly shortened and hence incomplete, resulting in migrants finding themselves warned to leave their homes only in the most urgent cases, even though the regulatory framework also allowed for recreational outdoor walks (Lorenz & Marchart, 2020).

In both Austria and Germany, several of the strategies suggested by international research on effective COVID-19 outreach for marginalized groups were hence not employed top-down by the national governments, but rather by migrant communities and NGOs in a bottom-up approach. For instance, the Vienna-based civil organization AFYA (denoting "health & well-being" in Arabic) coordinated online meetings via WhatsApp, rather than making clients register on yet another, unknown digital platform. Since most clients were already familiar with the social media app, this proved to be a low-threshold approach. Their report shows how relevant culture-sensitive health offers are: During Ramadan, online meetings were scheduled for late at night. The turnout for the virtual meetings was so positive because they proved to be less time-consuming than real ones (Khattab, 2020).

In Germany, COVID-19 health communication for asylum seekers became a much-mediatized topic due to an outbreak in a refugee shelter with more than 500 inhabitants. As the shelter was placed under quarantine, several asylum seekers were allegedly violating quarantine regulations, which led to heightened police presence to detain them. After the event, media reports speculated that residents were not sufficiently informed about the outbreak (Riese, 2020). At the same time, several other accommodations experienced similar Coronavirus clusters but reported high levels of cooperation from residents. Nevertheless, the incidence of infection in shared refugee accommodations (so-called "Sammelunterkünfte") was one of the highest in Germany, averaging about 21 infected persons per outbreak, well ahead of nursing homes and homes for the elderly. Despite containment and quarantine measures in some facilities, more than 50% of residents were found to be infected with COVID-19. Due to the shared dormitories, sanitary facilities and cooking facilities in these densely inhabited shelters, the general recommendations on hygiene and physical distancing are difficult or even seemingly impossible to implement (Biddle et al., 2021).

Overall, what emerged from incidents in shelters was that information strategies to reach humanitarian migrants in shared accommodation were highly heterogeneous and seldom coordinated. As a result, reception center authorities were forced to take on essential ad hoc tasks to provide and secure health interventions for which they did not receive sufficient specialized and practical support from local, regional, and national authorities (Biddle et al., 2021). Moreover, research shows that the situation of permanent control typical of such shelters, in combination with segregation from the general population of the host country, leads to a loss of a feeling of solidarity with the host population, which may indirectly negatively affect inhabitants' willingness to participate in social distancing and maintain quarantine regulations. Furthermore, cramped living conditions increase social tensions and domestic violence during quarantine.

A key learning that emerged from Coronavirus clusters in refugee shelters is that "it is not sufficient to hang posters and forward information" (Razum et al., 2020, p. 395). Rather, hygiene measures must be demonstrated and modeled by staff. Information is best spread either orally (Biddle et al., 2021) or virtually, for instance, via short videos that can be watched on mobile phone screens. This ensures that residents with low literacy skills can access information too, as do pictograms. In order to access virtual information, Wi-Fi connection in shelters proved key. Furthermore, measures must be adapted to the special circumstances of a shared accommodation, which differ substantially in almost all aspects from those of private households. This again highlights the needs for target-group-specific and culturally sensitive health communication. "One size fits all" does not apply in a pandemic situation.

Recommendations for Future Health Communication Addressed at Refugees and Migrants

Briefly before the onset of the global pandemic, both Austria and Germany had just gone through what was widely considered a major national emergency situation: the so-called European refugee crisis, which heavily affected the German-speaking countries. By the end of 2015, Germany had received roughly half a million first-time asylum applications, mostly from Syrians, Iraqis and Afghans. In Austria, first-time asylum applications reached 86,000 (Eurostat, 2016). Between 2015 and 2020, roughly 1 million individuals in Germany and 125,000 in Austria were officially granted asylum, including subsidiary protection and protection on humanitarian grounds (BMI, 2020; BAMF, 2021).

In response to the great summer of migration, several initiatives and programs were established in the area of refugee health and health communication. Furthermore, a variety of bottom-up civil society organizations were founded that continue to cater to refugees' social, economic, and cultural needs, for instance by providing buddy programs, housing, or language courses. All of these pre-existing initiatives proved to be of vital importance for coping with the Coronavirus pandemic in the Austrian and German refugee communities. Hence, as the first take-away from our analysis, we recommend including NGOs and migrant organizations in health communication. Especially in a crisis situation such as a global pandemic, small-scale initiatives can rely on established, trusted strategy and communication channels to reach their clients fast and efficiently.

Following the assessment of Maldonado and colleagues (2020) that "[f]or health communication to be a successful component of an outbreak response, entire populations of affected countries must be able to access, understand and comprehend the information being communicated," we recommend the early, accurate and culturally sensitive translation of health information in the host country's most relevant migrant languages. Secondly, national governments must ensure a low-threshold access to these translations, making sure that particularly vulnerable groups of migrants and refugees, such as illiterate persons or the elderly, have the ability and means to obtain information without external assistance. In addition to translations into migrants' first languages, providing information in plain language can also help to decrease language barriers.

In accordance with the *inclusive migrant-sensitive* approach outlined above, we furthermore recommend adapting health communication "to meet the needs of marginalized populations, such as migrants" (Maldonado et al., 2020). This goes much beyond mere linguistic needs, but includes the removal of cultural barriers and stigmatization, as well as awareness of socio-economic circumstances and legal status. Socio-demographic factors, such as country of origin, sex, age, and family status, must necessarily be taken into consideration when drafting communication strategies (WHO, 2020a): Communicating health information to a male 20-year-old Afghan refugee and frontline worker will necessarily read and sound very different than addressing a partially literate, elderly Turkish woman out of employment. In addition, addressing migrants and refugees can only be one side of the coin: In an integrated understanding of health communication, the whole population must be included, instilling a "the health of one is the health of all" mindset (Maldonado et al., 2020).

In order to maximize effectiveness and uptake, it is vital to involve migrants in all stages of the process, i.e. in "adapting, introducing and evaluating interventions designed to improve cross cultural communication in primary care settings" (Teunissen et al., 2017, p. 10). As a mid- to long-term goal, this can be assisted by increasing the percentage of migrant and refugee workers in health care, medical practice, and research. For the ongoing COVID-19 vaccination efforts in many countries, we recommend the inclusion of migrant and refugee workers as part of the vaccination staff and as national spokespeople. This will also be key in countering misinformation and conspiracy theories, and paving the way to a post-COVID-19 society with more equal health, living and employment conditions.

Notes

1 ATHIS is a social survey on physical and mental health, need for care and/ or support, and health determinants like drug consumption and physical activity, is a nationally representative study of persons aged 15 years and more living in Austria.
2 According to the Corona Panel's methodology, respondents had to be residents of Austria to take part in the study. In addition to socio-demographic information on age, gender, education, region, occupation, religion, and household structure, respondents' migration background was also assessed.
3 Mobile Health (mHealth) is a subset of Electronic Health (eHealth) and refers to medical services from prevention and diagnosis to treatment and aftercare provision accessible via mobile devices. With regard to the COVID-19 pandemic, so-called tracing/exposure notification apps are particularly relevant examples of mHealth services.

Recommended Readings

Kar, B., & Cochran, D. M. (Eds.). (2019). *Risk communication and community resilience*. Routledge.

Kohlenberger, J., Buber-Ennser, I., Rengs, B., Leitner, S., & Landesmann, M. (2019). Barriers to health care access and service utilization of refugees in Austria: Evidence from a cross-sectional survey. *Health Policy, 123*(9), 833–839.

Maldonado, B. M. N., Collins, J., Blundell, H. J., & Singh, L. (2020). Engaging the vulnerable: A rapid review of public health communication aimed at migrants during the COVID-19 pandemic in Europe. *Journal of Migration and Health, 1–2*, 100004.

OECD. (2020, October 19). What is the impact of the COVID-19 pandemic on immigrants and their children? *OECD Policy Responses to Coronavirus (COVID-19)*. https://www.oecd.org/coronavirus/policy-responses/what-is-the-impact-of-the-covid-19-pandemic-on-immigrants-and-their-children-e7cbb7de/

WHO – World Health Organization. (2020). *ApartTogether survey: Preliminary overview of refugees and migrants self-reported impact of COVID-19*. https://www.who.int/publications/i/item/9789240017924

References

Anzenberger, J., Bodenwinkler, A., & Breyer, E. (2015). *Migration und Gesundheit. Literaturbericht zur Situation in Österreich.* [Migration and Health. Literature review on the situation in Austria.] Im Auftrag der Arbeiterkammer Wien und des Bundesministeriums für Gesundheit. Wien: Gesundheit Österreich GmbH.

ATHIS – Austrian Health Interview Survey. (2019). *Österreichische Gesundheitsbefragung 2019.* http://www.statistik.at/web_de/services/publikationen/4/index.html?includePage=detailedView&sectionName=Gesundheit&pubId=794

BAMF – German Federal Office for Migration and Refugees. (2021). *Schlüssel-zahlen Asyl 2020* [Key Asylum Figures]. https://www.bamf.de/SharedDocs/Anlagen/DE/Statistik/SchluesselzahlenAsyl/flyer-schluesselzahlen-asyl-2020.pdf?__blob=publicationFile&v=3

Berens, E. M., Ganahl, K., Vogt, D., & Schaeffer, D. (2021). Health literacy in the domain of healthcare among older migrants in Germany (North Rhine-Westphalia). Findings from a cross-sectional survey. *International Journal of Migration, Health and Social Care, 17*(1), 62–74.

Bermejo, I., Hölzel, L., & Schneider, F. (2017). Transkulturelle Psychiatrie [Transcultural psychiatry]. In F. Schneider (Ed.), *Facharztwissen Psychiatrie, Psychosomatik und Psychotherapie* [Medical specialists' knowledge psychiatry, psychosomatic and psychotherapy] (pp. 605–613). Springer.

Bermejo, I., Hölzel, L. P., Kriston, L., & Härter, M. (2012). Subjektiv erlebte Barrieren von Personen mit Migrationshintergrund bei der Inanspruchnahme von Gesundheitsmaßnahmen [Subjectively experienced barriers of persons with a migration background in the utilisation of health measures]. *Bundesgesundheitsblatt-Gesundheitsforschung-Gesundheitsschutz, 55*(8), 944–953.

Biddle, L., Jahn, R., Perplies, C., Gold, A. W., Rast, E., Spura, A., & Bozorgmehr, K. (2021). COVID-19 in Sammelunterkünften für Geflüchtete: Analyse von Pandemiemaßnahmen und prioritäre Bedarfe aus behördlicher Sicht [COVID-19 in collective accommodation for refugees: Analysis of pandemic measures and priority needs from the authorities' perspective]. *Bundesgesundheitsblatt-Gesundheitsforschung-Gesundheitsschutz, 64*, 342–352.

BMA – Austrian Federal Ministry of Labour. (2021). *BALI. Beschäftigung-Arbeitsmarkt-Leistungsbezieherinnen-Informationen* [BALI. Employment-Labour-Market-Beneficiaries-Information] http://www.arbeitsmarktpolitik.at/

BMGF – Austrian Federal Ministry for Health and Women. (2014). *Gesundheitsziel 3- Gesundheitskompetenz der Bevölkerung stärken* [Health Goal 3- Strengthen the health literacy of the population]. https://gesundheitsziele-oesterreich.at/website2017/wp-content/uploads/2017/05/bericht-arbeitsgruppe-3-gesundheitsziele-oesterreich.pdf

BMI – Austrian Federal Ministry of Interior. (2020). *Statistiken Asyl* [Asylum Statistics]. https://www.bmi.gv.at/301/Statistiken/

Bozorgmehr, K., Nöst, S., Thaiss, H. M., & Razum, O. (2016). Health care provisions for asylum-seekers: A nationwide survey of public health authorities in Germany. *Bundesgesundheitsblatt-Gesundheitsforschung-Gesundheitsschutz, 59*(5), 545–555.

Braveman, P. A., Cubbin, C., Egerter, S., Williams, D. R., & Pamuk, E. (2010). Socioeconomic disparities in health in the United States: what the patterns tell us. *American Journal of Public Health, 100*(S1), 186–196.

Crossland, D. (2020, September 26). Coronavirus: Illegal wedding blamed for lockdown in German city of Hamm. *The Times.* https://www.thetimes.co.uk/article/coronavirus-illegal-wedding-blamed-for-lockdown-in-german-city-of-hamm-8t3wccl2s

EC - European Commission. (2021). *Innovative approaches to integration and inclusion of migrants.* [Synthesis report]. https://ec.europa.eu/social/main.jsp?langId=en&catId=1024&furtherNews=yes&newsId=9814

Elbert, T., Wilker, S., Schauer, M., & Neuner. F. (2017). Dissemination psycho-
therapeutischer Module für traumatisierte Geflüchtete. Erkenntnisse aus der
Traumaarbeit in Krisen- und Kriegsregionen [Dissemination of psychotherapy
modules for traumatized refugees. Experience gained from trauma work in
crisis and conflict regions]. *Der Nervenarzt, 88*(1), 26–33.

Eurostat. (2016, March 4). *Record number of over 1.2 million first time asylum seekers registered in 2015.* Syrians, Afghans and Iraqis: top citizenships.
[Press release]. https://ec.europa.eu/eurostat/documents/2995521/7203832/3
-04032016-AP-EN.pdf/790eba01-381c-4163-bcd2-a54959b99ed6

Fernández-Gutiérrez, M., Bas-Sarmiento, P., & Poza-Méndez, M. (2019).
Effect of an mHealth intervention to improve health literacy in immigrant
populations: A quasi-experimental study. *CIN: Computers, Informatics,
Nursing, 37*(3), 142–150.

Finset, A., Bosworth, H., Butow, P., Gulbrandsen, P., Hulsman, R. L., Pieterse,
A. H., Street, R., Tschoetschel, R., & van Weert, J. (2020). Effective health
communication–a key factor in fighting the COVID-19 pandemic. *Patient
Education and Counseling, 103*(5), 873–876.

Ford, T. N., Reber, S., & Reeves, R. V. (2020, June 16). Race gaps in
COVOD-19 deaths are even bigger than they appear. *Brookings.* https://
www.brookings.edu/blog/up-front/2020/06/16/race-gaps-in-covid-19
-deaths-are-even-bigger-than-they-appear/

Fuchs, J., Kubis, A., & Schneider, L. (2015). *Zuwanderung aus Drittstaaten in
Deutschland bis 2050* [Immigration from third countries to Germany until
2050]. Bertelsmann Stiftung. https://www.bertelsmann-stiftung.de/fileadmin/
files/BSt/Publikationen/GrauePublikationen/Studie_IB_Zuwanderungsbe-
darf_aus_Drittstaaten_in_Deutschland_bis_2050_2015.pdf

Ganahl, K., Dahlvik, J., & Pelikan, J. (2016, October 13). *Gesundheitskompetenz und Erleben von Kommunikation im System der Krankenbehandlung von
Personen mit Migrationshintergrund aus der Türkei und aus Ex-Jugoslawien*
[Health literacy and experience of communication in the health care system
of persons with a migration background from Turkey and former Yugoslavia]
[Conference Session]. ÖPGK-Conference, Vienna, Austria. https://oepgk.at/
wp-content/uploads/2018/10/tf-3-ganahl.pdf

German Federal Statistics Office. (2019). *Ausländische Bevölkerung nach Fam-
ilienstand und ausgewählten Staatsangehörigkeiten am 31.12.2019* [For-
eign population by marital status and selected citizenships as of 31.12.2019].
https://www.destatis.de/DE/Themen/Gesellschaft-Umwelt/Bevoelkerung/Mi-
gration-Integration/Tabellen/auslaendische-bevoelkerung-familienstand.html

German Federal Statistics Office. (2020, July 28). *Bevölkerung mit Migrationshintergrund 2019 um 2,1% gewachsen: schwächster Anstieg seit
2011* [Population with migrant background grew by 2.1% in 2019: weakest
increase since 2011] [Press release]. https://www.destatis.de/DE/Presse/
Pressemitteilungen/2020/07/PD20_279_12511.html

Hofer, H. & Weyerstraß, K. (2016). Der Beitrag der Migration zum Wachstums-
potenzial der österreichischen Wirtschaft [Migration's contribution to the
growth potential of the Austrian economy]. *Wirtschaftspolitischen Blätter,
2016*(3). https://www.wko.at/site/WirtschaftspolitischeBlaetter/Helmut-Hofer,
-Klaus-Weyerstrass:-Der-Beitrag-der-Migratio.html

Hurrelmann, K., & Richter, M. (2019). *Understanding Public Health. Productive Processing of Internal and External Reality.* Routledge.

IOM – International Organization of Migration. (n.d.). How to focus communication towards migrants during the COVID-19 outbreak? *Blog – On the Move.* https://rosanjose.iom.int/SITE/en/blog/how-focus-communication-towards-migrants-during-covid-19-outbreak

Islertas, Z. (2020). The Importance of New Media and eHealth Information in the Everyday Life of Female Adolescents with Turkish Migration Background in Germany. In L. A. Saboga-Nunes, U. H. Bittlingmayer, O. Okan & D. Sahrai (Eds.), *New approaches to health literacy* (pp. 203–222). Springer VS.

Kaestner, R., Pearson, J. A., Keene, D., & Geronimus, A. T. (2009). Stress, allostatic load, and health of Mexican immigrants. *Social Science Quarterly, 90*(5), 1089–1111.

Karl-Trummer, U., Novak-Zezula, S., & Metzler, B. (2009). Managing a paradox: health care for undocumented migrants in the EU. *Finnish Journal of Ethnicity and Migration, 4*(2), 53–60.

Khattab, O. (2020). Ein sicherer Ort in der Krise: Erfahrungen mit muttersprachlichen Online-Gesundheitskreisen. Praxisbericht [A safe place in crisis: _Experiences with mother-tongue online health circles. Practice report]. In Büro für Frauengesundheit und Gesundheitsziele (Ed.), *Frauengesundheit und Corona* (pp. 243–245). Stadt Wien.

Kittel, B., Kritzinger, S., Boomgaarden, H., Prainsack, B., Eberl, J., Kalleitner, F., Lebernegg, N. S., Partheymüller, J., Plescia, C., Schiestl, D. W., & Schlogl, L. (2020). *Austrian corona panel project* [Data set]. https://data.aussda.at/dataset.xhtml?persistentId=doi:10.11587/28KQNS

Klein, J., & von dem Knesebeck, O. (2018). Inequalities in health care utilization among migrants and non-migrants in Germany: a systematic review. *International Journal for Equity in Health, 17*(1), 1–10.

Koschollek, C., Kuehne, A., Müllerschön, J., Amoah, S., Batemona-Abeke, H., Dela Bursi, T., Mayamba, P., Thorlie, A., Tshibadi, C. M., Greiner, V. W., Bremer, V. & Santos-Hövener, C. (2020). Knowledge, information needs and behavior regarding HIV and sexually transmitted infections among migrants from sub-Saharan Africa living in Germany: Results of a participatory health research survey. *PLoS One, 15*(1), e0227178.

Lebernegg, N. S., Eberl, J., Boomgaarden, H. G., & Partheymüller, J. (2020). Alte und neue Medien: Informationsverhalten in Zeiten der Corona-Krise [Old and New Media: Information Patterns in Times of the Corona Crisis]. *VIECER Blog by the University of Vienna.* https://viecer.univie.ac.at/corona-blog/corona-blog-beitraege/blog04/

Lorenz, L., & Marchart, J. M. (2020, April 16). Integrationsfonds informiert Migranten unvollständig über Corona-Maßnahmen [Integration Fund provides incomplete information about Corona measures to migrants]. *Der Standard.* https://www.derstandard.at/story/2000116915568/integrationsfonds-informierte-unvollstaendig-ueber-corona-massnahmen

Maldonado, B. M. N., Collins, J., Blundell, H. J., & Singh, L. (2020). Engaging the vulnerable: a rapid review of public health communication aimed at migrants during the COVID-19 pandemic in Europe. *Journal of Migration and Health, 1–2,* 100004.

Marmot, M., Allen, J., Boyce, T., Goldblatt, P., & Morrison, J. (2020). *Health equity in England: The Marmot Review 10 years on.* Institute of Health Equity. http://www.instituteofhealthequity.org/resources-reports/marmot-review-10-years-on/the-marmot-review-10-years-on-full-report.pdf

Matlin, S. A., Depoux, A., Schütte, S., Flahault, A., & Saso, L. (2018). Migrants' and refugees' health: towards an agenda of solutions. *Public Health Reviews, 39*(1), 1–55.

Meeuwesen, L., Harmsen, J. A., Bernsen, R. M., & Bruijnzeels, M. A. (2006). Do Dutch doctors communicate differently with immigrant patients than with Dutch patients? *Social Science & Medicine, 63*(9), 2407–2417.

Moore, C. J., & Cunningham, S. A. (2012). Social position, psychological stress, and obesity: a systematic review. *Journal of the Academy of Nutrition and Dietetics, 112*(4), 518–526.

National Academies of Sciences, Engineering, and Medicine. (2017). *Health Communication with Immigrants, Refugees, and Migrant Workers* [Workshop Proceedings]. https://www.nap.edu/catalog/24796/health-communication-with-immigrants-refugees-and-migrant-workers-proceedings-of

OECD. (2020, October 19). What is the impact of the COVID-19 pandemic on immigrants and their children? *OECD Policy Responses to Coronavirus (COVID-19).* https://www.oecd.org/coronavirus/policy-responses/what-is-the-impact-of-the-covid-19-pandemic-on-immigrants-and-their-children-e7cbb7de/

Parker, R., & Ratzan, S. C. (2010). Health literacy: A second decade of distinction for Americans. *Journal of Health Communication, 15*(S2), 20–33.

Piga, A. (2007). Mediennutzung von Migranten: Ein Forschungsüberblick [Media Use by Migrants: A research overview]. In H. Bomfadelli & H. Moser (Eds.), *Medien und Migration [Media and migration]* (pp. 209–234). VS Verlag für Sozialwissenschaften.

Prugger, D. (2020, December 7). Austria: Anger as Kurz blames minorities for spreading COVID-19. *Aljazeera.* https://www.aljazeera.com/news/2020/12/7/austria-anger-as-kurz-blames-minorities-for-spreading-covid-19

Quenzel, G., Vogt, D., & Schaeffer, D. (2016). Unterschiede der Gesundheitskompetenz von Jugendlichen mit niedriger Bildung, Älteren und Menschen mit Migrationshintergrund [Differences in health literacy among young people with low education, older people and people with migration background]. *Das Gesundheitswesen, 78*(11), 708–710.

Razai, M. S., Kankam, H. K., Majeed, A., Esmail, A., & Williams, D. R. (2021). Mitigating ethnic disparities in covid-19 and beyond. *BMJ 2021,* 372:m4921.

Razum, O., Penning, V., Mohsenpour, A., & Bozorgmehr, K. (2020). Covid-19 in Flüchtlingsunterkünften [Covid-19 in refugee shelters]. *Gesundheitswesen, 82,* 392–396.

Razum, O., & Spallek, J. (2014). Addressing health-related interventions to immigrants: migrant-specific or diversity-sensitive? *International Journal of Public Health, 59*(6), 893–895.

Riese, D. (2020, March 18). Polizeieinsatz gegen Geflüchtete in Suhl: "Absolut chaotische Situation" [Police action against refugees in Suhl: "Totally chaotic situation"]. *taz.* https://taz.de/Polizeieinsatz-gegen-Gefluechtete-in-Suhl/!5668971/

Sauer, M. (2010). Mediennutzungsmotive türkeistämmiger Migranten in Deutschland [Media Use Motives of Migrants from Turkey in Germany]. *Publizistik, 55*(1), 55–76.

Schulz, P. J., & Nakamoto, K. (2013). Health literacy and patient empowerment in health communication: The importance of separating conjoined twins. *Patient Education and Counseling, 90*(1), 4–11.

Sørensen, K., Van den Broucke, S., Fullam, J., Doyle, G., Pelikan, J., Slonska, Z., & Brand, H. (2012). Health literacy and public health: a systematic review and integration of definitions and models. *BMC Public Health, 12*(1), 1–13.

Statistics Austria. (2020a). *Migration und Integration. Zahlen, Daten, Indikatoren 2020* [Migration and Integration. Figures, Data, Indicators 2020]. https://www.statistik.at/web_de/services/publikationen/2/index.html?includePage=detailedView&sectionName=Bev%C3%B6lkerung&pubId=621

Statistics Austria. (2020b). Mikrozensus-Arbeitskräfteerhebung Jahresdaten [Microcensus-Labour Force Survey Annual Data]. https://www.data.gv.at/katalog/dataset/d8d0f02d-8022-344b-9de7-b7af6ebdce01

Teunissen, E., Gravenhorst, K., Dowrick, C., van Weel-Baumgarten, E., Van den Driessen Mareeuw, F., de Brún, T., Burns, N., Lionis, C., Mair, F. S., O'Donnell, C., O'Reilly-de Brún, M., Papadakaki, M., Saridaki, A., Spiegel, W., Van Weel, C., Van den Muijsenbergh, M., & MacFarlane, A. (2017). Implementing guidelines and training initiatives to improve cross-cultural communication in primary care consultations: A qualitative participatory European study. *International Journal for Equity in Health, 16*(1), 1–12.

Viehmann, C., Ziegele, M., & Quiring, O. (2020). *Informationsnutzung in der Corona-Krise. Report zu ersten Befunden aus zwei Erhebungswellen.* https://www.kowi.ifp.uni-mainz.de/aktuelle-projekte/informationsnutzung-in-der-corona-krise/

White, A. I. (2020). Historical linkages: epidemic threat, economic risk, and xenophobia. *The Lancet, 395*(10232), 1250–1251.

WHO – World Health Organization. (2020a). *ApartTogether survey: Preliminary overview of refugees and migrants self-reported impact of COVID-19.* https://www.who.int/publications/i/item/9789240017924

WHO – World Health Organization. (2020b). *Risk communication and community engagement (RCCE) action plan guidance COVID-19 preparedness and response. Interim Guidance.* https://www.who.int/publications/i/item/risk-communication-and-community-engagement-(rcce)-action-plan-guidance

Williams, D. R. (2012). Miles to go before we sleep: Racial inequities in health. *Journal of Health and Social Behavior, 53*(3), 279–295.

8 Segregation within Welfare Societies – Communication Barriers to Migrants' Healthcare in Scandinavia

Elisabeth Mangrio and Michael Strange

The Scandinavian countries are often ranked highest amongst global health indicators, with a reputation as advanced welfare states with universal healthcare coverage free at the point of use. However, does this coverage extend to migrants resident within the region? During 2015–2016, the Scandinavian countries received a high proportion of refugees in comparison with many other European countries and in the context of their relatively small populations (Nordic Council of Ministers, 2018). Denmark, Norway, and Sweden have quite distinct histories with respect to the extent of residency rights given to asylum seekers and other vulnerable migrants. This chapter compares the three Scandinavian countries in terms of what healthcare coverage is available to asylum seekers and refugees. In so doing, it highlights an important distinction between formal rights and actual access to healthcare and identifies the key communication barriers limiting refugee and migrants' access to healthcare in Sweden. We know that such migrants often experience health challenges related not only to their migratory journey, but often the precarious situation in which they are placed upon arrival in host countries (Eckstein, 2011).

Past studies show significant challenges in obtaining care, and diffi-culties with communication, including cultural awareness. In addition, after arrival in Scandinavia, refugees and asylum seekers are known to suffer from different social issues such as crowded and insecure housing, missing family members after arrival in the host country and striving towards integration with the aim of trying to find a job, with negative effects on their mental and physical health (Johnson & Thompson, 2008; Mangrio et al., 2019; Mangrio & Zdravkovic, 2018; Savin et al., 2005). Since access to healthcare is crucial for good health among refugees (An-derson et al., 2003), it is important to investigate the experiences among refugees and asylum seekers in regard to healthcare access. Where health communication fails to meet the needs of a diverse population, we see growing societal segregation that follows often-racialized structures with long-term consequences for society.

DOI: 10.4324/9781003230243-8

Communication Barriers to Migrants' Healthcare in Scandinavia

This section provides a brief overview comparing Denmark, Norway and Sweden in terms of the formal access to healthcare for migrants, and the importance of health communication in explaining some of the most significant barriers limiting access.

Norway

After asylum seekers arrive in Norway, they are entitled to receive essential healthcare. They will also receive professional medical assistance if they have experienced war, conflicts, torture, violence, abuse or female genital mutilation (HelseNorge, 2021). When asylum seekers arrive in Norway, they must be tested for tuberculosis if they come from a country with a high incidence of tuberculosis and have to do so within 14 days after arrival (HelseNorge, 2021). All asylum seekers have the right to be assigned a general practitioner and have the right to get mental health care when needed. Interpreters are hired where required (HelseNorge, 2021). Even when asylum seekers receive a final refusal of asylum, they have the right to be examined at a hospital, to receive medical assistance when urgent, and if they are identified as suffering from mental illness, they have the right to mental health service care (HelseNorge, 2021).

In Norway, the municipalities are responsible for providing health-care suitable for early identification of somatic and mental health (Laue & Risor, 2018). Even if all but undocumented migrants have the right to healthcare in line with the Norwegian population, a report from the International Organization for Migration questions the degree to which access to care is given in relation to what rights they have (Laue & Risor, 2018). A scoping review was done in Norway, focused on migrants' access to primary healthcare (Debesay et al., 2019). Migrants, in general, have been found to use primary healthcare less than Norwegians, and the utilization has been found to be positively associated with length of stay and to vary depending on the individual's reason for migrating. Rates are typically higher for refugees but lower for labor migrants as compared to those migrating for family reunification. The review also showed that, although migrants from high-income countries presented a similar number of diagnoses when in contact with primary health-care, they used it less than Norwegians (Debesay et al., 2019; Diaz et al., 2015). A survey on the use of hospitals and specialist healthcare services among Norwegians and migrants in the period of 2008–2011 showed that the migrant population, in total, had a lower use of so-matic hospitals and mental health services than their proportion in the entire population (Elstad, 2016). Conversely, there were also reports that a greater proportion of migrants report mental health issues compared to the rest of the population in Norway (Vrålstad, 2016), but few visits to the psychologists or psychiatrists. Migrants from Iran had the most contacts and migrants from Eritrea had the least share of contacts regarding mental health issues (Vrålstad, 2016).

A recent study on how Ethiopian refugees perceive health and healthcare in Norway (Schein et al., 2019) concluded that their healthcare access improved after gaining residence permits and they thought that, while most of them were able to converse in English and now also spoke Norwegian, many discussed prior or current language barriers. Interpreters were not always reliable, and once participants learned Norwegian, many felt a new sense of autonomy and control over their healthcare experiences. They also talked about issues of race and differences in sociocultural backgrounds that complicated interactions with doctors. Several of the participants described better healthcare interactions with doctors who were perceived as also not Norwegian and thought that they understood them better (Schein et al., 2019).

In relation to the recent and ongoing Covid-19 pandemic, Norway has supplied migrants with information letters and videos in several languages (Norweigan Institute of Public Health, 2021). The information has covered topics such as basic information about the virus, social distancing and isolation, routines for self-isolation when symptomatic, as well as testing and mask-wearing (Norweigan Institute of Public Health, 2021). When it comes to supplying vaccinations for migrants in Norway, they have agreed on supplying vaccinations to asylum seekers with the same priority as the rest of the population in the country (EASO, 2021).

To conclude, Norway has liberal and extensive healthcare options for migrants, but although they have this right, they use it to a lesser extent than the rest of the population. And research shows that access improved after a while when language ability increased, since translators were not always reliable.

Denmark

The Danish healthcare system is characterized by universal coverage and financed mainly through taxes. For all persons with residence permits in Denmark, access to the healthcare system is free except for services such as dentistry and prescription medicine requiring some payment (Nielsen et al., 2012). Nielsen et al. conducted a survey, with the aim of investigating the use of healthcare services in different immigrant groups and whether differences in healthcare use could be explained by health status, socioeconomic factors, and integration (Nielsen et al., 2012). All migrant groups reported worse health symptoms than ethnic Danes, whereas descendants reported fewer physical health problems, but more mental health symptoms (Nielsen et al., 2012). Compared with ethnic Danes, most migrant groups had similar contacts to hospitals, increased contacts to emergency hospital care, general practitioners, and specialists in private practice, but fewer to dentists (Nielsen et al., 2012). Increased physical health symptoms were associated with increased hospitalization among all groups except Iraqi and Somali migrants where no effect was found. Likewise, for GPs, physical health symptoms had a positive explanatory effect on all groups, except Somali. Integration indicators (length of stay and Danish language proficiency) had no statistically significant effect on the level of use by most groups (Nielsen et al., 2012).

Another Danish study investigated general practitioners' experiences with providing care to refugees with mental health problems, and highlighted the importance of good communication; defined not only in terms in terms of language, but also cultural understanding (Jensen et al., 2013). Some of the general practitioners expressed that the patient and the health professional did not have the same understanding of health and disease, and some of the professionals expressed that refugee patients may have difficulties understanding that psychological and social problems may also lead to the presentation of physical symptoms. The general practitioners also explained how they had to handle patients when presenting problems outside their area of expertise and that they were not always able to live up to patients' expectations, with difficulties communicating these issues (Jensen et al., 2013).

In Denmark, a nationwide registry-based study was conducted to determine whether inequality exists regarding access to anti-dementia treatment and care between migrant and Danish-born patients with dementia (Stevnsborg et al., 2016). The migrant background was associated with a significantly lower likelihood of receiving anti-dementia drug therapy (Stevnsborg et al., 2016). Language problems and unfamiliarity with the health system structure may create difficulties navigating the system, leading to dissatisfaction and resulting in a lack of compliance with treatment (Franca Felix, 2017).

In relation to Covid-19, despite there being a high proportion of migrants not speaking Danish, the country was very slow in translating information about the virus, including precautions and restrictions (European Commission, 2021). When it comes to supplying vaccination for migrants in Denmark, however, the national program is supplying vaccinations to asylum seekers with the same priority as the rest of the population (EASO, 2021). To conclude, migrants in Denmark have worse health symptoms compared to the native Danes and seek healthcare in some instances more frequently. There are also significant communication issues that undermine migrants' access to, and understanding of, the Danish healthcare system.

Sweden

Asylum seekers and undocumented migrants in Sweden are entitled to both emergency care and dental care and healthcare that is identified as urgent (Migrationsverket, 2021). In practice, the decision over what this covers is made at the regional governmental level. Asylum seekers are also entitled to childbirth care, abortion care, advice on contraception, maternity care and healthcare under the Swedish Communicable Diseases Act (Migrationsverket, 2021).

New research in Sweden investigating access to health- and dental care in Sweden (Mangrio et al., 2018, 2020a; Zdravkovic et al., 2020), shows that hindrances to healthcare include upfront costs, mistrust in doctors and language issues (Mangrio et al., 2018). Around 70% of the migrants had been in need of healthcare but not sought care due to these factors (Mangrio et al., 2018). Qualitative research from the same research group shows that migrants are discontent, some had been denied healthcare when they sought it, which was due to their refugee status, and some had been lost in the referral of healthcare between different healthcare settings (Mangrio et al., 2018).

In another Swedish study, over a third of the refugees surveyed reported having refrained from seeking healthcare in the most recent three months. The most common reasons for this were: language problems (40%), did not think that help could be obtained (24%), would wait for a while (19%), and did not know where to go (19%) (Wångdahl et al., 2018). The lower the comprehensive health literacy was, the more the respondents reported having refrained from seeking healthcare. Other factors associated with having refrained from seeking healthcare were education level, not having participated in the health assessment after arrival, and having a long-term illness (Wångdahl et al., 2018). Another Swedish study on the experience of Somali and Arabic refugees regarding health-related information (Mårtensson et al., 2020), showed that the information, in general, was sufficient but lacked guidance about how to handle specific health issues. There was also a desire for knowledge about the healthcare system in Sweden and how it is organized and regulated, what rights and charges there are to the use of healthcare, and specific routines related to the provision of health care. They also expressed that health information was not available and applicable to everyone because of analphabetism, deficient language skills or lack of knowledge of where to find the information (Mårtensson et al., 2020).

Due to the increased migration into Sweden, a cross-sectional study was conducted evaluating the use of interpreters within healthcare in a certain part of Sweden (Hadziabdic & Hjelm, 2019). The study showed that the highest number of incidents between 2012 and 2016 was reported in local healthcare and the reason for the adverse incidents was mainly related to the absence of an interpreter at the agreed time. Also, 80% of interpretation assignments were mostly performed by non-authorized in-person interpreters and Arabic was the most requested interpreter language (Hadziabdic & Hjelm, 2019).

In the case of Covid-19, Sweden has supplied migrants with information about the virus, precautions and restrictions, and such information has been translated into different languages (Swedish Migration Agency, 2021; The Public Health Agency of Sweden, 2021). In addition, there has been a telephone line supplying information and contacts for different languages (The Public Health Agency of Sweden, 2021). Although the information was supplied, a recently published paper highlights the need that the information could have come quicker and bearing in mind that migrants have different levels of health literacy, which could affect the information understood (Mangrio, 2020b). When it comes to supplying vaccination for migrants, Sweden has agreed to supply vaccinations to asylum seekers with the same priority as the rest of the population in the country (EASO, 2021).

To conclude, Sweden has liberal and extensive services for migrants, but in spite of the generous rights, several studies show that migrants have difficulties accessing healthcare and that they face different barriers in order to obtain healthcare and that more information is needed.

Health Literacy, Cultural Competence, & Intersectionality

The aspect of health literacy

A key aspect determining migrants' access to different healthcare settings is their level of health literacy. To be health literate means to be able to access, understand, value, and use health information (Delmi, 2020). There are two different kinds of health literacy: complex health literacy and functional health literacy. Complex health literacy means to independently get hold of, value, and use health information (Delmi, 2020). On the other hand, functional health literacy means being able to passively receive health information and being able to read the information (Delmi, 2020). When functional health literacy is limited, migrants could have a limited ability to receive instructions during health visits, ask fewer questions and participate to a lesser extent in health-promoting actions (Delmi, 2020). Health practitioners need to be trained to identify wherever there is health literacy, since it is a significant barrier to healthcare as well as undermining the effectiveness of health interventions.

Cultural Competence

Cultural competence is defined as an approach, knowledge and skills that are needed in order to deliver healthcare with good quality to people with different cultural backgrounds (Kersey-Matusiak, 2013). The approach needed for giving culturally competent healthcare is to be open-minded and keep reflecting on your own values, opinions, and stereotypes and to be able to consider another person's opinion or outlook on life. Healthcare professionals need to increase their knowledge about themselves and their patients. They need to get knowledge about the history of the patient, their country of origin, and cultural and ethnic background when they consider all this information. It becomes easier to get a holistic view of the patient that you care for. When it comes to needed and required skills, healthcare professionals need good communication skills that improve the relationships between professionals and patients, and there needs to be reflective listening and communication in a language that the patient understands. An active listening, which means both listening and asking questions in order to increase understanding and communication, is also essential as an approach for providing culturally competent healthcare (Kersey-Matusiak, 2013).

Intersectionality

Although health inequities, including issues around access and literacy, can often appear marked along certain social boundaries (e.g., race, gender, class, sexuality), insight from Intersectional theory shows that there is also a danger if policies intended to enhance health equity focused solely on any single category (Weber & Parra-Medina, 2003). Health communication that excludes migrants, for example, may even be worsened if remedial policies focus exclusively on a top-down identification of individuals as 'migrants.' As intersectional approaches to the societal determinants of health show, social markers like 'race' or 'gender' do not exist in isolation but operate within a dynamic context in which individuals must navigate multiple societal positions in which they find themselves. One of the most important insights from this perspective is that effective health communication cannot rely on an apriori categorization of individuals, but needs to be developed in relation to the 'personal narratives' of those living on the margins of society (Hankivsky & Christoffersen, 2008; McCall, 2005). The alternative is to attempt to somehow unravel the complex knot of multiple societal positions from the top-down, which would ultimately result in missing some important information determining health inequity. To obtain rich information on the structures that impact societal health, it is necessary to consult directly with those individuals most negatively affected by those structures.

Recommended Strategies

Community Engagement

During the present and ongoing pandemic of Covid-19, during 2020–2021, it has been evident how important community engagement has been for reaching migrants with information during the pandemic. This is important because migrants already face challenges to access to healthcare and information and challenges to comply with the given information (Unicef et al., 2020). In crises such as the recent pandemic, it is important to engage with all actors and to make sure that all voices are heard and that all practices promoted are understood. It is crucial to ensure that national strategies are developed to include refugees, migrants and vulnerable people in the affected communities, and to ensure that information is adapted to their needs so that it can be utilized effectively. It is also important to address communication issues such as language issues, access to media and mobile technology, and to ensure that information is accessible to those with physical, psychosocial, sensory and intellectual impairments. Another aspect that is important is to investigate what channels of information are trusted amongst the refugees and migrants in different communities, and then work through those channels. Further on, collaboration and coordination with involved stakeholders can improve communication and avoid duplication. Considering partnering with local government, civil society organizations, community and religious leaders, and influencers is crucial in order to reach migrants with important information.

For example, in recent research on different national approaches to migrants during the first wave of the Covid-19 pandemic, data from Sweden showed the importance of work by society and health communicators who were able to understand both the different languages and community organizations utilized by different migrant communities (Dalingwater et al., 2021).

Cultural Competence and Cultural Sensitivity

It is important to highlight cultural competence and cultural sensitivity for improving health communication for migrants. Cultural competence refers to having respect for people with different cultural backgrounds and, through this respect, fostering an atmosphere that is non-discriminating (Finnish Institute for Health and Welfare, 2021). Cultural competence includes cultural awareness, knowledge, skills and mirroring one's own cultural habits and values with the habits and values of other cultures. Cultural sensitivity is closely linked to cultural competence but means to have respectful interpersonal skills and respectful verbal and non-verbal encounters and communications between a professional and patient in a manner that involves the right of each party to express their culture and be accepted and heard in that context. To be culturally sensitive within a healthcare setting means to be flexible to the needs of different people.

The premises for cultural sensitivity within healthcare settings include perceiving one's own cultural background, manners and using that as a foundation for increasing the understanding of other cultures (Finnish

Institute for Health and Welfare, 2021). It also means respecting diversity, showing interest in different cultures, and finding the courage to meet patients as individuals rather than representatives of a specific culture. To ask patients about their values, habits and culture instead of just assuming and generalizing some facts about a certain culture is _important. Whenever language issues are faced, working with an interpreter is crucial (Finnish Institute for Health and Welfare, 2021).

A Swedish study investigated the impact that training within cultural competence could have on the work with migrants within the child health care settings (Berlin et al., 2010), evaluating the extent to which specific training affected how nurses rated their own cultural competence, difficulties, and concerns and to study how the nurses evaluated the training. They concluded that the training was appreciated and had positive effects on their cultural competence, difficulties and concerns (Berlin et al., 2010).

Health Literacy

Health literacy, as explained above, is important in order for migrants to understand and apply information given within health care settings. A recent survey among newly arrived migrants in Sweden showed that a majority (80%) of the migrants showed limited functional health literacy, and a quite smaller extent (62%) showed limited complex health literacy. This means that around 20% of the migrants had sufficient complex health literacy while they at the same time had limited functional health literacy. The same survey showed that limited functional health literacy was more common among migrants with a low educational level and also showed that functional health literacy was more common among migrants from Somalia than Iraq (Delmi, 2020). The aspect of health literacy is important to keep in mind when discussing health care access among migrants residing in the Nordic countries, since these countries have quite liberal rights for migrants to receive healthcare, but substantial research shows difficulties for migrants in obtaining care. One possible solution is suggested in a study on the effectiveness of an application for mobile devices – a so-called 'mHealth intervention program' (Fernández-Gutiérrez et al., 2019). The intervention showed that a program of mHealth intervention for health literacy that is culturally competent and based on community action and participation, can improve the cognitive and social skills required to access and use health services in participating migrants (Fernández-Gutiérrez et al., 2019).

Interpretation

A recent systematic review on challenges and facilitators for health-care encounters showed that language barriers were widely cited as a barrier during encounters with refugees or asylum seekers (Robertshaw et al., 2017). The included studies elaborated that language barriers presented challenges while assessing case histories, gaining consent, and ensuring that patients understood the given treatment (Robertshaw et al., 2017). On the other hand, the included papers showed that the use of interpreters was a great facilitator in communication and was much better when interpreters were familiar with medical terminology and were well trained. It was also noted that continuity of the same interpreter fostered good communication and increased the confidence in the integrity of the interpreter. The challenges that were associated with the use of interpreters were that it required additional time and financial expense. When suitable translators were not available, it led to delayed, extended or rearranged appointments. The use of telephone interpreters had mixed experiences, being that the teleservice offered both extended availabilities but gave an impersonal impression, and sometimes there were technical hinders (Robertshaw et al., 2017). In a scoping review, where the experiences of refugees encounter with health-care settings were investigated, it revealed similar results as above regarding the language and interpretation, but also lifted a challenge with interpreters mostly being from the same communities as the migrants themselves, and they were afraid that personal information would be disclosed within the communities (Mangrio & Forss, 2017).

Conclusion

Health communication is at the core of ensuring health equity, and in the case of migrants' health – particularly those living in a precarious situation – it is important to ensure that the communication strategies are sensitive to their needs. As the chapter has argued, that cannot be limited to pre-existing assumptions of their needs, but as with any marginalized group it is necessary to work with them directly to understand the obstacles they face when attempting to access healthcare. Cultural competence and sensitivity need to be achieved through an intersectional approach interested in personal narratives. Whilst that might not be realistic for each individual, it is very clear that healthcare provision for migrants in Scandinavia largely almost completely ignores their perspective such that the access of migrants to healthcare is greatly curtailed. This is of particular concern given wider pressures also placed on migrants, and the risk that growing health inequity points to wider segregation in the Scandic welfare model based on an individuals' status as foreign-born. In a world in which migration remains a fact regardless of political attitudes, emergent segregation is unsustainable but can be remedied with more effective health communication strategies that are developed in tandem with those currently excluding migrants.

Recommended reading

Hankivsky, O., & Christoffersen, A. (2008). Intersectionality and the determinants of health: a Canadian perspective. *Critical Public Health*, 18(3), 271–283.

Mangrio, E., Carlson, E., & Zdravkovic, S. (2018). Understanding experiences of the Swedish health care system from the perspective of newly arrived refugees. *BMC Research Notes*, 11(1), 616. https://bmcresnotes.biomedcentral.com/articles/10.1186/s13104-018-3728-4

Mangrio, E., & Forss, K. S. (2017). Refugees' experiences of healthcare in the host country: A scoping review. *BMC Health Services Research*, 17(1), 814. https://bmchealthservres.biomedcentral.com/track/pdf/10.1186/s12913-017-2731-0.pdf

Weber, L., & Parra-Medina, D., (2003). Intersectionality and women's health: Charting a path to eliminating health disparities, In V. Demos, & M. T. Segal (Eds.), *Advances in gender research: Gendered perspectives on health and medicine* (Vol. 7A, pp. 183–226). California: Elsevier.

Wångdahl, J. (2017). *Health literacy among newly arrived refugees in Sweden and implications for health and healthcare.* [Doctoral Dissertation Uppsala University] https://uu.diva-portal.org/smash/get/diva2:1158668/FULLTEXT01.pdf

References

Anderson, L. M., Scrimshaw, S. C., Fullilove, M. T., Fielding, J. E., Normand, J., & Task Force On Community Preventive Services. (2003). Culturally competent healthcare systems: A systematic review. *American Journal of Preventive Medicine*, 24(3), 68–79.

Berlin, A., Nilsson, G., & Törnkvist, L. (2010). Cultural competence among Swedish child health nurses after specific training: A randomized trial. *Nursing & Health Sciences*, 12(3), 381–391.

Debesay, J., Arora, S., & Bergland, A. (2019). 4. Migrants' consumption of healthcare services in Norway: Inclusionary and exclusionary structures and practices. In A. Borch, I. Harsløf, I. G. Klepp, & K. Laitala (Eds.), *Inclusive consumption* (pp. 63–78). Norway: Universitetsförlaget.

Delmi. (2020). *Migranters möte med svensk hälso- och sjukvård: Avhandlingsnytt 2020:7.* https://www.delmi.se/samhalle#!/xxx-avhandlingsnytt-20207-1

Diaz, E., Kumar, B. N., & Engedal, K. (2015). Immigrant patients with dementia and memory impairment in primary health care in Norway: A national registry study. *Dementia and Geriatric Cognitive Disorders*, 39(5–6), 321–331.

EASO. (2021, August 25). *COVID-19 vaccination for applicants and beneficiaries of international protection.* https://www.easo.europa.eu/sites/default/files/publications/EASO_Situational_Update_Vaccination31March..pdf

Eckstein, B. (2011). Primary Care for refugees. *Am Fam Physician*, 83(4), 429–436.

Elstad, J. I. (2016). Register study of migrants' hospitalization in Norway: World region origin, reason for migration, and length of stay. *BMC Health Services Research*, 16(1), 1–12.

European Commission. (2021, August 25). *European website on integration: Denmark: How has COVID-19 affected migrants?* https://ec.europa.eu/migrant-integration/news/denmark-how-has-covid-19-affected-migrants

Fernández-Gutiérrez, M., Bas-Sarmiento, P., & Poza-Méndez, M. (2019). Effect of an mHealth intervention to improve health literacy in immigrant populations: A quasi-experimental study. *CIN: Computers, Informatics, Nursing*, 37(3), 142–150.

Finnish Institute for Health and Welfare. (2021 August 25). *Migration and cultural diversity: Cultural competence and cultural sensitivity.* https://thl.fi/en/web/migration-and-cultural-diversity/support-material/good-practices/cultural-competence-and-cultural-sensitivity

Felix, F., (2017). *Barriers to access to healthcare services by immigrants population in Scandinavia: A systematic scoping review* [Matser dissertation, The Arctic university of Norway]. https://munin.uit.no/bitstream/handle/10037/12212/thesis.pdf?isAllowed=y&sequence=2

Hadziabdic, E., & Hjelm, K. (2019). Register-based study concerning the problematic situation of using interpreting service in a region in Sweden. *BMC Health Services Research*, 19(1), 1–8.

Hankivsky, O., & Christoffersen, A. (2008). Intersectionality and the determinants of health: A Canadian perspective. *Critical Public Health*, 18(3), 271–283.

HelseNorge. (2021, August 25). *Healthcare for asylum seekers and refugees in Norway.* https://www.helsenorge.no/en/foreigners-in-norway/asylum-seekers/#upon-arrival-in-norway

Jensen, N. K., Norredam, M., Priebe, S., & Krasnik, A. (2013). How do general practitioners experience providing care to refugees with mental health problems? A qualitative study from Denmark. *BMC Family Practice*, 14(1), 1–9.

Johnson, H., & Thompson, A. (2008). The development and maintenance of post-traumatic stress disorder (PTSD) in civilian adult survivors of war trauma and torture: A review. *Clinical Psychology Review*, 28(1), 36–47.

Kersey-Matusiak, G. (2013). *Delivering culturally competent nursing care.* Springer Publishing Company.

Laue, J., & Risor, T. (2018). Refugees and healthcare services. *Tidsskrift for den Norske laegeforening: tidsskrift for praktisk medicin, ny raekke*, 137(1), 1–5.

Mangrio, E., Carlson, E., & Zdravkovic, S. (2018). Understanding experiences of the Swedish health care system from the perspective of newly arrived refugees. *BMC Research Notes*, 11(1), 616.

Mangrio, E., Carlson, E., & Zdravkovic, S. (2019). Newly arrived refugee parents in Sweden and their experience of the resettlement process: A qualitative study. *Scandinavian Journal of Public Health*.

Mangrio, E., Carlzén, K., Grahn, M., & Zdravkovic, S. (2020a). *Kartläggning av nyligen nyanländas hälsa, levnadsvanor, sociala relationer, arbetsmarknad och boendemiljö efter etableringen.: Delrapport från MILSA 2.0.*

Mangrio, E., & Forss, K. S. (2017). Refugees' experiences of healthcare in the host country: A scoping review. *BMC Health Services Research*, 17(1), 814.

Mangrio, E., Maneesh, P. S., & Strange, M. (2020b). Refugees in Sweden during the Covid-19 pandemic – The need for a new perspective on health and integration *Frontiers in Public Health*. https://www.frontiersin.org/articles/10.3389/fpubh.2020.574334/abstract

Mangrio, E., & Zdravkovic, S. (2018). Crowded living and its association with mental ill-health among recently-arrived migrants in Sweden: a quantitative study. *BMC Research Notes*, 11(1), 609.

McCall, L. (2005). The complexity of intersectionality. *Signs: Journal of Women in Culture and Society*, 30(3), 1771–1800.

Migrationsverket. (2021, August 25). *Health care for asylum seekers*. https://www.migrationsverket.se/English/Private-individuals/Protection-and-asylum-in-Sweden/While-you-are-waiting-for-a-decision/Health-care.html

Mårtensson, L., Lytsy, P., Westerling, R., & Wångdahl, J. (2020). Experiences and needs concerning health related information for newly arrived refugees in Sweden. *BMC Public Health*, 20(1), 1–10.

Nielsen, S. S., Hempler, N. F., Waldorff, F. B., Kreiner, S., & Krasnik, A. (2012). Is there equity in use of healthcare services among immigrants, their descendents, and ethnic Danes? *Scandinavian Journal of Public Health*, 40(3), 260–270.

Nordic Council of Ministers. (2018). *State of the Nordic Region 2018. Immigration and integration edition*. https://norden.diva-portal.org/smash/get/diva2:1192284/FULLTEXT01.pdf

Norweigan Institute of Public Health. (2021, August 25). *Coronavirus disease—Advice and information*. https://www.fhi.no/en/id/infectious-diseases/coronavirus/

Robertshaw, L., Dhesi, S., & Jones, L. L. (2017). Challenges and facilitators for health professionals providing primary healthcare for refugees and asylum seekers in high-income countries: A systematic review and thematic synthesis of qualitative research. *BMJ Open*, 7(8), e015981. doi: 10.1136/bmjopen-2017-015981

Savin, D., Seymour, D. J., Littleford, L. N., Bettridge, J., & Giese, A. (2005). Findings from mental health screening of newly arrived refugees in Colorado. *Public Health Reports*, 120(3), 224–229.

Schein, Y. L., Winje, B. A., Myhre, S. L., Nordstoga, I., & Straiton, M. L. (2019). A qualitative study of health experiences of Ethiopian asylum seekers in Norway. *BMC Health Services Research*, 19(1), 1–12.

Stevnsborg, L., Jensen-Dahm, C., Nielsen, T. R., Gasse, C., & Waldemar, G. (2016). Inequalities in access to treatment and care for patients with dementia and immigrant background: A Danish nationwide study. *Journal of Alzheimer's Disease*, 54(2), 505–514.

Swedish Migration Agency. (2021, August 25). *Information regarding COVID-19*. https://www.migrationsverket.se/English/About-the-Migration-Agency/COVID-19.html

The Public Health Agency of Sweden. (2021, August 25). *COVID-19*. https://www.folkhalsomyndigheten.se/the-public-health-agency-of-sweden/communicable-disease-control/covid-19/

Unicef et al. (2020, August 25). *Practical guidance for risk communication and community engagement (RCCE) for refugees, internally displaced persons (IDPs), migrants, and host communities particularly vulnerable to COVID-19 pandemic*. https://www.unodc.org/documents/drug-prevention-and-treatment/Practical-Guidance-RCCE-Refugees-IDPs-Migrants.pdf

Vrålstad, S., & Wiggen, K. (2021, August 25). *Levekår blant innvandrere i Norge 2016.* https://www.kompetansenorge.no/statistikk-og-analyse/publikasjoner/levekar-blant-innvandrere-i-norge-2016/

Weber, L, & Parra-Medina, D. (2003). Intersectionality and women's health: charting a path to eliminating health disparities. In V. Demos & M. T. Segal (Eds.), *Advances in gender research: Gendered perspectives on health and medicine.* New York: Elsevier.

Wångdahl, J., Lytsy, P., Mårtensson, L., & Westerling, R. (2018). Poor health and refraining from seeking healthcare are associated with comprehensive health literacy among refugees: a Swedish cross-sectional study. *International Journal of Public Health*, 63(3), 409–419.

Zdravkovic, S., Carlzén, K., Grahn, M., & Mangrio, E. (2020). *Kartläggning av hälsa, levnadsvanor, sociala relationer, arbetsmarknad och boendemiljö bland arabisktalande nyanlända inom etableringen: Delrapport från MILSA 2.0.*

9 Diffusion of Information and Influence for Promoting Health among *Joseon-Jok* Workers in South Korea

Do Kyun David Kim, Eun-Jeong Han, and Seulgi Park

The number of foreign workers in South Korea (Korea hereafter) has significantly increased since the 1990s due to a variety of domestic and international factors, such as increasing domestic wages, Korean workers' avoidance of 3D (dirty, dangerous, demeaning) jobs, vibrant trend of globalization, and global diffusion of Korean pop culture (e.g., K-pop, K-TV dramas, K-movies, etc.) (Kim, 2015; Kim, 2016; Park, 2014; Yoon & Kim, 2011). The Asian Games in 1986 and the Olympics in 1988 also contributed to enhancing international awareness of Korea's successful economy and democratization efforts, which attracted people in other Asian countries to have a Korean dream (Kim, 2016). As a result, the influx of Asian migrant workers to Korea increased exponentially, and one of the major migrant worker groups is ethnic Koreans from mainland China, so-called *Joseon-Jok* (조선족) (Lee, Kim, & Yang, 2011; Seo, 2014; Yoon & Kim, 2011).

Joseon-Jok is the group name of Chinese nationals of Korean descent who migrated from Korea to China mostly in the Japanese colonial era (1910–1945) and remained in ethnic enclaves in northeast China (Kim, 2019; Piao, 2017). As one of the officially recognized minorities in China, the Chinese government granted them Chinese citizenship and allowed them to form an autonomous prefecture in a northeast area close to the border with North Korea (Kim, 2019). This transnational Korean ethnic group began to return to Korea for guest labor work in the 1980s after Deng Xiaoping initiated the reformation of the Chinese economy and gradually eased international trade (Kim, 2019). Although the influx of *Joseon-Jok* had notably increased since then, the Korean government had not granted them any visa category to facilitate their migration until the mid-2000s (Kim, 2019; Seol & Skrentny, 2009). Before then, *Joseon-Jok* who wished to visit Korea were required to obtain an invitation from their distant relatives in Korea, which often cost a large amount of documentation fee charged by commercial immigration brokers (Kim, 2019).

In order to recognize and legalize ethnic Koreans abroad who wished to work in Korea, the Korean government created a work visa category

DOI: 10.4324/9781003230243-9

(H-2, or the Work and Visit program) in 2007 and tried to embrace *Joseon-Jok* and ethnic Koreans from the post-Soviet Union (*Koryo-saram*), such as Kazakhstan and Uzbekistan (Lim & Seol, 2018). However, the immigration law limited employment for H-2 visa holders only within designated industrial sectors including agriculture, construction, and the service industry (Seol & Skretny, 2009). Most Joseon-Jok have supplied low-wage labor to these industrial sectors in which Korean natives are not in favor of working (Seol & Skretny, 2009).

For example, one of the jobs permitted for *Joseon-Jok* workers is the caregiver job. According to a recent report by the Ministry of Public Health and Welfare (Shin & Chae, 2021), approximately 16,400 *Joseon-Jok* out of 40,000 caregivers are working in nursing homes/hospitals. Some news reports estimate a much higher number of *Joseon-Jok* caregivers, accounting for as much as 80–90% of total caregivers in nursing homes and hospitals (e.g. Kang, Jeong, & Jung, 2019; Park, 2016). While working under a high physical demand and poor work conditions, *Joseon-Jok* workers often experience social stigma that considers them as uneducated and undisciplined and makes them often the most vulnerable among the vulnerable and socially marginalized people in Korea (Park, 2016; Shin, 2019). This chapter investigates problems and difficulties in promoting public health among *Joseon-Jok* workers and recommends theory- and evidence-based health communication strategies that can guide them to scientific public health information and accessible healthcare facilities.

Health Challenges of Migrant Workers in a Low-Wage Labor Market

Migrant workers who fill the gap in the international labor market have often experienced many challenges, including labor exploitation, discrimination, and contract violation, while working under unprotected and poor work conditions (Norredam & Agyemang, 2019). Particularly, most foreign migrant workers from Asian countries are employed in low-paid, physical labor jobs with long work hours. In terms of public health, Kim (2009) argued that major causes of migrant workers' health problems include long and excessive work hours, and poor working and housing conditions. Different climate, food, lifestyle, and eating habits should also be considered when examining foreign migrant workers' health conditions (Jeong, Lee, & Kim, 2019). Such harsh work situations and living conditions often become major hurdles for these migrant workers to maintain their physical and mental health (Jeong et al., 2019; Kim, 2014; Lim & Kim, 2014; Noh & Ko, 2013).

In fact, a high number of migrant workers in Korea experience several different health problems. According to Lim and Kim (2014), a majority of migrant workers who visited local healthcare centers had chronic diseases such as diabetes and high blood pressure. In addition, several studies found that the most common health problems from which foreign migrant workers suffer are muscular skeletal diseases, particularly rheumatism, and other major diseases including respiratory, digestive, and circulatory system disorders (Choi, 2011; Jeong et al., 2019). Many migrant workers experience pain from muscular skeletal diseases on a daily basis because of intensive physical labor that they rarely did in their home countries (Kim, 2014). Lee (2014)'s study also found that most middle-aged female migrant workers suffer from muscular skeletal diseases, such as shoulder pain, intervertebral disk pain, and knee joint pain. These major health problems are strongly related to their long work hours in physical labor jobs such as construction, restaurant work, caregiving, and housekeeping (Lee, 2014).

Migrant workers experience not only physical health problems but also various mental health problems. Previous studies (e.g., Jeong et al., 2019; Kim, 2015) have revealed that mental health problems that many migrant workers in Korea experience were related to stress from cultural differences, insecure legal status, language barriers, and discrimination. Precarious employment, which can be defined with one of the following words – temporary, atypical, contingent, or non-standard work, job insecurity, lack of work rights; and inadequate salary – are also major factors that can lead to migrant workers' mental health problems (Ornek et al., 2020). Common mental health problems among migrant workers include anxiety, depression, alcoholism, insomnia/sleep disorder, post-traumatic disorder, memory loss, and aggression (Pocock et al., 2018; Mucci et al., 2020). According to the Jeong et al. (2019) study, the most common mental or psychological problems of migrant workers in Korea are depression, sleep disorders, anxiety, and homesickness.

Some migrant workers now prepare for anticipated health problems as awareness has grown about existing and potential health problems among international migrant workers. For example, most *Joseon-Jok* female migrant workers who migrate to Korea bring a variety of medicines with them, mostly painkillers, that they previously used in China. Even after they come to Korea, many of them regularly refill those medicines through their family members or friends in China (Lee, 2014). Many *Joseon-Jok* female migrant workers also take several dietary supplements (e.g., Vitamins) to maintain their health as advised by their Korean employers or informed by mass media. Some Korean co-workers and employers take care of migrant workers' health problems. According to Jeong et al. (2019)'s study, Nepalese migrant workers in farming areas of the *Jeju* island often get information about daily diet and exercise as well as available healthcare services from their Korean employers who spend much time with them at their workplaces. Similarly, some *Joseon-Jok* female migrant workers often receive medicines they used in China through the help of their Korean employers (Lee, 2014). Although some migrant workers take care of themselves with the help of their Korean employers, co-workers, and even family members and friends in their home countries, most do not receive the appropriate healthcare services that they need (Kim, 2015; Noh & Ko, 2013; Park, 2004).

Legal and Systematic Barriers

According to the Labor Standard Act in Korea, any workers, regardless of their legal status and country of origin, can receive healthcare services when they are injured at their workplace as long as their employers have industrial accident compensation insurance, and most of the companies have it because it is mandated by law (Choi, 2011; Noh, 2015; Noh & Ko, 2013; Yoon & Kim, 2011). Based on that law, migrant workers are also supposed to be covered by the industrial accident compensation insurance and the national health insurance system, which is critical especially for migrant workers as many of them work under 3D (dirty, dangerous, demeaning) environments. In reality, however, many migrant workers do not receive proper healthcare services because of legal and systematic limitations and suffer from isolation and ignorance when they are physically and mentally ill (Choi, 2011; Noh & Ko, 2013).

First, industrial accident compensation insurance is not required for individuals who hire domestic workers (e.g., babysitters, housekeepers, cooks), small business owners with less than five regular employees in agriculture, fishing, and the forestry industry, and employers of small-sized construction projects (Kim, 2014; Lee, 2014; Noh, 2015; Noh & Ko, 2013). Ironically, most migrant workers work at the small businesses listed above and, therefore, are not eligible to be beneficiaries of industrial accident compensation insurance (Kim, 2014; Lee, 2014; Noh, 2015; Noh & Ko, 2013). For example, the majority of female *Joseon-Jok* migrant workers do not have employment-based health insurance because they are employed as domestic workers (e.g., babysitters, housekeepers, etc.), caregivers for the sick or servers at small restaurants (Lee, 2014).

Secondly, large businesses that have industrial accident compensation insurance for their employees are reluctant to report their accidents to the Ministry of Labor due to a fear of receiving a penalty for frequent accidents. When migrant workers are injured by accidents at their workplaces, it is common that employers cover medical and healthcare expenses (e.g., emergency treatment, surgery, rehabilitation, etc.) by themselves without reporting to their insurance and the Ministry of Labor. Therefore, migrant workers in large businesses often do not receive proper medical treatments for full recovery from accidents and, most times, go back to work before they are fully recovered (Choi, 2011; Noh, 2015; Noh & Ko, 2013; Yoon & Kim, 2011). In the case of migrant workers who have serious or permanent disabilities from an industrial accident, some employers do not compensate them, trying to take advantage of migrant workers' lack of knowledge of labor law in Korea (Choi, 2011; Noh & Ko, 2013; Yoon & Kim, 2011).

Documented migrant workers who are not covered by employment-based health insurance are eligible to buy public health insurance. However, it is much more expensive than employment-based health insurance, and individual workers have to pay for all without their employers' co-payment. Most migrant workers cannot afford it (Kim, 2014; Kim, 2015; Lee, 2011; Noh & Ko, 2013; Seo, 2014). Another challenge of buying public health insurance is that it requires many documents to verify a migrant worker's income stability. Since most of the migrant workers work at small service businesses paying cash for work or are temporary construction workers, they do not receive regular paystubs, and it is hard for them to prove their financial stability (Yoon & Kim, 2011). Additionally, migrant workers who have stayed in Korea less than 90 days are not even eligible to apply for public health insurance (Kim, 2014).

Many undocumented migrant workers, due to fear of deportation, tend to refuse necessary medical treatment (Noh, 2015; Noh & Ko, 2013; Yoon & Kim, 2011). In fact, in 2000, the Korean government implemented a policy that grants healthcare services even for undocumented migrant workers through local healthcare centers. In addition, since 2005, the Korean Ministry of Health and Welfare has started to offer free healthcare services for migrant workers through several designated hospitals (Choi, 2011). However, due to fear of losing jobs and deportation, these undocumented workers rarely visit the government-supported local healthcare centers (Choi, 2011; Lim & Kim, 2014). Because of all these legal and systemic barriers, many documented and also undocumented migrant workers usually take over-the-counter medicines instead of visiting a doctor's office when they are sick or injured (Kim, 2015).

Social, Cultural, and Individual Barriers

As another major barrier to access healthcare services, migrant workers in Korea often face social, cultural, and individual constraints. The first constraint is migrant workers' lack of information about healthcare services. The Korean government provides various services for migrant workers through local healthcare centers, but few workers use them due to a lack of awareness of the services (Kim, 2015). Most of the migrant workers are not aware that they are entitled to receive various healthcare services. Some understand that they are covered by health insurance, but they have little knowledge about what kinds of services are available through health insurance and how to use them (Kim, 2015). Some others do not even know they have health insurance, despite the fact that they regularly pay for it (Choi, 2011; Choi & Kim, 2011; Kim,

2015). Kim (2015) found that a majority of migrant workers have little understanding or wrong information about the (emergency) health services or free health services they can receive from their health insurance plans.

Insufficient Korean language proficiency is another barrier for migrant accessing healthcare facilities and improving their medical literacy. Furthermore, few hospitals offer translation services for foreigners in Korea (Kim, 2015; Lim & Kim, 2014). Thus, most migrant workers have difficulty understanding critical information about treatments or medication provided by healthcare providers (Kim, 2014; Lee & Lee, 2013). Lee and Lee (2013) found that most migrant workers' average medical literacy level is lower than that of Korean senior citizens, and they hardly understand healthcare manuals and patient information forms that they have to fill out at their healthcare centers. Because of language incompetence, many migrant workers prefer local churches or other faith-based non-profit organizations to get health and medical information and simple treatments (Kim, 2015). Even when using healthcare services, they tend to select health services by following their friends' personal advice rather than carefully reviewing official information (Kim, 2015). Not surprisingly, those migrant workers with a high level of language proficiency and medical literacy tend to call 119 (911 in the U.S), while those with a low level of these abilities usually call their friends in emergency situations (Lee & Lee, 2013).

Migrant workers' work conditions and environments are other barriers that reduce their accessibility to healthcare services. Specifically, Kim (2015) has pointed out the problem with lack of time, facilities, and transportation. First, under the traditional organizational culture in Korea, it is not easy for employees to visit a doctor's office during work hours or weekdays regardless of possession of health insurance (Lim & Kim, 2014). Several studies (e.g., Kim, 2015; Lee, Bae, & Kim, 2016) reported that migrant workers are not allowed or do not have time available to visit a doctor's office during work hours. Therefore, they often use free healthcare services that are offered by non-profit organizations, including local churches and temples, during weekends. Coupled with the lack of approval from employers, another problem is for few healthcare facilities in rural areas where many migrant workers live and work. To make matters worse, the public transportation system in rural areas is not convenient enough to allow these workers to easily access many health care facilities. In order to visit necessary healthcare services, migrant workers in rural areas may have to use a taxi service, which is expensive, hence, becomes a financial barrier (Kim, 2015).

Different belief systems and perceptions about healthcare services are also serious barriers that impede migrant workers to receive adequate healthcare services in a foreign country. According to Kim (2015), most migrant workers' decisions about choosing healthcare services are not based on the results of medical examinations or a doctor's advice, but are based upon their own belief systems and self-perceptions. Some migrant workers from non-western countries do not trust biology-based western medical treatments. As a result, they often miss appropriate or timely treatments and visit doctors when these workers' ailments have reached an advanced degree of seriousness. Related to their different belief systems and perceptions of health, migrant workers often trust oriental medicine services more than Western medicine (Kim, 2015). It is not unusual for migrant workers from non-western countries to decline to take prescribed medicines due to limited trust in western medicine and medical treatments. Some migrant workers even visit shamans instead of doctors for their pain. Middle-aged female *Joseon-Jok* migrant workers often used moxa cautery (a form of heat therapy where dried plants are burned close to the skin) to reduce muscle pain which is unproven for its effectiveness (Lee, 2014).

Organizations Supporting Joseon-Jok Workers and Their Services

Although the Korean government offers several healthcare services for migrant workers, the services are not widely or effectively used because of many of the reasons described above. Instead, various non-profit organizations, particularly faith-based organizations, and several private health organizations have played key roles in supporting migrant workers' health (Atteraya et al., 2015; Choi, 2011; Kim, 2016; Lee, 2011; Lim & Kim, 2014; Noh & Ko, 2013; Park, 2011; Park, 2014). Broadly speaking, there are two types of healthcare services for migrant workers in Korea: (1) free healthcare service centers run by various non-profit organizations and (2) healthcare services for members of mutual aid associations for migrant workers (Kim, 2015). Approximately, there are more than 50 healthcare centers that migrant workers can use for free throughout the country (Park, 2004). The majority of volunteers at such healthcare service centers are members of faith-based organizations, members of clubs in colleges, public health practitioners, medical doctors, and students from medical or nursing schools (Park, 2004). Most of these free healthcare service centers are open every Sunday at various local public places, such as churches, temples, schools, civic/community centers, and public health centers (Park, 2004). Due to financial limitations, these free-of-charge healthcare centers only offer basic medical examinations, but some provide advanced treatments in consultation with their hospital networks (Park, 2004).

Recently, migrant workers have started to organize mutual aid associations to provide healthcare services for their members. Two well-known mutual aid associations are the Health Insurance Union for Migrant Workers and *Hee-Nyeon* (희년), a health insurance union

(Park, 2004). The Health Insurance Union for Migrant Workers was established for the purpose of helping undocumented migrant workers who are not eligible to buy national health insurance (Choi, 2011). Its services include (1) basic medical examination services at Sunday health centers, (2) local/community mobile clinic services, and (3) financial support for migrant workers' major surgical operations and treatments at the general hospitals (Choi, 2011).

A number of studies (e.g., Atteraya et al., 2015; Kim, 2009, 2015; Lim & Kim, 2014) have explained why migrant workers tend to use the healthcare services offered by non-profit organizations rather than using government-supported healthcare services with employment-based or public health insurance. First, a major benefit of the healthcare service centers for migrant workers is that they provide multiple services at the same place. Therefore, patients do not need to travel to different hospitals to have different healthcare services and medical treatments. Knowing the migrant workers' limited mobility due to time constraints, financial hardships, and limited Korean language proficiency, most healthcare service centers for migrant workers offer diverse health services, including dental services and even oriental medicines and treatments (Lim & Kim, 2014). Another benefit of these healthcare service centers is that migrant workers can easily access interpretation/translation services (Lim & Kim, 2014). Most health care practitioners and even patients in general hospitals in Korea are native Korean speakers. Therefore, it is very difficult for foreign language speakers to find translators to communicate with doctors and other health practitioners. Meanwhile, at healthcare service centers run by non-profit organizations to help migrant workers, there are often people available from the same countries to enhance communication (Lim & Kim, 2014).

Most migrant workers feel safer and much more comfortable when they meet other migrant workers of the same nationality at a healthcare service center for migrant workers (Lim & Kim, 2014). At the healthcare centers, they can receive strong psychological support, share their challenges with others in their languages, and learn how other migrant workers deal with the same or similar challenges (Atteraya et al., 2015; Lee, Lee, Kim, & Kim, 2009). Furthermore, migrant workers believe that the volunteers at the healthcare service centers run by non-profit organizations are friendlier and more genuinely interested in helping them than the healthcare practitioners at the general hospitals (Lim & Kim, 2014).

Faith-based organizations, such as churches and temples, play multiple roles for migrant workers, offering diverse services such as emergency shelters, counseling/consulting services on legal or human rights issues, Korean language and culture classes, and basic healthcare services. More importantly, migrant workers receive not only these practical services but also spiritual and social support from religious leaders and other members of religious organizations (Kim, 2009). According to Kim (2015), most migrant workers reported that they did not have a reliable source of information for help except a few close friends and, therefore, sought services from faith-based organizations when they needed help. Similarly, Atteraya et al. (2015) has found that most undocumented migrant workers in Korea visited faith-based organizations when they cannot get help from their own networks.

Communication Strategies for Promoting Joseon-Jok Workers' Health and Well-Being: Diffusion of Information and Influence

As the number of foreign migrant workers increases, the Korean government and civil society provide several public health services for migrant workers. However, information about public health services does not seem to be effectively delivered to the migrant workers. There is a strong need to effectively diffuse important health information to *Joseon-Jok* migrant workers. Related to this task, the theory of diffusion of innovations (DOI) has been applied to numerous health communication projects internationally (Haider & Kreps, 2004). An innovation in DOI can be understood as an object, idea, practice, program, policy, or anything that is perceived as new by a unit of adoption, such as an individual, organization, community, or even bigger social unit (Rogers, 2003). Diffusion projects for promoting public health typically aim to design communication strategies that disseminate health innovations (e.g., health information, practices, policies, and other health-related innovation) through certain channels over time among the members of a target population (Kim & Dearing, 2014; Kreps & Neuhauser, 2015). Rogers (2003) viewed that the ultimate purposes of diffusion projects were to reach critical mass (about 85% adoption of innovation) and implement and routinize an innovation until it becomes part of adopters' daily lives. Moreover, a consequence of the diffusion of innovations can be not only the adoption of an innovation by an individual, but also social change once a majority of the population adopts the innovation.

From the DOI perspective, a diffusion process can be activated and accelerated through two means of communication: mass communication (including new media) and interpersonal communication (Dearing & Kim, 2008). Mass communication includes public speech situations and technology-mediated communication that refers to information delivery through traditional media (e.g., television, radio, and print-newspapers) and the Internet-based media (e.g., online news sites, blogs, and social media). Interpersonal communication indicates direct communication between two people or in a small group setting where communicators are exposed to one another. Generally speaking, the use of mass communication channels is a good choice for fast and wide information diffusion, while interpersonal communication channels are most effective in promoting behavior change (Kim, Kee, & Dearing, 2020; Kreps, 2012). In other words, the use of mass media would not be sufficient alone for making a deterministic impact on behavior change, and diffusion projects using interpersonal communication alone would be slower in delivering information and influence than using mass media.

When DOI is employed for a real-world project, formative research is recommended to gather information about the target population's communication attributes and social culture that affect their behavioral decision because different groups may have different decision-making mechanism (Kreps, 2012; Rogers, 2003). DOI identifies three factors that affect the adoption of an innovation: an individual's independent consideration (optional innovation-decision), a collective decision (collective innovation-decision), and an authoritative power (authority innovation-decision). In a democratic society, these three factors are not mutually exclusive, but interplay for a unit of adoption to determine whether they adopt an innovation or not. Based on these theoretical knowledge and applicable principles of the diffusion of innovations, what would be effective communication strategies that spread accurate and helpful information to *Joseon-Jok* workers and promote their health in Korea?

First, in terms of the need for information, it is important to disseminate information about the accessibility to over-the-counter medicines and their evidence-based effectiveness to Joseon-Jok workers. Although *Joseon-Jok* are Korean-speaking people, they have strong accents that mainstream Koreans can easily notice. Therefore, because of people's gaze and existing stigmas on *Joseon-Jok*, they are reluctant to actively seek or visit medical services they need. This is one of the reasons why many *Joseon-Jok* bring their medicines, mostly scientifically unproven folk/traditional medicines, from their hometown in China (Lee, 2014). In fact, Korea has a very convenient pharmaceutical system and produces globally competitive pharmaceutical products. Pharmacies can be easily found everywhere, and almost all convenience stores sell a variety of over-the-counter medicines. Therefore, if *Joseon-Jok* are aware of the easy accessibility to the over-the-counter medicines and their scientifically proven effectiveness, they will have less concern about finding right medicine in Korea and do not have to bring unproven medicines from China at their entry to Korea and even while they stay in Korea.

Second, it is strongly recommended to design an opinion leader-based communication strategy to diffuse health information and guide *Joseon-Jok* to make evidence-based behavioral decisions for their health treatments. Although Korea is their ancestors' homeland, Korea is alien to *Joseon-Jok* since they were born outside of Korea and were educated in China. In addition, because of their insufficient levels of health literacy, migrant workers often have difficulties understanding the local health care landscape and accessing needed care (Kreps & Sparks, 2008). *Joseon-Jok* tend to share information among themselves without appropriate advice from health care professionals due to constraints associated with people's gaze, stigma, and miscommunication (Kim, 2015; Noh & Ko, 2013; Park, 2004). Theoretically, because of such limitations in communication and interaction in a foreign country, immigrants' communication networks are often limited to small personal interlocking networks – networks that consist of a limited set of similar individuals (often co-workers) who interact with one another within a group (Kim, Kreps, & Shin, 2015; Lee, 2014; Rogers, 2003). An opinion leader-based diffusion strategy is particularly advantageous for this type of communication network organized with internal group members (Kelley, Hannans, Kreps, & Johnson, 2012; Kim & Dearing, 2014).

Opinion leaders in DOI are not necessarily individuals who hold high positions or status at workplaces or communities, but are most likely those who are more accessible from others, have technical competence, and show conformity to norms of their social system (Rogers, 2003). Coupled with these characteristics, opinion leaders from the diffusion perspective are a small group of people who are at the center of interpersonal communication networks and tend to be informal opinion leaders rather than formal leaders (Kim & Dearing, 2014, 2016). According to Kim and Dearing's (2015) study on the diffusion of information regarding health service for international migrant workers in South Korea, an opinion leader-based diffusion strategy can be effectively used to design health promotion projects targeting migrant workers because of peer effect, persuasiveness in interpersonal communication, observability of decision making, and easy accessibility to ask questions and seek answers. Opinion leaders who have similar backgrounds and experiences with migrant workers can serve as behavioral and social models, showing how to seek guidance for making appropriate health decisions.

Third, simultaneously with the use of opinion leader-based health communication strategy, a mobile health information service can be very effective, since almost all adult migrant workers use smartphones (Kim, Singhal, & Kreps, 2014). Technologically, Korea has one of the most effective Internet and social network service infrastructures in the world and also has a very advanced ability to design mobile apps. The general public also use many mobile apps for their works and personal purposes in their daily lives (Ramirez, 2017). This well-established mobile communication infrastructure can greatly help the Korean government provide *Joseon-Jok* with information and communication services. For example, if the Korean government develops an app to deliver information about available health services and other necessary health information, Korean-speaking foreign workers can instantly seek health (service) information that they need to make the best possible decisions and address their health needs, especially at dire health situations. In fact, it is important for the government to centralize its communication channels for disseminating scientific health information, especially when unscientific misinformation is prevalent (Kim & Kreps, 2020). This type of mobile health information service can be an effective tool to disseminate information about health services and knowledge to *Joseon-Jok* workers and also contribute to public health in general as *Joseon-Jok*, in most cases, work together with native Korean workers.

Conclusion

Joseon-Jok workers are apparently the largest group of foreign migrant workers in Korea. The number of *Joseon-Jok* in Korea is expected to continuously increase as international migration has constantly increased over time. As the number of migrant workers has increased significantly, and all countries are densely weaved under the influence of globalization, host countries should prepare for proactive plans to take care of foreign workers' health and well-being. For *Joseon-Jok*, since they can be considered as historically marginalized ethnic Koreans who have experienced continuous diaspora between China and Korea, the Korean government should provide them with well-organized health services to promote their well-being in Korea. Recommended communication strategies in this chapter for Joseon-Jok workers can produce great economic, social, and multicultural outcomes, contributing to the diversification of social capital in Korea and also helping promote peace in the Asia/Pacific region in the age of globalization.

Recommended Readings

Jang, S., & Oh, J. (2020). *Health disparities in contemporary Korean society: Issues and subpopulations.* Lexington Books.

Lee, K. H. (2018). *Between foreign and family: Return migration and identity construction among Korean Americans and Korean Chinese.* Rutgers University Press.

Shin, H. (2021). The precarity and strategic navigation of Chosonjok migrant in South Korea. *European Journal of Korean Studies, 20*(2), 7–35.

References

Atteraya, M. S., Jung, J., Lee, D., Jun, H., & Gnawali, S. (2015). Social adjustment for undocumented migrant workers in South Korea: Role of religious institutions. *Journal of International Studies, 23*(4), 53–80.

Choi, J. (2011). Research on the condition of free medical treatment and secondary treatment for foreign workers: Focused on the Ansan city. *Journal of Multi-Cultural Contents Studies, 10*, 301–339.

Choi, J. & Kim, S. (2011). Use of dental institutions among foreigners in Korea. *Journal of the Korea Contents Association, 11*(11), 253–263.

Dearing, J. W., & Kim, D. D. (2008). Diffusion of information and innovations. *International Encyclopedia of Communication.* Blackwell Publishing.

Haider, M., & Kreps, G. L. (2004). Forty years of diffusion of innovations: Utility and value in public health. *Journal of Health Communication, 9*(Supplement 1), 3–11.

Jeong, S., Lee, C., & Kim, J. (2019). Ambiguous boundary, transference sacrifice – Health behavior and socio-cultural dynamics of Nepalese migrant workers in Jeju. *Journal of Local History and Culture, 22*(2), 387–447.

Kang, J., Jeong, M., & Jung, M. (May 8, 2019). Nobody seems to care for Korea's caregivers, *Korea JoonAng Daily.* https://koreajoongangdaily. joins.com/2019/05/08/socialAffairs/Nobody-seems-to-care-for-Koreas-caregivers/3062802.html

Kelley, R., Hannans, A., Kreps, G. L., & Johnson, K. (2012). The Community Liaison Program: A health education pilot program to increase minority awareness of HIV and acceptance of HIV vaccine trials. *Health Education Research, 27*(4), 746–754, doi10.1093/her/cys013.

Kim, H. (2016). The impact of Korea's immigration policy on Korean-Chinese community. In *Proceedings of Research Group for Global Korean Business & Culture*, Gwangju: Chonnam National University.

Kim, J. (2019). 'Ethnic capital' and 'flexible citizenship' in unfavourable legal contexts: Stepwise migration of the Korean Chinese within and beyond northeast Asia. *Journal of Ethnic & Migration Studies, 45*(6), 939–957.

Kim, M. (2014). Health conditions of migrant workers. *Monthly Social Welfare, 190*, 15–22.

Kim, S. (2009). The effect common health disorders of foreign workers: Focused on Daegu and Kyungpook region. *Journal of the Korea Contents Association, 9*(9), 268–277.

Kim, S. (2015). The conception and factors that affect the utilization of health care services among foreign migrant workers in Korea. *Journal of Multi-Cultural Contents Studies, 18*, 255–297.

Kim, D. D., & Dearing, J. W. (2014). Communication network analysis for the diffusion of health: Identifying key individuals. In D. D. Kim, A. Singhal, & G. L. Kreps. *Health communication: Strategies for developing global health programs.* Peter Lang Publishing Group.

Kim, D. D., & Dearing, J. W. (2015). The use of informal opinion leaders-based strategy for the diffusion of public health services among international workers in South Korea. *Health Communication Research, 12*, 115–148.

Kim. D. D., & Dearing, J. W. (2016). Opinion leader identification. In D. D. Kim, & J. W. Dearing. *Health communication research measures.* Peter Lang Publishing Group.

Kim, D. D., Singhal, A., & Kreps, G. (2014). *Health communication: Strategies for developing global health programs.* New York, NY: Peter Lang Publishing.

Kim, D. D., Kee, K. K., & Dearing, J. W. (2020). Applying the communication theory of diffusion of innovations to economic sciences: A response to the '*Using gossips to spread information*' experiments conducted by the 2019 Nobel Laureates. *Journal of Applied Communication Research, 48*(2), 157–165.

Kim, D. D., & Kreps, G. L. (2020). An analysis of government communication in the United States during the COVID-19 pandemic: Recommendations for effective government health risk communication. *World Medical & Health Policy, 12,* 398–412.

Kim, W., Kreps, G. L., & Shin, C.-N. (2015). The role of social support and social networks in health information-seeking behavior among Korean Americans: A qualitative study. *International Journal of Equity in Health, 14*(40). DOI 10.1186/s12939-015-0169-8.

Kreps, G. L. (2012). Strategic communication for cancer prevention and control: Reaching and influencing vulnerable audiences. In A. Georgakilas (Ed). *Cancer prevention* (pp. 375–388). Vienna: Intech Publishers.

Kreps, G. L., & Neuhauser, L. (2015). Designing health information programs to promote the health and well-being of vulnerable populations: The benefits of evidence-based strategic health communication. In C. A. Smith & A. Keselman (Eds.), *Meeting health information needs outside of healthcare: Opportunities and challenges* (pp. 3–17). Waltham, MA: Chandos Publishing.

Kreps, G. L., & Sparks, L. (2008). Meeting the health literacy needs of vulnerable populations. *Patient Education and Counseling, 71*(3), 328–332.

Lee, H. (2014). Study on middle-aged joseonjok (Korean-Chinese) women migrants illness experience. *Korean Association of Women's Studies, 30*(1), 213–252.

Lee, J. (2011). The cultural politics of communication and the difference in the Korean-Chinese society: Structure and exchanges in the Korean-Chinese community in Korea. *Journal of Democracy and Human Rights, 11*(3), 213–247.

Lee, J., Bae, S., & Kim, H. (2016). Subjective oral health status and unmet dental needs of migrant workers. *Journal of the Korea Entertainment Industry Association, 10*(2), 209–218.

Lee, J., & Lee, E. (2013). Factors influencing level of health literacy of migrant workers in Korea. *Journal of the Korean Academy of Fundamentals of Nursing, 20*(3), 269–277.

Lee, S., Lee, Y., Kim, S., & Kim, S. (2009). Social support and acculturative stress in migrant workers. *Journal of Korean Academy of Nursing, 39*(6), 899–910.

Lee, J., Kim, H., & Yang, Y. (2011). Investigation on the social status of Korean Chinese migrant labors in the Korean multi-cultural era. In *Proceedings of Research Group for Global Korean Business & Culture*, 389–405, Gwangju: Chonnam National University.

Lim, S., & Kim, K. (2014). Ethnographic research on Gwangju migrant workers clinic center. *Journal of Diaspora Studies, 8*(2), 257–282.

Lim, T., & Seol, D. (2018). Explaining South Korea's diaspora engagement policies. *Development and Society, 47*(4), 633–662.

Mucci, N., Traversini, V., Giorgi, G., Tommasi, E., De Sio, S., & Arcangeli, G. (2020). Migrant workers and psychological health: A systemic review. *Sustainability, 12.* file:///C:/Users/C00251946/Downloads/sustainability-12-00120-v2%20(5).pdf

Noh, H. (2015). A study on the problems of reciprocity in the treatments for foreigners under the Korean social security system. *Social Security Law Review, 4*(1), 55–97.

Noh, J., & Ko, J. (2013). Problems and improvements on social insurance act for foreign workers. *Han Yang Law Association, 43,* 121–158.

Norredam, M., & Agyemang, C. (2019). Tackling the health challenges of international migrant workers. *The Lancet Global Health, 7*(7), e813–e814. https://doi.org/10.1016/S2214-109X(19)30224-4

Ornek, O. K., Weinmann, T., Waibel, J., & Radon, K. (2020). Precarious employment and migrant workers' mental health: A protocol for a systematic review of observational studies. *Systematic Review, 9*(1), 50–56.

Park, H. (2004). Overview of the status of free healthcare services for migrant workers. *Research Institute for Healthcare Policy Korean Medical Association, 2*(1), 102–105.

Park, J. (2016, June 17). Tears of Korean Chinese caregivers. *The Kyunghyang Shinmun (Kyunghyang Daily)*. http://news.khan.co.kr/kh_news/khan_art_view.html?art_id=201606172122005

Park, K. (2014). Transnational migrant workers and the politics of culture: Conceptual discussion. *Contemporary Society and Multi-Culture, 4*(2), 90–121.

Park, Y. (2011). A study on the transition of Korean-Chinese organization and struggle for recognition in Korea. *Economy and Society*, 241–268.

Piao, Y. (2017). Hierarchical citizenship in perspective: South Korea's Korean Chinese. *Development and Society, 46*(3), 557–589.

Pocock, N. S., Nguyen, L. H., Lucero-Prisno Iii, D. E., Zimmerman, C., & Oram, S. (2018). Occupational, physical, sexual and mental health and violence among migrant and trafficked commercial fishers and seafarers from the Greater Mekong Subregion (GMS): Systematic review. *Global Health Research and Policy, 3*, 28. https://doi.org/10.1186/s41256-018-0083-x

Ramirez, E. (January 31, 2017). Nearly 100% of households in South Korea now have Internet Access, thanks to seniors. *Forbes*. https://www.forbes.com/sites/elaineramirez/2017/01/31/nearly-100-of-households-in-south-korea-now-have-internet-access-thanks-to-seniors/?sh=7f6e530a5572

Rogers, E. M. (2003). *Diffusion of innovations* (5th ed). New York, NY: Free Press.

Seo, J. (2014). The return of Korean-Chinese and Korean society issue to be solved: Beyond Chaoxian minority of China and Chinese brethren of Korea. *Journal of Diaspora Studies, 8*(1), 71–94.

Seol, D.-H., & Skrentny, J. D. (2009). Ethnic return migration and hierarchical nationhood: Korean Chinese foreign workers in South Korea. *Ethnicities, 9*(2), 147–174.

Shin, K. (2019). *Near yet far: Co-existing with ethnic Korean neighbors*. Seoul: The Seoul Institute.

Shin, S., & Chae, H. (2021, January 26). One caregiver cares for 8 patients around the clock… "I don't have enough time even to change their diapers". *JoongAng Ilbo*. https://news.joins.com/article/23979225

Yoon, H. & Kim, H. (2011). Legal status and economic status of the labor migrants of Korean Chinese in Korea. *Journal of Diaspora Studies, 5*(1). 37–60.

10 Immigration, Social Support, and Well-Being

A Case Study of Immigrants in Hong Kong

Leanne Chang

Migration involves losing some parts of connections with home countries and rebuilding social relationships in the host society. Social support presents the social resources critical to immigrants' adaptation to a new environment that impacts their health (Kuo & Tsai, 1986). Social support includes tangible and intangible resources derived from a person's social relationships that are meant to be helpful. It is communicated through verbal and nonverbal cues that help reduce uncertainty and enhance personal control over problematic situations (Goldsmith & Albrecht, 2011). Much literature suggests that social support has buffering and direct impacts on health (Uchino et al., 2018). The buffering model holds that social support mitigates the adverse effects of stress on health by reducing stress strength. Alternatively, the main effect model holds that social support can enhance psychological states (e.g., sense of connection, recognition of self-worth, and awareness of health norms) and directly affect health, regardless of the stress level. Immigrants, particularly new arrivals, are likely to encounter a lack of social support in the host society. Extant studies have suggested three approaches – structural, functional, and perceptual – to examine the role of social support in immigrants' health.

Structural Approach

The structural approach to social support focuses on the physical attributes of support systems. This approach links social support to the scope of social networks and the level of social integration. Network size, composition, frequency of contact, and the strength of social ties are measures reflecting the quantity of an immigrant's support networks. Alternatively, the diversity of social relationships and the range of social activities an immigrant can engage in reflect the degree of social integration in a support network (Goldsmith & Albrecht, 2011).

From a structural perspective, immigrant deficiency in social support is apparent. Immigrants commonly leave their established social relationships in their homelands. For immigrants who migrate alone, strong-tie support networks composed of family members and close

DOI: 10.4324/9781003230243-10

friends are absent in their physical world. Immigrants are likely to join ethnic support networks consisting of other immigrants from the same culture to build new support networks. Attachment to ethnic support networks may protect immigrants from discrimination and secure a sense of belonging. However, it can also discourage immigrants from expanding support networks with locals in the host society and result in reinforced perceptions of their unwillingness to fit in and more discrimination against them (Jasinskaja-Lahti et al., 2006).

Functional Approach

The functional approach focuses on different supportive functions that a person's social relationships can serve. The literature has identified four major types of supportive functions (Goldsmith & Albrecht, 2011). Physical or instrumental support encompasses material assistance. This type of support communicates how a person is being taken care of by providing tangible assistance, such as goods, services, and financial assistance. Informational support provides information related to a person's decision-making that is intended to be helpful. Examples of informational support include advice, guidance, and suggestions. Emotional support involves the expression of sympathy, affection, and acceptance, which generates a feeling of being cared for and loved. Esteem support refers to the availability of information for adding new perspectives on self-evaluation. This support is considered a specific form of emotional support (Cohen et al., 2000).

Immigrant studies indicated that different supportive functions may be emphasized in different resettlement phases (Stewart et al., 2008). New arrivals need help to find food, housing, services, and other necessities during the initial stage of migration. Thus, instrumental and informational support becomes critical. Emotional and esteem support needs may arise only after the initial survival needs are satisfied (Wong & Song, 2006). Alternatively, different sources may differ in their capacities to fulfill immigrants' support needs. Formal sources, such as the government, community-based agencies, and service providers, are best at providing instrumental support, such as medical aid, employment, and subsidies. In contrast, informal sources, such as family and friends, are best at offering emotional and esteem support (Stewart et al., 2008). The interplay of support sources and functions on immigrant health has been the focus of support research from a functional perspective.

Perceptual Approach

The perceptual approach to social support further differentiates the cognitive and behavioral aspects of supportive functions. This approach separates perceived and received support from the recipients' perspective

(Cohen et al., 2000). Perceived support refers to a person's perception of the availability of support resources, while received support refers to the actual receipt of support resources. Empirical evidence suggests that received support may buffer the negative impacts of stress on health by enhancing a person's coping performance. Contrarily, perceived support may improve a person's psychological well-being by changing perceptions of an event's stress based on the belief that support will be available (Uchino, 2009).

Results from meta-analyses and critical reviews indicated that perceived support is a more consistent predictor of physiological and psychological health than received support (Haber et al., 2007; Uchino, 2009). Some explanations include that perceived support is more stable and predictable, while received support is more contextual and could be experienced as unhelpful, condescending, and burdensome. Researchers have suggested that both aspects of support should be examined to compare differences in their impacts on health (Uchino, 2009). With these theoretical concepts in mind, the following sections review social support among two immigrant groups in Hong Kong.

Immigrants in Hong Kong

On July 1st, 1997, Hong Kong became a Special Administrative Region of the People's Republic of China, ending its status as a colony of the British Empire since 1842. Hong Kong is considered an immigrant society as 40% of the 7.5 million population was not born locally (Census and Statistics Department, 2017). More than 90% of the population is ethnic Chinese. The major ethnic minority groups include Filipino (2.5%), Indonesian (2.1%), White (0.8%), Indian (0.5%), Nepalese (0.3%), other Asian (0.8%), and others (0.9%). English and Chinese are the official languages. However, Hong Kong uses traditional Chinese in writing and Cantonese – a Chinese dialect – in speaking, which differs from the simplified Chinese and Mandarin used on the mainland. Immigrants in Hong Kong can generally be divided into three groups: foreign professionals, immigrants from mainland China, and migrant workers from low-income countries. As mainland immigrants and migrant workers are likely to be in the lower strata of society and vulnerable to discrimination, they are the focus of this chapter.

New Immigrants from the Mainland

Mainland immigrants are a major source of population growth in Hong Kong. In the past century, Hong Kong experienced few waves of immigrant influx from mainland China. The first wave occurred between the 1930s and the 1940s, during which China underwent the Anti-Japanese War and the Civil War. Between 1945 and 1946, the Hong

Kong population increased from approximately 500,000 to 600,000 to 1,168,000. The government initially opened the border for free entry but closed it in 1950, although the policy change could not stop the huge influx of refugees. The second wave of immigration occurred between the early 1960s and the late 1970s. Many mainland immigrants fled to Hong Kong to escape from the Great Chinese Famine between 1959 and 1961 and the Cultural Revolution between 1966 and 1976. Simultaneously, Hong Kong experienced rapid labor-intensive industrialization. Thus, the *touch-base* policy was implemented to allow those who successfully reached the urban areas to stay but repatriate those arrested at the border. This policy was a practical strategy for importing low-skilled workers (Law & Lee, 2006). The third phase of cross-border immigration began in the early 1980s and lasted until the present. In this wave, most mainland immigrants entered Hong Kong under the One Way Permit (OWP) scheme that allows mainland residents to enter Hong Kong for family reunions. Eligible OWP applicants include children of Hong Kong permanent residents holding certificates of entitlement, spouses, and other dependents. The OWP scheme imposes a daily quota system, which changed from 75 places in 1982, 105 in 1993, and 150 from 1995 until the present. Since 1997, over 570,000 mainland immigrants have entered Hong Kong through the OWP. Between 2015 and 2018, the new arrivals of OWP holders were equivalent to approximately 90% of the population growth. Between 2019 and 2020, when Hong Kong experienced population decline amid the devastation of social unrest, the number of new OWP holders was 49,200, compared to the net emigration of others of 59,000 (Census and Statistics Department, 2021a).

Other than the OWP scheme, mainland Chinese may legally enter Hong Kong as skilled workers, professionals, and graduates under the Admission Scheme for Mainland Talents and Professionals, Quality Migrant Admission Scheme, and Immigration Arrangement for Non-Local Graduates Scheme. Nevertheless, the proportion of these professionals is smaller than that of OWP holders.

Compared to international migrants to Hong Kong, Chinese immigrants should have minimal difficulties in acculturation, given their similarities in race and culture. However, mainland immigrants, particularly OWP holders, commonly experience settlement challenges due to economic disadvantages and social exclusion. From an economic perspective, new immigrants are likely to be disadvantaged in the labor market because of their lower educational attainment, limited language ability, and place of origin. For instance, fewer OWP holders have a post-secondary degree than local natives, which limits their occupation choices. Approximately 40% of the new arrivals cannot speak Cantonese. Most of the other 60% fluent in Cantonese came from Guangdong Province, where Cantonese is widely spoken (Home Affairs Department & Immigrant Department, 2021). However, their accent could mark their place of origin and result in discrimination and reduced job opportunities (Law & Lee, 2006). Moreover, the majority of OWP holders do not speak English, which is the language used in education systems and skilled jobs in Hong Kong. The initial conditions of new arrivals are likely to trap them in low-skilled jobs or unemployment. The disparity between new immigrants and natives is reflected in income attainment. In 2020, the median monthly family income of new arrivals was HK$12,700 (~US$1,600), which was much lower than the entire population's HK$26,500 (US$3,400) (Home Affairs Department & Immigrant Department, 2021). Although evidence suggests that new immigrants' economic disadvantages tend to improve over time, income inequality may never be overcome due to limitations on educational qualifications, social capital, and required skills (Zhang & Wu, 2011).

From a communal perspective, new immigrants are likely to be excluded from Hong Kong society and be treated as unwanted members. Social exclusion can be viewed from two opposing perspectives. Locals feel the historical differences between themselves and the mainlanders. The political systems and cultures they experienced differ distinctively. Over the years, Hong Kong people have developed a *Hongkonger* identity affiliated with the city. This social identity is intertwined with the experience of living in a highly competitive society with significant socioeconomic inequality and the perception of being forced to be integrated with China and sharing resources and opportunities with mainlanders (Leung, 2020). New immigrants could be perceived as threats to the already scarce resources of employment, housing, education, and health services and are easy targets to blame for economic problems.

Furthermore, new immigrants are perceived to have different ideological beliefs and living habits. Incidents of controversies such as public defecation, parallel trading, and birth tourism escalate tensions between Hongkongers and mainlanders. Recent events like the 2019 Anti-Extradition Bill Movement further widened rifts in society and prompted local antagonism toward mainlanders (Leung, 2020). These sociopolitical backgrounds contribute to the stereotypical perceptions of new immigrants. A survey conducted by the Hong Kong Council of Social Service (2003) showed that Hongkongers held mixed attitudes toward new immigrants. Although most locals reported their willingness to befriend new immigrants and agreed that new arrivals were motivated, diligent, and thrifty, they also acknowledged that new arrivals were greedy, selfish, and emotional. A recent survey indicated similar polarized attitudes toward new immigrants; 26% of Hongkongers accepted or rejected new immigrants, while the rest held neutral attitudes (Hong Kong Institute of Asia-Pacific Studies, 2016).

Alternatively, new immigrants feel that Hongkongers treat them with prejudice. Different survey studies indicated that new immigrants felt rejected because of their new arrival status (Hong Kong Council of Social Service, 2016; Ng et al., 2015). New immigrants reported experiencing disparaging comments, ignorance, and ridicule in public spaces and encountering insult and exclusion in the workplace and school. They also noted that discriminatory depictions of new immigrants as poor, uncivilized, and predatory prevail in local media and user-generated content platforms, cultivating stigmatization and deepening social division (Ng et al., 2015).

The negative association between perceived discrimination and new immigrants' well-being has received increased research attention. Studies found that perceived discrimination increases the depressive symptoms of new immigrants and reduces their self-esteem and beliefs in their capacity to change the status quo (Au & Zhu, 2020). Perceived discrimination also predicts lower life satisfaction and quality of life (Wong, 2008; Wong et al., 2012). Noting the negative influences of social exclusion, a growing body of literature has emerged concerning the role of social support in enhancing immigrants' well-being and resilience to discrimination.

Social Support for New Immigrants

Most new immigrants have families in Hong Kong. From a structural perspective, the existence of a strong-tie support network suggests the availability of social support to some extent (Chen, Li et al., 2019). However, new arrivals are likely to encounter difficulties in building weak-tie networks with locals because of language, sociopolitical, and economic barriers. Research indicates that new immigrants often receive discrimination from weak-tie relationships, such as employers, coworkers, classmates, and clients (Zhang & Wu, 2011). In recent years, tensions between Hongkongers and mainlanders have intensified, resulting in more distrust and biases toward each other rather than a community supportive of new immigrants' social integration. Various studies have indicated that most new immigrants feel isolated and lack a sense of belonging to the city. Those with smaller support networks and less frequent contact are likely to feel lonely and have lower life satisfaction (Au & Zhu, 2020; Chui, 2014).

From a functional perspective, research on immigrant youth indicates that peers are the most important support source that helps young immigrants withstand migration-related stress and buffer its adverse impacts on mental health (Wong, 2008). Surprisingly, family is not a significant source of social support. A possible explanation is that most immigrant youths are OWP holders from a family consisting of an older Hong Kong father in poor financial conditions and a much younger mainland mother. Marital conflicts associated with different cultural backgrounds and financial problems can grow into a source of distress rather than support for young immigrants (Chen, Xu et al., 2019). Accordingly, immigrant youths tend to seek peer support to deal with hardships in life. However, the importance of peer support also suggests that immigrant youths are likely to suffer an isolation crisis when fellow students and coworkers reject them.

In line with existing findings, research on adult Chinese immigrants indicates that the sources and types of social support change over time due to shifted support needs during the resettlement process (Wong & Song, 2006). In the initial phase of resettlement, adult immigrants need more physical aid, such as finances, food, and resettlement assistance, and informational aid, such as advice on housing, school placements, job opportunities, and facility utilization. Immediate family members in Hong Kong, including spouses and in-laws, and immigrant friends are primary sources of support in this phase. In later stages, emotional needs may arise after marital and other family conflicts begin to emerge. Evidence shows that adult immigrants prefer to seek emotional support from family and friends on the mainland via cross-border visits and mobile communication. Contrarily, they seldom seek help from coworkers and neighbors (Wong & Song, 2006). A pattern of relying on an ethnic support network is observed.

Finally, from a perceptual perspective, cross-sectional studies found that perceived support from family and friends has direct impacts on new immigrants' depressive symptoms and buffers the negative association between perceived discrimination and mental health (Wong et al., 2012). Perceived support is also positively associated with new immigrants' satisfaction with physical health, social relationships, and overall quality of life (Ng et al., 2015). These results are consistent with the extant understanding of the positive effect of perceived support on immigrant health (Kuo & Tsai, 1986). However, extant measures of perceived support seldom differentiate between strong-tie support networks in the homeland and host society. Additionally, there is a dearth of research comparing the capacity of received and perceived support in predicting immigrants' physiological and psychological health. More research can be conducted to compare their unique impacts on new immigrants' health.

In sum, new immigrants may have a thin support network in Hong Kong that offers instrumental and informational support and a stronger support network in their hometowns that offers emotional support. When building new social relationships in Hong Kong, new immigrants tend to connect with fellow immigrants. The in-group membership enhances their resilience to perceived discrimination and life satisfaction. However, as indicated in other immigration research, the ethnic homogeneity of support networks may also hinder their integration into Hong Kong society and risk mutual exclusion from local people (Jasinskaja-Lahti et al., 2006). Differing from other societies, mainland immigrants may reverse their marginalized position because of political reforms and policy changes that encourage more mainlanders to migrate to Hong Kong. How new immigrants adapt to a polarized society and mingle with locals to co-construct the Hong Kong identity will continue to be a significant challenge.

Migrant Workers in Hong Kong

Foreign domestic helpers (FDHs) are migrant workers who provide domestic services on a full-time basis. The government liberalized the employment of FDHs in 1974 in response to rapid economic growth and increased labor force participation of women. Probably because Hong Kong has other laborers (e.g., mainland immigrants) contributing to the industrial sectors, migrant workers in Hong Kong are predominantly FDHs. By 2020, FDHs constituted 5% of the population. They provided services to 327,700 households and accounted for approximately 10% of the overall workforce (Census and Statistics Department, 2021b).

Most FDHs are female workers hired from the Philippines (55.5%) and Indonesia (42.2%) to care for children and older adults. Their monthly wage ranges between HK$4,000 and HK$4,900 (about US$510–US$624). This amount is affordable for many Hong Kong families, considering that the median monthly household income for a domestic household of four is HK$42,000 (Census and Statistics Department, 2021c). Still, the wages are comparatively higher than the average wages in the Philippines and Indonesia and motivate many women to work as FDHs (Yap, 2015). In fact, many Filipina workers are college graduates but choose to work as FDHs because the wages are better than white-collar jobs back home. The trade-off for financial benefits, however, is the loss of social and ethnic status in a foreign land (Chiu & Asian Migrant Centre, 2005).

Research indicates that FDHs are discriminated against because of the combination of their occupation and race (Chiu & Asian Migrant Centre, 2005). FDHs' work contents and low wages reinforce negative stereotypes of them as second classes in society. Limited local language proficiency also marginalizes them into the cultural other in an ethnic Chinese-dominant society. While most Hongkongers speak Cantonese at home, most FDHs only have low to medium levels of Cantonese language proficiency, posing barriers to assimilation and job satisfaction (Liao & Gan, 2020). Moreover, FDHs' work permit requirements impede equal protection of their labor rights. FDHs are prohibited from getting permanent residency and family reunification as are other immigrants. The requirement of living in the employer's place also applies only to FDHs, but not to local domestic helpers. The round-the-clock presence and the expectation of service-on-demand create a work environment conducive to exploitation and abuse (Chiu & Asian Migrant Centre, 2005).

Exploitation

By law, FDHs are entitled to have daily food and traveling allowance of HK$100 per day, at least one rest day of no less than 24 hours in every period of seven days, statutory holidays, and free medical treatment. However, exploitation often occurs in ways that violate standard employment contracts. Time exploitation is most experienced by FDHs, which includes excessive working hours, interruptions during eating or rest, and shortened rest days. Specifically, having the rest days is critical to the well-being of FDHs. The off-days, which are commonly on Sundays, allow FDHs to relax and exchange support (Mok & Ho, 2020). A typical phenomenon observed on Sundays in Hong Kong is the gathering of many FDHs in open spaces, such as urban parks, pedestrian footbridges, and roadsides. Social space enables migrant workers to stay with peers, participate in recreational or religious activities, share home food, and talk to family back home. FDHs prefer to take their break outside the employer's house to escape from the expectation of on-demand services and satisfy their needs for privacy taken away by the mandatory live-in arrangement. However, research indicates that the days off are usually shortened by the need to attend to morning and evening duties, such as cooking breakfast, sending the children to extracurricular activities, cooking dinner, and finishing preparations for the next day. Long working hours and insufficient rest breaks have been identified as a significant source of workplace distress that adversely affects FDHs' health (Chiu & Asian Migrant Centre, 2005).

Other common forms of exploitation include economic exploitation (e.g., late payment or underpayment), food deprivation (e.g., not enough food, rotten food, or food violating religious requirements), and forced duties (e.g., working at the employer's shop as no-paid labor or for people outside the employer's household) (Amnesty International, 2014). Notably, although the government introduced a maximum commission of 10% of the first-month salary of an FDH, many agencies' commission, training, and placement fees could be up to HK$21,000. Excessive agency fees often put FDHs in debt and result in their endurance of exploitation because they cannot afford additional agency fees to change their employer (Chiu & Asian Migrant Centre, 2005).

Abuse

Abusive treatment of FDHs may be physical, psychological, or sexual (Ullah, 2015). Verbal abuse is the most common form of abuse, which includes shouting, threats of isolation and repatriation, and the use of degrading language. Some FDHs reported suffering physical abuse, such as being punched, kicked, slapped, and hit with objects. Disturbingly, incidences of sexual abuse have also been reported. Inappropriate sexual behaviors include talking to FDHs in sexual language, showing pornographic materials or nudity, touching and kissing, malicious watch, and requesting sex (Cheung et al., 2019; Chiu & Asian Migrant Centre, 2005).

Both employers and other family members could be perpetrators of workplace abuse. For instance, FDHs' instructions may be disobeyed by the children, for knowing the power difference between them. Small things like eating meals on time or refraining from watching TV could create emotional tension and result in verbal and physical abuse (Choy et al., 2020). FDHs who care for frail older adults, particularly those with dementia, are at risk of being physically and verbally abused because of the patients' functional and cognitive decline. The employer could also perpetrate abuse by taking FDHs as a convenient emotional outlet for their work- or life-related stress. Specifically, female employers are more likely to perpetrate verbal abuse, while male employers are more often the perpetrators of sexual abuse (Cheung et al., 2019). In incidences of sexual assaults, the FDHs often bear the blame even if the attempts were made by male family members (Ullah, 2015).

Each year, the Philippines and Indonesian consulates receive thousands of complaints from their citizens working as FDHs. However, it is estimated that abuse and exploitation cases remain largely underreported. Factors preventing help-seeking include a lack of legal knowledge, language insufficiency, isolation in the household, difficulties in collecting evidence, a low expectancy of positive responses to their complaints, fear of not being believed, fear of being punished, and fear of losing jobs (Cheung et al., 2019). Exploitation and abuse directly cause physical health problems, such as injuries, weakened immune systems, and dyspepsia (Ullah, 2015). They also evoke mental health problems, such as depression, delusions, loneliness, anxiety, psychiatric disorders, and suicide attempts (Malhotra et al., 2013). Social support is a means to cope with workplace distress. Unlike Chinese immigrants who move to reunify with family members, FDHs migrate alone. This suggests that their support challenges differ when dealing with hardships in Hong Kong society.

Social Support for FDHs

From a structural perspective, strong-tie support networks for FDHs are only available in virtual space. Benefiting from the reduced cost of data plans, nowadays FDHs can use mobile apps to communicate with family and friends back home and parent their children from a distance. Virtual interactions provide feelings of affection that contribute positively to

FDHs' well-being. However, research indicates that many FDHs avoid talking about work to families. Their concerns include not wanting family members to worry and not wanting to receive unhelpful advice, such as asking them to accept the hardships unconditionally (McKay, 2007). Accordingly, most social support from families is general affection rather than a perception of having someone to talk about work-related difficulties.

Peers, religion, and the employer constitute FDHs' new support networks in Hong Kong. Peers include fellow FDHs who come from the same country. From a functional perspective, peers are the primary sources of informational, emotional, and esteem support. When isolated, FDHs may normalize abuse and exploitation as part of work norms. The group counseling function of Sunday gatherings offers information about ways to deal with adverse work conditions and to locate health, welfare, and legal services. Emotional support from peers, such as companionship, empathy, and encouragement, is essential to alleviating work-related stress. Recreational activities, such as picnics, dancing, and singing, undertaken during Sunday gatherings directly impact the physical and mental health of FDHs. The presence of a community also promotes a sense of connection and self-worth beneficial to their psychological well-being (Mok & Ho, 2020).

Religion is another important source of social support. Most Filipina domestic workers are Catholic and most Indonesian workers are Muslim (Yap, 2015). Engaging in religious activities during Sunday gatherings is a way to expand support networks, strengthen social ties, and accumulate social capital. From a functional perspective, local religious groups can offer instrumental support, such as temporary shelters, physical assistance, and advocacy of FDH labor rights. They can also be sources of emotional support that offer comfort, courage, and a sense of empowerment (Cruz, 2006). Alternatively, personal religious practices, such as praying, enable the expression of ill feelings that cannot be shared with others. Qualitative research indicates that religious support reduces the negative impacts of stress by enhancing FDHs' sense of hope, resistance to oppression, and identity negotiation (Cruz, 2006). Religion's ability to change perceptions of problems and control over life also directly affects their well-being and life dissatisfaction (Yap, 2015). The buffering and main effects of religion on health can be further validated through quantitative testing.

As FDHs spend most of their time in the household, employers shape their work experiences and could be an important source of support. In the incidences of conflicts with family members, such as children or older adults, the employer's support is critical to alleviating caregiver burden and stress (Choy et al., 2020). Many FDHs caring for older adults with dementia suffer psychological and physical abuse. Emotional support from the employer is vital for them to endure hardships at work. Recognition and appreciation from employers also offer important esteem support that enhances FDHs' sense of self-worth and life satisfaction (Choy et al., 2020). Medical care and extra financial support are tangible aids welcomed by FDHs. Finally, employers could serve as a source of informational support that provides suggestions about health, daily living, and assimilation helpful for FDHs' adaptation to life in Hong Kong.

In sum, extant research on FDHs in Hong Kong focuses more on received support. FDHs received affection and motivation from strong ties in their home countries. In the host society, Sunday gatherings are the primary sites of support exchange. FDHs obtain informational, emotional, and esteem support from fellow FDHs. Public gatherings also present a home-like community that mitigates the feeling of alienation and enhances identity negotiation. Religious support is a less studied area that may involve functions of perceived support. Initial findings show that religiosity helps FDHs make sense of and cope with hardships. Finally, employers are double-sided swords who can be the source of distress or support that fulfills FDHs' needs for survival and recognition. Other than their employment agencies, many FDHs are unaware of the availability of support organizations (Choy et al., 2020). The promotion of community-based support services and education on labor rights against abuse and exploitation may help enhance FDHs' coping with migration challenges and quality of life.

Conclusion

Social support is pivotal for mainland immigrants and domestic workers in the adaptation process. Both communities prefer informal sources, such as peers and family, rather than formal sources, such as organizations and government bodies. Among the informal sources, each source may play a distinct role in fulfilling a specific support need. Race, access to strong-tie networks, and immigration status shape different settlement experiences between new immigrants and FDHs. New immigrants migrate to settle on a permanent basis. Despite the initial socioeconomic disadvantages, immigration policy does not impose limitations on their integration into society. In contrast, FDHs bond to the employment contract and their migration is deemed transitional. Accordingly, the two communities encounter different acculturation challenges and show different patterns of support exchange. For FDHs, social support helps them withstand hardships during the contract period. As immigration policy restricts their eligibility for the Right of Abode in Hong Kong, they are likely to form isolated communities supporting each other with minimal engagement with locals. New immigrants have greater opportunities to assimilate into Hong Kong society, but their social relationships with the locals could be a major acculturative stressor. In both communities, locals' acceptance is critical to their adaptation to the new environment. However, while supportive communication between FDHs and locals mostly happens in the private domain, which varies from one household to another, supportive communication between new immigrants and Hongkongers is embedded in macro-level tensions that remain unsolved in Hong Kong society. The research directions differ accordingly.

Recommended Readings

Chen, J., Li, Z., Xu, D., & Wu, X. (2019). Effects of neighborhood discrimination towards mainland immigrants on mental health in Hong Kong. *International Journal of Environmental Research and Public Health*, 16(6), 1025. https://doi.org/10.3390/ijerph16061025

Law, K. Y., & Lee, K. M. (2006). Citizenship, economy and social exclusion of mainland Chinese immigrants in Hong Kong. *Journal of Contemporary Asia*, 36(2), 217–242. https://doi.org/10.1080/00472330680000131

Liao, T. F., & Gan, R. Y. (2020). Filipino and Indonesian migrant domestic workers in Hong Kong: Their life courses in migration. *American Behavioral Scientist*, 64(6), 740–764. https://doi.org/10.1177/0002764220910229

Mok, K. H., & Ho, H. C. (2020). Finding a home away from home: An explorative study on the use of social space with the voices of foreign domestic workers in Hong Kong. *Annals of the American Association of Geographers*, 111(5), 1403–1419. https://doi.org/10.1080/24694452.2020.1813542

Yu, X., Stewart, S. M., Liu, I. K., & Lam, T. H. (2014). Resilience and depressive symptoms in mainland Chinese immigrants to Hong Kong. *Social Psychiatry and Psychiatric Epidemiology*, 49(2), 241–249. https://doi.org/10.1007/s00127-013-0733-8

References

Amnesty International. (2014). *Submission to the legislative council's panel on manpower – Policies relating to foreign domestic helpers and regulation of employment agencies.* https://www.legco.gov.hk/yr13-14/english/panels/mp/papers/mp0227cb2-870-3-e.pdf

Au, R. K., & Zhu, C. (2020). Unmet need for belonging and loneliness in determining life satisfaction of mainland Chinese new immigrants in Hong Kong. *Psychologia*, 62(3–4), 270–288. https://doi.org/10.2117/psysoc.2019-A118

Census and Statistics Department. (2017). *2016 population by-census technical report.* https://www.censtatd.gov.hk/en/data/stat_report/product/B1120099/att/B11200992016XXXXB0100.pdf

Census and Statistics Department. (2021a). *Table 2: Population growth by component.* https://www.censtatd.gov.hk/en/web_table.html?id=2#

Census and Statistics Department. (2021b). *Thematic household survey report No. 72.* https://www.censtatd.gov.hk/en/data/stat_report/product/C0000016/att/B11302722021XXXXB0100.pdf

Census and Statistics Department. (2021c). *Table E034: Median monthly domestic household income of economically active households by household size.* https://www.censtatd.gov.hk/en/EIndexbySubject.html?scode=500&pcode=D5250038

Chen, J., Li, Z., Xu, D., & Wu, X. (2019). Effects of neighborhood discrimination towards mainland immigrants on mental health in Hong Kong. *International Journal of Environmental Research and Public Health, 16*(6), 1025. https://doi.org/10.3390/ijerph16061025

Chen, J., Xu, D., & Wu, X. (2019). Seeking help for mental health problems in Hong Kong: The role of family. *Administration and Policy in Mental Health and Mental Health Services Research, 46*(2), 220–237. https://doi.org/10.1007/s10488-018-0906-6

Cheung, J. T. K., Tsoi, V. W. Y., Wong, K. H. K., & Chung, R. Y. (2019). Abuse and depression among Filipino foreign domestic helpers. A cross-sectional survey in Hong Kong. *Public Health, 166*, 121–127. https://doi.org/10.1016/j.puhe.2018.09.020

Chiu, S. W. K., & Asian Migrant Centre. (2005). *A stranger in the house: Foreign domestic helpers in Hong Kong.* http://www.hkiaps.cuhk.edu.hk/wd/ni/20181024-101559_1_hkiaps_op162_secure.pdf

Choy, C. Y., Chang, L., & Man, P. Y. (2020). *How does social support help foreign domestic helpers cope with abuse and exploitation in Hong Kong?* Paper presented at the annual conference of the International Communication Association, May 21–25, Gold Coast, Australia.

Chui, C. F. (2014). *Survey on life satisfaction of new arrivals 2014* (in Chinese). Windshield Charitable Foundation. http://www.windshieldcharitable.org/download/report(2014-1).pdf

Cohen, S., Gottlieb, B. H., & Underwood, L. G. (2000). Social relationships and health. In S. Cohen, B. H. Gottlieb, & L. G. Underwood (Eds.), *Social support measurement and intervention: A guide for health and social scientists* (pp. 3–25). Oxford University Press.

Cruz, G. T. (2006). Faith on the edge: Religion and women in the context of migration. *Feminist Theology, 15*(1), 9–25. https://doi.org/10.1177/0966735006068847

Goldsmith, D. J., & Albrecht, T. L. (2011). Social support, social networks, and health: A guiding framework. In T. L. Thompson, R. Parrott, & J. F. Nussbaum (Eds.), *The Routledge handbook of health communication* (pp. 335–348). Routledge.

Haber, M. G., Cohen, J. L., Lucas, T., & Baltes, B. B. (2007). The relationship between self-reported received and perceived social support: A meta-analytic review. *American Journal of Community Psychology, 39*(1), 133–144. https://doi.org/10.1007/s10464-007-9100-9

Home Affairs Department and Immigrant Department. (2021). *Statistics on new arrivals from the mainland (Fourth quarter of 2020).* https://www.had.gov.hk/file_manager/tc/documents/public_services/services_for_new_arrivals_from_the_mainland/2020%20Q4%20Report.pdf

Hong Kong Council of Social Service. (2003). *Research report of cross-cultural perception and acceptance between local residents and new arrivals* (in Chinese). http://webcontent.hkcss.org.hk/fs/er/Reference/NA03Full.pdf

Hong Kong Council of Social Service. (2016). *New immigrants discrimination survey 2016* (in Chinese). https://soco.org.hk/wp-content/uploads/2014/10/new-immigrants-discrimination-survey-2016_11.pdf

Hong Kong Institute of Asia-Pacific Studies. (2016). *Views on new immigrants from Mainland China* (in Chinese). https://www.cpr.cuhk.edu.hk/wp-content/upload/resources/press/pdf/582568e8b35c5.pdf

Jasinskaja-Lahti, I., Liebkind, K., Jaakkola, M., & Reuter, A. (2006). Perceived discrimination, social support networks, and psychological well-being among three immigrant groups. *Journal of Cross-Cultural Psychology*, *37*(3), 293–311. https://doi.org/10.1177/0022022106286925

Kuo, W. H., & Tsai, Y. M. (1986). Social networking, hardiness and immigrant's mental health. *Journal of Health and Social Behavior*, *27*(2), 133–149. https://doi.org/10.2307/2136312

Law, K. Y., & Lee, K. M. (2006). Citizenship, economy and social exclusion of mainland Chinese immigrants in Hong Kong. *Journal of Contemporary Asia*, *36*(2), 217–242. https://doi.org/10.1177/0002764220910229

Leung, T. Y. (2020). Mapping the matrix of nationalisms in Hong Kong: On the six generations of Hongkonger identities from the 1920s to 2020 and their generational conflicts. In L. Greenfeld & Z. Wu (Eds.), *Research handbook on nationalism* (pp. 290–311). Edward Elgar.

Liao, T. F., & Gan, R. Y. (2020). Filipino and Indonesian migrant domestic workers in Hong Kong: Their life courses in migration. *American Behavioral Scientist*, *64*(6), 740–764. https://doi.org/10.1177/0002764220910229

Malhotra, R., Arambepola, C., Tarun, S., de Silva, V., Kishore, J., & Østbye, T. (2013). Health issues of female foreign domestic workers: A systematic review of the scientific and gray literature. *International Journal of Occupational and Environmental Health*, *19*(4), 261–277. https://doi.org/10.1179/2049396713Y.0000000041

McKay, D. (2007). 'Sending dollars shows feeling' – Emotions and economies in Filipino migration. *Mobilities*, *2*(2), 175–194. https://doi.org/10.1080/17450100701381532

Mok, K. H., & Ho, H. C. (2020). Finding a home away from home: An explorative study on the use of social space with the voices of foreign domestic workers in Hong Kong. *Annals of the American Association of Geographers*, *111*(5), 1403–1419. https://doi.org/10.1080/24694452.2020.1813542

Ng, I. F., Lee, S. Y., Wong, W. K., & Chou, K. L. (2015). Effects of perceived discrimination on the quality of life among new Mainland Chinese immigrants to Hong Kong: A longitudinal study. *Social Indicators Research*, *120*(3), 817–834. https://doi.org/10.1007/s11205-014-0615-9

Stewart, M., Anderson, J., Beiser, M., Mwakarimba, E., Neufeld, A., Simich, L., & Spitzer, D. (2008). Multicultural meanings of social support among immigrants and refugees. *International Migration*, *46*(3), 123–159. https://doi.org/10.1111/j.1468-2435.2008.00464.x

Uchino, B. N. (2009). Understanding the links between social support and physical health: A life-span perspective with emphasis on the separability of perceived and received support. *Perspectives on Psychological Science*, *4*(3), 236–255. https://doi.org/10.1111/j.1745-6924.2009.01122.x

Uchino, B. N., Trettevik, R., Kent de Grey, R. G., Cronan, S., Hogan, J., & Baucom, B. R. (2018). Social support, social integration, and inflammatory cytokines: A meta-analysis. *Health Psychology*, *37*(5), 462–471. https://doi.org/10.1037/hea0000594

Ullah, A. A. (2015). Abuse and violence against foreign domestic workers: A case from Hong Kong. *International Journal of Area Studies, 10*(2), 221–238. https://doi.org/10.1515/ijas-2015-0010

Wong, D. F. K. (2008). Differential impacts of stressful life events and social support on the mental health of mainland Chinese immigrant and local youth in Hong Kong: A resilience perspective. *British Journal of Social Work, 38*(2), 236–252. https://doi.org/10.1093/bjsw/bcl344

Wong, D. F. K., & Song, H. X. (2006). Dynamics of social support: A longitudinal qualitative study on mainland Chinese immigrant women's first year of resettlement in Hong Kong. *Social Work in Mental Health, 4*(3), 83–101. https://doi.org/10.1300/J200v04n03_05

Wong, W. K., Chou, K. L., & Chow, N. W. (2012). Correlates of quality of life in new migrants to Hong Kong from mainland China. *Social Indicators Research, 107*(2), 373–391. https://doi.org/10.1007/s11205-011-9853-2

Yap, V. C. (2015). The religiosity of Filipina domestic workers in Hong Kong. *Asian Anthropology, 14*(1), 91–102. https://doi.org/10.1080/16834 78X.2015.1025600

Zhang, Z., & Wu, X. (2011). Social change, cohort quality and economic adaptation of Chinese immigrants in Hong Kong, 1991–2006. *Asian and Pacific Migration Journal, 20*(1), 1–29. https://doi.org/10.1177/011719681102000101

11 Covid-19 Pandemic Experienced by Migrant Workers in Densely Populated Singapore

Case Perspectives for Health Communication

May O. Lwin, Chitra Panchapakesan, and Hedwig Alfred

Singapore, a densely populated island nation with only 726 square kilometers (Singapore Land Authority, 2020), is a continuously growing urban economy in Southeast Asia. Migrant workers have been an integral part of Singapore's infrastructural developments in recent decades. The current migrant worker population in Singapore stands at approximately 1.3 million, which includes nearly 1 million lower-wage workers on work permits (Ministry of Manpower, 2021b). This number is relatively large when compared to the total local population of approximately 5.7 million (National Population and Talent Division, 2020).

Hosting such a large migrant worker community has led Singapore to face many unique difficulties amongst the migrant workers as the Covid-19 pandemic hit the country and reached this particular group. In this chapter, we narrate Singapore's experiences and use secondary data to reflect and synthesize the role of communication and the health communication strategies used by various entities during the unprecedented Covid-19 outbreak among the migrant worker communities in 2020.

Figure 11.1 details the timeline of events of the Covid-19 pandemic in Singapore in 2020. Detailed in the chart are the various phases of the outbreak which illustrate how the pandemic unfolded and the resultant government policies to manage the crisis. At the current time of writing, Singapore has reported 62,216 cases of Covid-19 and 33 deaths – the lowest Covid-19 case fatality ratio globally (Johns Hopkins University, 2021).

The migrant worker episode in the overall national experience occurred in April 2020 to December 2020 and involved an unexpected swift surge in Covid-19 infections among migrant workers living in dormitories and other types of housing. The number of cases escalated daily, reaching

DOI: 10.4324/9781003230243-11

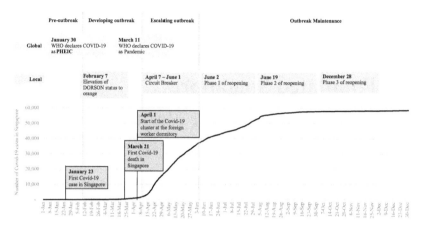

Figure 11.1 Timeline of the Covid-19 pandemic in Singapore in 2020
Reference: (Lwin et al., 2021)

over 1,000 new cases per day at the peak (Yong, 2020a). The number of cases among migrant workers outnumbered community cases manifold during this particular period.

Migrant Worker Living Conditions

In Singapore, migrant workers are typically housed in large purpose-built dormitories which can accommodate large numbers of workers. Some of the largest are vast compounds that accommodate around 25,000 people while others stay in shared accommodation in government Housing and Development Board (HDB) flats or smaller factories-converted housing arrangements. Depending on the housing type, migrant workers typically share their room with other workers, some in-dorm rooms with as many as 10–12 roommates. The dormitories, however, make up the major component of migrant worker housing. In total, there are 51 dormitories in Singapore that accommodate a large number of the migrant worker population (Ministry of Manpower, 2021c).

On a typical day, most migrant workers work long 10–11-hour shifts and return to their rooms to rest, shower and sleep. During lunchtimes, workers take a break at worksites. On a typical weekday, workers in local communities can be seen eating packed meals in the shade of trees or covered areas near their workplaces. For dinner, some rooms in dormitories have in-built kitchens within rooms or communal kitchens where the workers can cook, and others offer canteens for meals. On weekends, most workers go out to various venues in the city which cater to their grocery needs and meal tastes. Such enclaves in the city areas include Little India for South Asian workers, Peninsula Plaza for Burmese workers and the Golden Mile Complex for Thai workers.

Timeline of Surge in Migrant Worker Cases

When the pandemic hit Singapore, it became clear the migrant workers' working and living conditions were not ideal for battling the infectious disease outbreak. The first Covid-19 case among the migrant worker community was identified just two weeks after the first imported case arrived in Singapore (08 February 2020) (Chang, & Tjendro, 2020). By the end of April 2020, nearly 1,000 migrant workers were testing Covid-19 positive each day (Yong, 2020a), making this situation a nationwide health concern. By early May 2020, the migrant worker cases had reached 88% of the total number of Covid-19 positive cases in Singapore (Koh, 2020). At this time, the government decided to put the migrant worker population under lockdown along with parallel restrictions for the entire nation. This led to a large number of men being kept restricted in close quarters, where at first they congregated for meals and other daily activities. As more men became sick, more curbs were placed on the workers' movement, and many were placed in confined spaces of their rooms. With only basic facilities, this proved stressful for the workers who had little to do in a limited space.

"I know our living and working conditions; if a migrant worker gets infected, then it'll spread very fast because our dormitories have a lot of people living together inside a room. It means we will get sick together," said a 41-year-old construction safety coordinator to Channel News Asia (CAN) (Phua & Min, 2020).

As the number of cases surged and the men had to be safely distanced from one another, the authorities sought to find more space for the workers, including housing those recovering from the Coronavirus. These included expanding residential spaces to other types of housing via the creative utilization of large housing areas. For instance, the SuperStar Gemini and the SuperStar Aquarius cruise ships were used to house some 2,000 recovering migrant workers. Meanwhile, those who tested positive for Covid-19 but who were not seriously ill were housed at a community care facility, in the form of the repurposed Changi Exhibition Centre.

By October 2020, the Covid-19 cases among migrant workers in dormitories reduced (Yong, 2020b). Later in the year, as the number of Covid-19 cases declined, the government conducted tests in December 2020 and found that almost half of the 323,000 migrant workers living in the dormitories have had a Covid-19 infection (Lim, 2020). One of the major positives during the entire episode, however, was the very low mortality rate among Covid-19 positive migrant workers (Ministry of Manpower, 2020).

Method

This chapter narrates the experiences of migrant workers using secondary data obtained from information gathered for an advanced journalism academic module which focused on how the pandemic affected workers who had travelled from far away countries to earn a living in Singapore. We examine the modes of communication utilized by the community, and how communication played a role in supporting the men's needs and well-being. We also gathered and examined data from government press releases, video conference reports and published newspaper articles.

The primary source of data was the publication entitled Invisible Men (Chua et al., 2020), which details the narratives from interviews and observations conducted by 14 advanced journalism students and two faculty members at the Wee Kim Wee School of Communication and Information. The team attended briefings with 10 experts, from infectious diseases specialists to dormitory operators, before conducting intensive interviews with migrant workers, employers, agents, canteen operators, volunteer organizations, and government officials over a period of three months, from July to September 2020. About 780 hours of interviews were conducted in total. And a significant number of hours was spent on social media monitoring posts of migrant workers and other stakeholders. The students' efforts culminated in news stories, which in this chapter, provide data used for insights for thematic analysis.

All secondary data were pooled and analyzed using thematic analysis. In-depth familiarization was done by going through the quotes first before coding them. The quotes were subsequently coded and categorized into themes that emerged from the data. Our thematic analysis surfaced cluster the quotes into themes pertaining to the entire episode as follows: (a) Swift government responses and online communication dependence (b) Digital communication tools for workers' health (c) Support by external groups, particularly NGOs and community initiatives (d) Communication contributing towards bettering migrant workers' mental health (e) Communication amongst migrant workers via social media.

Findings and Perspectives

The following details the five key themes that surfaced during the course of our analysis.

Swift Government Responses and Online Communication Dependence

The Singapore government ministries and health authorities acted quickly to control the spread of Covid-19 among the migrant workers, first targeting the dormitories and then the other types of accommodations. The role of managing the outbreak amongst migrant workers fell mainly on the Ministry of Manpower (MOM). The inter-agency task force (ITF) included more than 2,000 officers and were from the MOM, Ministry of Health (MOH), National Environment Agency (NEA), the Singapore Armed Forces (SAF), the Singapore Police Force (SPF) and the Migrant Workers' Centre, and this group set out the communication response network and immediately created channels of communication with dorm operators, NGOs, employers, medical authorities, and other organizations during the pandemic to reduce the spread of the virus within the dorms (Ministry of Manpower, 2021a). Within one week (by mid-April 2020) all dorms were put on lockdown and within each dorm, each group of workers in rooms was placed in isolation to contain the spread of the virus. On the population front, parallel restrictions were put in place. The nationwide lockdown was introduced from 7 April 2020 to 4 May 2020 to control the Covid-19 spread as the number of cases per day peaked. Most workplaces were closed, except for those providing essential services, and schools moved to home-based learning (Singapore Government, 2020).

On the migrant worker communication front, the governmental task force used several parallel measures and multi-modal communication strategies using mobile technology to spread health messages within the dorms. The ITF gathered a team of translators to assist with the translation of messaging and information in the various languages used by the migrant workers. The ITF moved from printed material to WhatsApp messages, and began to include podcasts and videos as well, some featuring migrant workers themselves. The MOM distributed free SIM cards and set up free Wi-Fi in the dorms to establish direct communication with migrant workers to disseminate information and advice regarding Covid-19 safety protocols and gather information from the workers. The MOM also used social media as a communication tool to share information with the migrant worker population and to reassure each worker they would be taken care of and would be given medical treatment if they needed it.

"Anyone who is tested positive will be taken care of. We will help you to recover. In fact, many of the workers we have treated have fully recovered," said Manpower Minister Josephine Teo, through a Facebook post on 18th April 2020 (Ang, 2020).

On its part, the government also swiftly tested workers, confined positive cases in the dorms and cared for the migrant workers' health. The government also isolated and treated any migrant worker who reported feeling ill or showed flu-like symptoms. The government actions aimed to clear the dorms of Covid-19 as soon as possible so the migrant workers could get back to work safely.

Digital communication tools for workers' health

To monitor any new suspected cases, the government provided thermometers and oximeters so that migrant workers living in dorms could self-report their temperature and oximeter readings regularly. Medical teams oversaw these and acted when they identified irregularities in the reports. At the same time, ITF set up a medical team that consisted of doctors, nurses and technicians in the dormitories to care for the unwell and monitor the health of others. The presence of doctors in the dorms reassured migrant workers that they would get medical care if they needed it.

> *"I think above all, we served as a comforting presence to these workers - when the entire dormitory is locked down, people are scared and anxious, so having the medical post there reminded them that we're there for them and we will attend to their needs to the best of our efforts."*
>
> said Dr. Chen Yongsheng (Tan, 2020).

ITF mounted several technologically streamlined solutions through the use of mobile applications to make getting back to work for the migrant workers as easily as possible. The SGWorkPass app was introduced to the migrant workers and this app informed them, their employers and the dorm operators to check if the workers had received a *"green status"* and could leave the dorm for work (Ho, 2020).

   "This new access code feature will allow the workers themselves, their employers as well as the dormitory operators to have clarity about who can exit the dormitories to work," said Manpower Minister Josephine Teo at a virtual media conference on 1 June 2020 (Ho, 2020).

   Each migrant worker was also asked to use the FWMOMCare app to report their temperature, heart rate and flu-like symptoms, if any, on a daily basis and they could also check their Covid-19 test results through this app. By 19 June 2020, all migrant workers in the dorms were asked to install and use the national contact training app "TraceTogether". It provided another layer of checks, as it detected those who may have been close to other positive Covid-19 cases, and they could be isolated and tested more quickly than before (Ministry of Health Singapore, 2020).

   Even though the worker dormitories had medical teams on hand to monitor the Covid-19 situation among workers, there were hurdles to overcome: language barriers, chronic illnesses and mental health issues. A group of doctors made cards to help workers with symptoms they might be experiencing, and the cards became a tool that was used in several dormitories to help workers explain what they were feeling. At some dorms, workers who were well were asked to help patients explain their symptoms to the medical team present.

There were also workers who had chronic illnesses but were now unable to make their regular hospital visits because of the lockdown. Teleconsultation services from a mobile application were set up for them to update their health status daily, and which could connect them to a doctor within 30 minutes. The teleconsultation service made getting medical attention easier for workers and medicine was delivered within a few hours.

"Last time if there is any problem, I must inform the employer. Now, I can call a doctor anytime," said a 31-year-old male Bangladeshi migrant worker.

The Importance of NGOs and Community Initiatives

Migrant workers were under extreme stress during this uncertain time and wanted answers to their concerns regarding their salary, their future work and how things were going to unfold. There were already several long-running non-governmental organizations with volunteers who worked specifically with migrant workers. Groups, such as Transient Workers Count Too (TWC2), Humanitarian Organization for Migration Economics and HealthServe, stepped up services to help workers they could reach. Instead of workers coming to them on their off days, the volunteers had to now find ways to reach workers quarantined in the dorms and flats across the island. Among their initiatives, they also trained migrant workers to act as ambassadors to their fellow workers. These migrant workers were trained to read health directives, information and educational materials from the Ministry of Health and the Ministry of Manpower. They were then equipped to convey health information to fellow workers through podcasts and videos shared on social media.

"Spoken Tamil is so different from written Tamil and getting information simply and clearly, about your salary and that you would be taken care of if you got sick, was critical for the workers," said Mrs Christine Pelly, an executive committee member of TWC2.

Meanwhile, as many as 20 new volunteer groups surfaced in the local community. They offered an array of services including money, gift baskets, meals, masks, prayer mats and kettles to workers. To ensure the good intentions were not misdirected, the NGOs and new groups decided to coordinate their efforts through a WhatsApp group. By April 2020, they were holding regular meetings via video conferencing to identify overlaps in providing the same type of help to one location.

"The pandemic was a humanitarian disaster. So the communication was essential to know which areas were looked after and which areas needed to be looked after more," said a male civic group leader.

The NGOs also worked closely with the Ministry of Manpower (MOM), developed joint communication and on 12 August 2020 issued

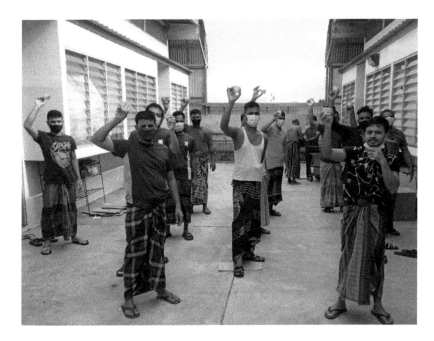

Figure 11.2 Migrant workers in a dormitory show ice-cream treats sent by NGOs during the lockdown. *Photo by: Shamin Ahmed (Permission obtained for the publication)*

a joint statement outlining the measures for dormitory residents to enjoy safe rest days.

> *"I certainly look forward to more of these types of sessions where MOM not only asks for our opinions, but also listens to our concerns and suggestions. And I believe that MOM has recognised that they will need us to support their efforts."*
>
> said a female NGO leader.

Communication towards Bettering Migrant Workers' Mental Health

Most of the migrant workers were confined in dormitories and other migrant worker living spaces, except for those providing essential services, such as in the shipyards and as housing estate cleaners. During this time, migrant workers were regularly tested for Covid-19. As their number was large test results were often delayed leaving many men anxious. At times, a few men from the room would be removed with no explanation, leaving everyone fearful, even though this could have been done to remove older more susceptible workers from the group. Migrant workers also had other worries during a lockdown: would they continue getting their salaries, who would pay for the treatment if they got Covid-19, how would they send money home, how were their families back home and what would happen next (Figure 11.3).

The mental strain on workers in lockdown was a concern well noted by the government and NGOs. In particular, the lack of interpersonal communication especially for those in confinement was clear. To mitigate this communication gap, more experienced migrant workers with leadership qualities were identified asked to act as ambassadors to help identify and support those who needed help. Meanwhile volunteers from the NGO coalition, such as one headed by social entrepreneur Cai Yinzhou, began to produce 15–30 minutes educational videos that workers could access online. These included language tutorials and lessons on photography and art. The group also set up health and well-being helplines that the men could contact.

"Being confined with 10–20 workers will have a huge mental impact on them. An idle mind is a dangerous place," said Mr Cai Yinzhou to CNA on 10 April 2020 (Phua, 2020).

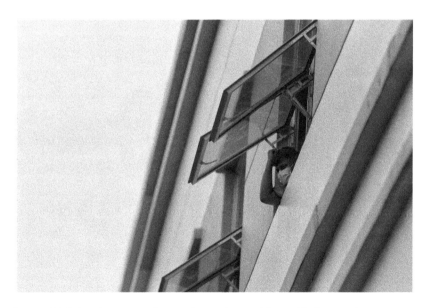

Figure 11.3 A migrant worker peeks at the world outside from a factory converted dormitory during lockdown. *Photo by Joel Chan (Permission obtained for the publication)*

Communication amongst Migrant Workers Via Social Media

Being idle without work and in lockdown was new to this group of men. The situation created ample free time and the men had to come up with ways to spend it. Many migrant workers shared that during this time, they understood the need to support each other and found they could do this by either in person with roommates (e.g. talking about what they knew about Covid-19, things back home, sharing jokes, playing board games and watching videos) or with the larger community online (e.g. connecting with hobby interest groups, seeking entertainment). Social and mobile media was already a critical link between the men and families and friends in home countries. However, it played an added role in enabling new support structures. Connections with others in similar situation was enabled mainly by chat apps (e.g. WhatsApp, Viber, Telegram) and served as an invaluable network of mutual support. Many migrant workers came up with creative ways to use social media channels for communication and to support one another during the lockdown and Covid-19 pandemic. Organically, groups with similar interests, such as virtual musical groups were formed and sustained mutual interests online (Figure 11.4).

TikTok became one of the social media platforms for the migrant workers to share information, show a glimpse into their daily life, communicate, be social support for one another and even make friends

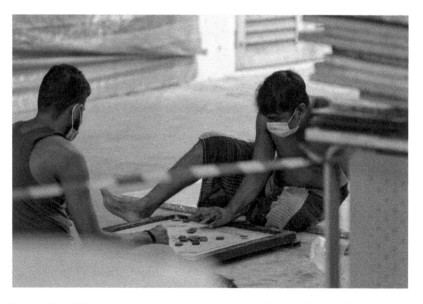

Figure 11.4 Migrant workers play carrom to pass the time during the lockdown. *Photo by Joel Chan (Permission obtained for the publication)*

during the lockdown period. For example, a migrant worker shared a video clip of long queues of masked workers waiting to get their free mobile top-up cards at a dormitory carpark. There were also videos expressing gratitude towards the Singapore government for the care and treatment they received during this time.

"No matter how big the tension, making TikTok videos helps us feel jolly," said a 34-year-old male Indian migrant worker.

Another Bangladeshi worker made nearly 80 videos. The content of these videos was of daily activities, such as his roommates exercising or him singing during the lockdown. The majority of his followers were fellow migrant workers. The migrant workers said they received an unexpectedly large number of viewers and good wishes through social media.

One such example is the story of a Bangladeshi worker (Billal Khan, 28-years-old) who created a Facebook page in April 2020. He created the page to share updates and news the regarding Covid-19 pandemic and initiatives. Every day after work he checks for new information and news to be shared. He reviews the articles that are translated to Bengali and sometimes translates them himself before posting them on his Facebook page, which has more than 5,000 followers. These social media pages also act as social support from within the migrant workers' group to reassure them they are going through the pandemic together (Chua et al., 2020).

Another interesting use of social media was the sharing of specific experiences and encounters surrounding how migrant workers with Covid-19 were being treated in health facilities, with regular recovery updates by them. When Mr. Zasim turned out to be Covid-19 positive, he recorded his recovery and shared it via social media while he was in the hospital.

"Everyone will believe me since I'm the person with Covid-19," said the 27-year-old male Bangladeshi migrant worker.

Through his videos, this worker wanted to reassure other migrant workers that if they got Covid-19, they would be well looked after. Later, the Ministry of Manpower used this particular video on their Facebook communication page.

"Using TikTok made me feel less lonely, especially during the month when I stayed alone in the hotel," said 34-year-old male Bangladeshi migrant worker.

Communication Strategies Used and Recommendations

The study findings of migrant workers' experiences in Singapore during Covid-19 have implications for government, health authorities and policymakers. In particular, our assessment highlights the importance of communication during the surge of Coronavirus cases among hundreds of thousands of migrant workers in lockdown situations. Regular and rapid communication was even more critical as fear, worry and confusion dominated the emotions of the men in lockdown in dormitories. In hindsight, this case study revealed several important lessons for authorities and communication planners at both strategic and tactical levels.

a   **Utilization of multimodal communication:** The Singapore Covid-19 task force, government and migrant workers used numerous communication channels including traditional, online and social media to reach out during the Covid-19 episode. It was critical that messaging was available both on the physical front in the dormitories (for example, via posters, physical mail, pamplets) as well as the digital front. In this regard, the spectrum of communication tools needed in the migrant worker case was very wide, and included translated texts, language cue cards, podcasts, videos and social media apps. This showcases the importance and need of using multifaceted communication strategies to cover all the bases during a public health emergency.

b   **Deployment of engagement via mobile devices:** Mobile devices were the single major tangible connection between the workers and the outside world. They were indispensable on three fronts. Firstly, the mobile platform served to connect the men to regular local news and behavior directives (e.g. safe distancing and mask-wearing) which helped the men get information about their circumstances. Second, the mobile device connected the men to home news and loved ones and their communities which kept them updated about what was happening back home. Finally, the mobile phone connected the men to one another, providing opportunities to share and peer support those facing similar circumstances. A turning point during this period was the migrant workers themselves making podcasts and videos, which were widely circulated. Particularly, social media groups that connected amongst groups of men through the use of their favorite apps, such as TikTok and Facebook, proved beneficial.

c   **Communication speed and adaptability to the fast-unfolding situation:** Crisis communication from various organizations including government agencies and NGOs to contain the spread of the disease and give the men as much help as possible evolved at a rapid pace during the entire lockdown period. It was apparent that both the authorities and the dormitory operators, faced an unprecedented set of circumstances and had to swiftly respond to changing scenarios of the disease spread. The speed of information also helped to reduce anxiety and concerns amongst all stakeholders. The sooner good information got to the migrant workers, the better they felt about their situation. Hereafter, health authorities should prepare in advance and to mount regular crisis response teams within organizations that are well networked with all stakeholders and trained in crisis management to enable rapid responses for all forms of health emergencies.

d   **Presence and connectivity to medical and support structures:** The presence of medical teams in the dormitories also reassured the migrant workers. In addition, most of the migrant workers were able to seek medical information on online platforms as needed. These lessons indicate the importance of using online media including social media in health crisis situations, not just for sharing information but for influencing worker sentiments, addressing concerns and providing social and peer support. Additionally, communication helplines such as those set up by NGOs and community groups helped to tackle the tremendous strain faced by the men of being locked in close quarters with half a dozen or so others for weeks. Local community groups in Singapore should better connect with the migrant communities beyond the pandemic so that community assistance and support, as well as connections across the population groups can be more forthcoming, and rapidly mounted in the future. How such communication can further connect across groups may need considerations regarding the multilingual nature of the worker population. Future response strategies may draw upon smart technology such as AI and Chatbots to provide concurrent translations in relevant languages to connect across linguistically diverse populations.

In summary, the Covid-19 migrant worker episode in Singapore provides substantial support pertaining to the need to utilize many available media to reach and connect with every worker affected in emergency. Digital media, in particular, is clearly necessary and plays a critical role in offering one-way, two-ways and group communication functions to all stakeholders and those affected. With the Covid-19 and pandemic threats still very salient internationally, the lessons from the pandemic messaging and communication across vulnerable communities warrant further close study and discussion. Our case assessment of the migrant worker community clearly demonstrates the unique effects on the community which may not parallel the experiences in the mainstream society. Understanding the needs of the communities and the effective communication strategies for these groups will allow stakeholders in various communities to be better prepared for future health events.

Acknowledgements

The authors thank:

- Wee Kim Wee School of Communication and Information (WKWSCI) Legacy Fund and the Go-Far 2020 Team at the WKWSCI, Nanyang Technological University Singapore.
- Singapore Ministry of Health's National Medical Research Council under its COVID-19 Research Fund (COVID19RF-005).

Recommended Readings

Koh, D. (2020). Migrant workers and COVID-19. *Occupational and Environmental Medicine* 2020;77:634–636.

WHO. (2020). The Migrant Worker Whose COVID-19 Story Inspired Singapore, News Clip 17 Dec 2020, https://www.who.int/singapore/news/feature-stories/detail/the-migrant-worker-whose-covid-19-story-inspired-singapore

References

Ang, P. [Prisca] (2020, April 19). Coronavirus: We will look after you, ministry assures foreign workers. *Straits Times*. Retrieved from https://www.straitstimes.com/singapore/we-will-look-after-you-ministry-assures-foreign-workers

Chang, N. [Nicole], & Tjendro. J. [Johannes] (2020, February 09). Coronavirus outbreak: 3 new cases confirmed in Singapore, 4 more discharged. *Channel News Asia*. Retrieved from https://www.channelnewsasia.com/news/singapore/wuhan-coronavirus-singapore-new-confirmed-cases-feb-9-12412622

Chua, E., Chew, J., Lee, M., Loh, M., Ganesan, N., ... & He, S. (2020). *Invisible Men: NTU Go-Far 2020*. Retried from https://ebook.ntu.edu.sg/go-far-2020.html

Ho, O. [Olivia] (2020, June 2). Which workers can leave dorms for work? Find out with new app. *Straits Times*. Retrieved from https://www.straitstimes.com/singapore/manpower/which-workers-can-leave-dorms-for-work-find-out-with-new-app

Johns Hopkins University. (2021, January 17). *Mortality Analyses*. Retrieved from https://coronavirus.jhu.edu/data/mortality

Koh, D. (2020). Migrant workers and the Covid-19 pandemic. *Occup Environ Med*, 1–3. https://doi.org/10.1136/oemed-2020-106626

Lim, M. Z. (2020, December 15). 47 Per Cent Of Migrant Workers In S'pore Dorms Have Had A Covid-19 Infection, Say Manpower And Health Ministries. *The Straits Times*. Retrieved from https://www.straitstimes.com/singapore/47-per-cent-of-migrant-workers-in-dorms-have-had-a-covid-19-infection-say-manpower-and

Lwin, M. O., Panchapakesan, C., Sheldenkar, A., Tandoc Jr, E. C., Hye, K. K., Yang, S., Ong, Z., Lee, S. Y., & Kwan, M. R. (2021). Battling Covid-19 pandemic in a densely populated Island nation: The Singapore experience. In *Community, the Economy, and COVID-19: Lessons from Multi-Country Analyses of the* SARS-CoV-2 *Pandemic*. Springer.

Ministry of Health Singapore. (2020, September 9). TraceTogether and SafeEntry to be enhanced in preparation for further opening of the economy. *Ministry of Health Singapore*. Retrieved from https://www.moh.gov.sg/news-highlights/details/tracetogether-and-safeentry-to-be-enhanced-in-preparation-for-further-opening-of-the-economy

Ministry of Manpower. (2020, December 14). Measures to contain the Covid-19 outbreak in migrant worker dormitories. *Ministry of Manpower, Singapore*. Retrieved from https://www.mom.gov.sg/newsroom/press-releases/2020/1214-measures-to-contain-the-covid-19-outbreak-in-migrant-worker-dormitories

Ministry of Manpower. (2021a, January 5). Inter-agency taskforce to support foreign workers and dormitory operators during circuit breaker period. *Ministry of Manpower, Singapore*. Retrieved from https://www.mom.gov.sg/newsroom/press-releases/2020/0407-inter-agency-taskforce-to-support-fws-and-dormitory-operators-during-circuit-breaker-period

Ministry of Manpower. (2021b, March 30). Foreign workforce numbers. *Ministry of Manpower, Singapore*. Retrieved from https://www.mom.gov.sg/documents-and-publications/foreign-workforce-numbers

Ministry of Manpower. (2021c, April 9). List of foreign worker dormitories. *Ministry of Manpower, Singapore*. Retrieved from https://www.mom.gov.sg/passes-and-permits/work-permit-for-foreign-worker/housing/foreign-worker-dormitories#/?page=3&q=

National Population and Talent Division. (2020, September 24). Population in brief 2020: Key trends. *National Population and Talent Division, Prime Minister's Office Singapore*. Retrieved from https://www.population.gov.sg/media-centre/articles/population-in-brief-2020-key-trends

Phua, R. [Rachel] (2020, April 10). NGOs launch initiatives to help migrant workers amid COVID-19 outbreak. *Channel News Asia*. Retrieved from https://www.channelnewsasia.com/news/singapore/covid19-migrant-foreign-workers-dormitory-food-coronavirus-12627032

Phua, R. [Rachel] & Min, A. H., [Ang Hwee] (2020, September 12). IN FOCUS: The long, challenging journey to bring COVID-19 under control in migrant worker dormitories. *Channel News Asia*. Retrieved from https://www.channelnewsasia.com/news/singapore/in-focus-covid19-singapore-migrant-worker-dormitories-lockdown-13081210

Singapore Government. (2020, April 3). PM Lee: The Covid-19 situation in Singapore (3 Apr). *Singapore Government*. Retrieved from https://www.gov.sg/article/pm-lee-hsien-loong-on-the-covid-19-situation-in-singapore-3-apr

Singapore Land Authority. (2020, September 18). Total land area of Singapore. *Data.gov.sg*. Retrieved from https://data.gov.sg/dataset/total-land-area-of-singapore?view_id=e6e37f25-01ef-4c23-a7cb-5682ab5edb75&resource_id=f4bbfac9-c3ed-4f71-9b9a-238517b214ef

Tan, C. [Cheryl] (2020, June 20). Doc stayed away from family to volunteer at dorms. *Straits Times*. Retrieved from https://www.straitstimes.com/singapore/doc-stayed-away-from-family-to-volunteer-at-dorms

Yong, M. (2020a, April 18). Timeline: How the Covid-19 outbreak has evolved in Singapore so far. *Channel News Asia*. Retrieved from https://www.chan-nelnewsasia.com/news/singapore/singapore-covid-19-outbreak-evolved-coro-navirus-deaths-timeline-12639444

Yong, M. (2020b, October 13). Timeline: No new Covid-19 case in Singa-pore's dormitories for the first time in more than 6 months. *Channel News Asia*. Retrieved from https://www.channelnewsasia.com/news/singapore/covid-19-cases-singapore-dormitory-zero-six-months-13271976

12 Health Communication Barriers Faced by Rohingya Refugees During COVID-19

Muhiuddin Haider, Sameen Ahmed, and Jamal Uddin

While COVID-19 has proven to be a threat for all humans, regardless of race, age, or gender, some groups are at a greater risk of contracting the virus due to poor living conditions and pre-existing health conditions. As of January 18th, 2021, there have been approximately 93,611,355 confirmed cases of COVID-19 and 2,022,405 deaths globally.[1] In order to reduce these numbers, people must follow WHO guidelines including social distancing, consistent hand washing, and the use of face masks, however, for refugees, following these guidelines is incredibly difficult. The limited access to healthcare and personal protection equipment has left refugee communities unguarded and at great risk of an unmanageable outbreak.

As of December 2020, approximately 79.5 million people who are fleeing persecution due to political and religious unrest live as refugees in various host countries.[2] Almost 90% of refugees live in developing countries that do not have the resources and financial means to provide basic needs, including water, food, and protection.[3] Host countries are struggling to provide for and protect their own citizens from the COVID-19 virus, further leaving refugees unprotected. While the host countries mentioned throughout this chapter are open to accepting refugees in need of help, the pandemic has caused refugee populations to exist as a threat to various host countries' public health safety.[2] Communication barriers between refugees and their host country's health care providers make it difficult for them to understand how to protect themselves, leaving a large portion of the population uninformed of the severity of the COVID-19 virus and its symptoms.

To develop a deeper understanding and analysis of communication barriers existing among refugee populations, a systematic search of various literature was conducted and compiled. Through this research, this chapter aims to analyze the population characteristics of refugee populations, especially Rohingya refugees, and the dangers posed by their living conditions. Disease epidemiology, of both communicable and noncommunicable illnesses, and their effects on the overall health of Rohingya, as well as Syrian and South Sudanese refugees, was also studied.

DOI: 10.4324/9781003230243-12

A substantial amount of data and analytic research was collected from scientific journals and reports from organizations such as The World Health Organization (WHO), The UN Refugee Agency (UNHCR), and The International Federation of Red Cross and Red Crescent Societies (IRFC). The research includes both quantitative and qualitative data from reliable primary and secondary sources. The focus of this research is to analyze various health communication barriers and the ways they have further impacted the wellbeing and health of the vulnerable population of the Rohingya Refugees, who are working to combat a pandemic. Syrian and South Sudanese refugee populations are also discussed in this chapter to further explain the problem.

Rohingya and Other Refugee Population Characteristics

As the number of refugees continues to grow due to civil unrest in many developing countries, the pandemic is becoming a greater threat for displaced people looking to seek asylum in neighboring countries. With over 5.6 million refugees, most of which are women and children, Syria has become one of the top countries with the most people fleeing civil unrest.[3]

Over 5 million of 5.6 million Syrian refugees seeking asylum, primarily in Turkey and Europe, are out of work or school.[4] Syria was once a flourishing state with a highly effective healthcare system, however, the violent and long civil war has demolished it, leaving millions of people displaced.[5] Syrian refugees are exposed to war, death, family separations, forced child recruitment, sexual harassment, and unsanitary living conditions, causing severe mental health issues and poverty.[6] Due to the state of the country, health care providers, doctors, and pharmacists have fled the nation.[7] In conjunction with the unsanitary conditions, famine brought upon by war, and the lack of healthcare, many once treatable diseases have progressed and spread, creating more serious and fatal issues.

A similar civil war persists in South Sudan. As of December 2013, violent government and civilian conflict in South Sudan has caused approximately 4 million people to lose their homes with over 2.2 million people fleeing the country as refugees, it has been identified as Africa's largest refugee crisis.[8] Many South Sudanese refugees seek asylum in neighboring countries, such as Kenya and Uganda. The majority of South Sudanese refugees are women and children, and 63% are under the age of 18.[9] Refugees travel across the border in hot and dry climates, arriving at their destinations malnourished and dehydrated due to food insecurity and homelessness. This journey leaves them with weakened immune systems and little strength, making it unlikely they can combat the symptoms of the COVID-19 virus.[78]

While most refugee camps have similar living conditions, those more densely populated are more susceptible to a COVID-19 outbreak, such as those in Bangladesh. Rohingya refugees are primarily Muslim refugees from Rakhine State, Myanmar who are fleeing religious persecution and political unrest. Civil unrest has caused refugee families to lose their homes, jobs, resources, and rights, as they are considered a stateless population targeted by the government-funded Buddhist military.[7 10] A 2018 study of the Rohingya refugees in Cox's Bazar found that around 76% of Rohingya refugees at the camp reported having no education because of the past seven years of political unrest and destruction in Myanmar.[11]

About 1,118,576 forcibly displaced Rohingya refugees are living in Bangladesh, a South Asian country east of India.[11] 860,175 of the displaced Myanmar nationals are taking shelter in Cox's Bazar, a city located in southeastern Bangladesh and named the largest refugee camp in the world.[12 13] Each of the 187,530 families living in the camps has 4–6 members on average and most live in a single room per family, making it difficult to socially distance.[11] Bangladesh has been ranked one of the top 17 countries with the highest COVID-19 cases and controlling the spread of the virus has become problematic for the densely populated country.

As resources have become especially limited and the residents living near and in the camp lack public health guidance that they can comprehend, the virus has quickly spread while the access to treatment remains insufficient. As reported in June 2020, Cox's Bazar District has approximately 1,900 beds for refugee patients with COVID-19 including those in four quarantine centers and four acute respiratory infection isolation treatment centers.[12] The country has 29 labs across the country, however refugees do not have access to them, limiting the number of COVID-19 tests available for suspected carriers living at the camp and preventing contact tracing and risk management.[14]

As of June 6, 2020, the Bangladeshi government labeled the areas surrounding the camp as red zones due to the vulnerability of the area.[11] The government has also started charging for tests completed at any government facility, despite 25% of the population living below the federal poverty line.[15] This has left the natives of the host country struggling to control the virus, and the proximity of refugee camps further adds to the threat of epidemic. Reported as of November 11th, 2020, Bangladesh confirmed 5,000 positive COVID-19 cases and 72 deaths, numbers experts say are likely less than accurate due to difficulties in collecting data from the region.[16] Among the Rohingya refugee camps, 348 cases of the virus and ten deaths were reported, figures that are predicted to be much larger, however difficult to estimate due to communication barriers with the locals of the region.[15] Apart from living incredibly close to each other, Rohingya refugees living in Cox's

Bazar also live near the residents of the city. Despite the travel regulations in and out of the camp, the proximity of people makes it difficult to prevent the spread of the virus, particularly because most people are not receiving adequate health education on risk management and disease prevention.[17]

While taking on the responsibility of more than 860,000 Rohingya refugees, Bangladesh has struggled with the quality and accessibility of healthcare provided for the entire country. Only 0.69% of the country's gross domestic product, or GDP, is spent on healthcare and the pandemic has further exposed weaknesses within the existing healthcare system.[18] Prior to the pandemic, 14.2% of Rohingya refugees living at Cox's Bazar reported that healthcare facilities were too far from their homes and that they could not afford the cost of transportation or medication.[19] Unattainable healthcare and the government's decision to levy for COVID-19 tests has left many natives unable to receive testing, leaving them unaware of their health status, and likely to spread the virus in their community.[20] The inaccessibility of healthcare is a problem for Bangladeshi citizens, let alone the refugees seeking asylum in Cox's Bazar.

Most refugee camps are densely populated grounds made up of tents or makeshift shelters made of materials such as bamboo and tarpaulin.[21] The camps lack clean drinking water, food, warm clothing, and sanitation/hygiene supplies such as soap, face masks, gloves, etc.[22] A study published in The Journal of Global Health states that only 30% of the Rohingya refugees have access to water, sanitation, and hygiene services, making it difficult to keep themselves and their families safe from contracting the virus.[23] Due to the large number of people, social isolation is a significant problem for migrants at Cox's Bazar. According to a study published in The Lancet Global Health Journal, the average population density at the camps is close to 40,000 people per km^2, a number greater than most other refugee camps around the world.[24] The unhygienic living conditions and lack of clean water at the camps have also made it incredibly difficult for refugees to maintain minimal hygiene. The camps have become the ideal environment for infectious viruses and diseases to spread and become an outstanding threat.

Noncommunicable Diseases Common among Refugee Populations

Due to the difficult journey most refugees endure before reaching their host country, they are known to have poor health and most lack immunity to vaccine-preventable illnesses. Their weak immune systems and limited information about how to combat the virus make it unlikely that refugees can combat the threat of COVID-19. The journey and life at the camps often cause adults and children to suffer from severe malnutrition due to food insecurity and scarcity, further deteriorating their health.[25] According to an article in the European Journal of Clinical Nutrition, malnutrition and various nutritional deficiencies have been proven to be a severe risk factor for the severity and long-term effects of COVID-19, a problem faced by all refugees.[26]

The death, violence, and inhumane living conditions refugees endure due to political unrest and religious persecution, often leads to severe and irreversible psychological distress. According to a study conducted by Dr. Harem Nareeman Mahmood, more than 60% of Syrian refugees living in Kurdistan, Iraq suffered from PTSD and 59.4% suffered from depression.[27] For children, extended absence from school can further influence these mental health illnesses.[28] In a report conducted by Save the Children, an organization that conducts global research and provides help for children in need, 71% of Syrian national interviewees said that Syrian children suffer from bedwetting and involuntary urination- both of which are common symptoms of severe stress and PTSD.[29] Such severe stress makes it hard for people to recover from illnesses such as the common cold and simple viruses, increasing the likelihood of more profound complications.[30]

Among Rohingya refugees, pregnant and lactating women need health care assistance, however, struggle to receive it and 78% of women are having to give birth at home.[31] Due to the lack of prenatal care risk of infection, developmental issues, and neonatal disorders have become common among the community. In Syrian refugee camps, children are suffering from similar developmental issues due to prolonged chemical exposure from chemical warfare and malnutrition. The mental trauma in conjunction with harmful chemical toxins can cause severe developmental and learning defects or speech impediments among children.[32] The physical and mental stress of living among chemical warfare has also increased the likelihood of patients suffering from underlying chronic conditions including cancer, heart disease, diabetes, substance abuse, and depression.[29]

Communicable Diseases Common among Refugee Populations

Diseases such as HIV and AIDS, tuberculosis, malaria, and respiratory illnesses linked to travel or inadequate living arrangements are also common among refugee communities. Water contamination and faulty sewage systems within conflict-stricken nations has also led to communicable diseases such as the poliovirus and cholera becoming common among asylum seekers.[33] Amidst Rohingya refugees, a Diphtheria outbreak has further contributed to the fragility of the general health of the community. With over 5,800 suspected cases of

Diphtheria and 38 deaths as of February 2020, people are facing extreme respiratory weakness.[34] Many of these illnesses persist after migration, and the lack of treatment and minimal vaccinations can cause the diseases to spread.[35][36] In 2016, out of 1,764 migrant children (mostly of Syrian descent) seen in medical clinics in Europe and Turkey, 30–40% were not vaccinated against tetanus, hepatitis B, mumps, measles and rubella, and whooping cough.[36] Pre-existing concerns that are not properly treated due to constrained healthcare services can make COVID-19 fatal for refugees.[37]

Currently, COVID-19 is the biggest communicable threat for displaced people as depleted resources in addition to the absence of public health guidance prevent them from defending their health. The easily transmitted disease is exceptionally challenging to track, and the novel vaccine is not readily available for refugee communities. The World Health Association has classified refugees as a vulnerable population and plans to reserve doses of the COVID-19 vaccine for them under the Humanitarian Buffer, however, communication barriers and lack of health care personnel may make it difficult for enough vaccines to be delivered fast enough to prevent an outbreak.[38]

Health Communication Barriers Faced by Refugees

The biggest problem refugees and their host populations face is communication. According to a study conducted in London by Dr. Behrouz Maldonado and colleagues, no government, of the 47 states of the Council of Europe included in the study, "produced risk communications on disease prevention targeting people in refugee camps or informal settlements."[39] The lack of comprehendible risk communication, exchange of time-sensitive information regarding one's health and safety, prevents refugee communities from receiving vital health guidance. Risk communication regarding the importance of social distance, washing hands, and avoiding large gatherings is necessary to protect communities from contracting the virus, and without it, refugees are in great danger. Communication barriers also inhibit the ability of host countries to collect vital information about the health of refugees and the number of COVID-19 cases at the camps, preventing accurate and up to date reporting of data.

One of the most challenging barriers in health communication is language. The inability of health care providers and government workers to communicate with refugee communities can lead to extreme confusion and hysteria.[40] The IRFC, working with Translators without Borders, has found that communities, including humanitarian NGOs, do a poor job of meeting the language needs of refugees. They reported that in Italy and Turkey, hosts to thousands of Syrian refugees, none of the 46 humanitarian organizations interviewed consistently asked refugees of their native language or the languages they understood.[40] Many translators and interpreters, who previously worked to alleviate language barriers, are unable to assist due to travel restrictions and the risk of physical interaction.[40] By not having updated language data, information shared with refugees often excludes a large number of people, preventing them from receiving life-saving information and minimizing trust between patients and physicians.

Lack of culturally appropriate services is another health communication barrier that exists among refugee populations, as it can prevent comfort and openness in patients.[41] In many cultures, such as those of the Syrian and Rohingya refugees, gender roles make it difficult for women to be treated by male doctors and they may feel more restricted when addressing their concerns.[41] Without anyone to advocate for them, women in these camps are often withheld from information and with limited health care providers, it has become increasingly difficult to fulfill the request of refugees who may want the same gender doctor or therapist.[42] For Rohingya women and children, COVID-19 has made these gender disparities much more extensive, further deteriorating their overall health. Additionally, domestic and sexual violence has significantly increased at Cox's Bazar, leaving women afraid and at risk of trauma and sexually transmitted diseases.[41][42] The pandemic has also made it challenging to employ health care providers who are trained to deal with patients who have suffered severe trauma.[41] The absence of culturally appropriate interaction skills has made communication between refugees, specifically women and children, and health care providers exceedingly difficult, leaving patients hesitant to open up to their physician.[43]

The growing use of technology and virtual communication is another problem persisting for refugee communities. Many healthcare services such as check-ups, psychiatric therapy, and public health reports and guidelines have shifted online via telemedicine and telecommunication. However, for refugees living in camps, this information is unattainable because of inaccessibility of computers, Wi-Fi, or even electricity.[44][45] Due to a ban placed on their devices in 2017 by the Bangladeshi government, Rohingya refugees at Cox's Bazar have constrained access to mobile phones.[16] Usage of mobile phones has been key in disseminating public health knowledge through social media and communication platforms, however, the ban has prevented crucial information from being dispersed at the camp.[47] This has made it difficult for refugees to access information regarding public health safety, as well as about local medical treatment facilities for pre-existing conditions. Even though the shift to telemedicine serves those with access to computers and mobile phones, absence of technology has caused refugees to face the same healthcare challenges they did prior to the pandemic.

Access to Comprehensive Risk Communication

Organizations such as UNHCR have developed messages on hand-washing, physical distancing, self-isolation, and locations of healthcare facilities in various languages to help refugees of different backgrounds and ethnicities. However, many of these messages are shared through hotlines and web-based platforms.[48] Community outreach workers have been trained to teach these messages, however, COVID-19 regulations and travel restrictions have hindered them from reaching many isolated asylum-seeking communities.[49] At Cox's Bazar, the few health care providers stationed at the camp have limited access to telecommunication and the Rohingya refugees have none due to the government ban on SIM cards and mobile phones.[50] [51] However, a strong social network between Rohingya refugees has allowed them to rely on each other for information. The Jordan Red Crescent Societies have established a similar system through a COVID-19 awareness campaign. The campaign provides video and infographics through social media, targeting a small group of Syrian refugees who have access to the information, and relying on them to spread the information to the rest of their community.[52]

Hostility from the host country's natives can also result in communication challenges between refugees and healthcare providers. Discrimination towards refugees, may prevent them from asking for help or clarification about risk communication, leaving them uninformed and defenseless. Fear of arrest or deportation may also prevent refugees from telling their healthcare provider that they have symptoms of the COVID-19 virus, potentially putting thousands of lives at risk.[53] Obstacles in communication and health literacy have also allowed rumors to spread among refugees. A rumor circulated at Cox's Bazar causing many Rohingya refugees to believe that in reporting COVID-19 like symptoms, they face the risk of being killed to prevent further infection.[54] In some cases, refugees are perceived as carriers of the virus, and in others, host natives may view refugees as a threat to their resources and safety.[55] Hostility and rumors result in fear and distrust among refugee communities, making it difficult for them to assimilate to their host country's customs, and further influencing health communication obstacles.

Refugees have always faced cultural and economic barriers when accessing immunization services from their host countries, who often lack the resources and programs to initiate an adequate immunization record collection system. According to a study discussed in a WHO article, refugees and asylum seekers show inadequate immunity to various vaccine-preventable diseases when compared to the native people of their respective host countries, suggesting that they receive far fewer vaccinations.[56] During the pandemic, these issues have worsened as the few refugees who may have been receiving medical treatment have had to refrain from seeing physicians. The need for proper immunization and vaccine administration has significantly increased as the COVID-19 vaccine becomes obtainable, and suboptimal medical records will not be enough for physicians to determine the eligibility and dose of medications to administer to each patient. Patients in need of the vaccine may not receive it or may miss their second dose and booster shots due to the failure of accessible medical history. This will make it difficult for health care providers to know exactly what the patient requires.[56] Previously discussed communication barriers such as language, culture, and gender roles, could further prevent healthcare workers from receiving essential information directly from the patient.

Discussion

Risk communication and assessment is the key to preventing a COVID-19 outbreak among densely populated countries. Vulnerable populations are at a much greater risk of contracting COVID-19 due to the lack of comprehensive information about risk management. By partnering with global health initiatives and health programs, host countries can work to establish accessible and affordable resources that combat existing communication barriers such as language, cultural competency, technology, and discrimination. Management Sciences for Health (MSH), a nonprofit organization partnering with governments and private sectors globally to build stronger health systems, has worked with The Rockefeller Foundation to prepare COVID-19 diagnostic resources including interactive dashboards and landscape analysis for low-income countries.[57] By establishing partnerships with organizations such as MSH, host countries can disseminate public health information regarding contagious diseases in diverse ways, helping to strengthen their healthcare systems. In addition to the safety threats posed by the living conditions at refugee camps, communication barriers make risk management even more important, but difficult. However, by partnering with NGOs, private sectors, and local communities, host country governments can work to eliminate communication barriers with risk assessment, management, and communication that meet the needs of refugees.

Overall, the inability of refugees to stay healthy and safe has been a problem for their communities and their host country's governments for years. However, the lack of comprehendible resources and high cost of healthcare pose a greater threat for refugee populations as nations are working toward combating a global health crisis. To prevent an outbreak of COVID-19 and future communicable viruses, health communication must be improved to account for the various communication differences discussed. Language, culture, gender, discrimination, education, access to technology, and health literacy are all variables that prevent health-care providers from providing adequate and accessible treatment for refugee populations, further increasing their vulnerability. These health communication barriers must be addressed and resolved to ensure the safety and survival of millions globally.

Recommendations

To combat the challenges brought upon by the COVID-19 pandemic, new implementation methods regarding dissemination of diversely understood public health information must be prepared and readily distributed. The threat of the COVID-19 pandemic must prepare governmental and healthcare agencies to deal with future global health threats. Government funding must be provided to healthcare agencies to make infographics and health literacy guidelines in a magnitude of languages and formats to serve all people.

The governments of refugee host countries must protect susceptible populations by providing accessible health care that meets the cultural needs of refugees. Healthcare providers should be trained with cultural and racial training to eliminate the risk of discrimination against migrant patients. This training should prepare doctors and healthcare service providers with knowledge of how to treat their patients without judgment of their gender, culture, or religion. Racial and implicit bias training will improve the quality of care as well as increase trust between the patient and physician, influencing patients to share their health concerns more openly regarding illnesses and symptoms.[58]

Healthcare clinics and facilities should be more accessible for those living at refugee camps and should provide affordable treatment for pre-existing illnesses. An assessment conducted by Truelove and colleagues suggests that with support and collaboration from governmental and healthcare agencies, the repurposing and emergence of cholera treatment centers and accessible psychological treatment for those suffering from depression and PTSD could lead to improvement in the overall health of the refugee population.[59] Providing treatment for pre-existing conditions, including both communicable and noncommunicable illnesses, will better equip refugee populations to combat the symptoms of novel viruses such as COVID-19.

Government and non-profit organizations must guarantee that refugees have access to timely and accurate information in their native languages regarding COVID-19 and the location of health facilities. This information should be prepared in various forms including both written and pictorial, shared both virtually and physically. Risk communication should be available to refugee communities regardless of their economic status, education level, or native language. Comprehendible information about social isolation, the importance of sanitation, usage of masks, and common COVID-19 symptoms, will equip communities with information necessary to protect themselves and their families from contracting and spreading the virus.

Telecommunication and cell service should be readily available in refugee communities to allow the spread of public health information and data. The usage of platforms such as Facebook and WhatsApp among the refugee population of Cox's Bazar can help reduce language and cultural communication barriers faced by the population.[60] The re-establishment of cell service by the Bangladeshi government will allow risk communication to increase in ways more likely to be understood by the refugee populations. Those who can afford mobile phones will have access to public health information in their native language and will be able to share it with others in their community.[61] The increased usage of mobile phones and social media has allowed for a timely and internationally available network of communication, one that should be utilized among vulnerable communities.

Rigorous efforts on risk assessment and management should receive increased attention and funding. Government agencies must prepare their healthcare systems to assess the health climate of vulnerable populations and treat those with pre-existing conditions. Once these risks are analyzed, proper actions should be taken to prepare refugee populations with public health information. Through partnerships between global health organizations and government agencies, the creation and dissemination of public health information that meets the communication needs of these populations will be encouraged. As the threat of communicable viruses has damaged the stability of most nations, risk management must be utilized to reduce the vulnerability of densely populated countries. Precautions must be taken to combat health communication barriers and ensure the safety and survival of millions of vulnerable lives.

Thank you, Anjali Mullor and Meshael Abusalem for review of the manuscript and editorial assistance.

Notes

1 *WHO Coronavirus Disease (COVID-19) Dashboard.* (2020). WHO. https://covid19.who.int/
2 Lee, S., Wehrli, Z., U.S. Global Leadership Coalition. (2020, December 14). COVID-19 Brief: Impact on Refugees –. USGLC. https://www.usglc.org/coronavirus/refugees/
3 Lee, S., Wehrli, Z., U.S. Global Leadership Coalition. (2020, December 14). COVID-19 Brief: Impact on Refugees –. USGLC. https://www.usglc.org/coronavirus/refugees/

4 Reid, K. (2020, June 11). Syrian refugee crisis: Facts, FAQs, and how to help. https://www.worldvision.org/refugees-news-stories/syrian-refugee-cri-sis-facts#:~:text=The%20majority%20of%20Syria's%205.6,limited%20access%20to%20basic%20services

5 Lee, S., Wehrli, Z., U.S. Global Leadership Coalition. (2020, December 14). COVID-19 Brief: Impact on Refugees –. USGLC. https://www.usglc.org/coronavirus/refugees/

6 Mahmood, H. N., Ibrahim, H., Goessmann, K., Ismail, A. A., & Neuner, F. (2019). Post-traumatic stress disorder and depression among Syrian refugees residing in the Kurdistan region of Iraq. *Conflict and Health*, 13(1). https://doi.org/10.1186/s13031-019-0238-5

7 Baker, A. (2014, March 14). *The Cost of War: Syria, Three Years On*. Time. http://time.com/24741/the-cost-of-war-syria-three-years-on/

8 United Nations High Commissioner for Refugees. (2020). *South Sudan emergency*. UNHCR. https://www.unhcr.org/en-us/south-sudan-emer-gency.html

9 *South Sudan Refugee Crisis: Aid, Statistics and News*. (2020). UNHCR. https://www.unrefugees.org/emergencies/south-sudan/

10 BBC News. (2020, January 23). *Myanmar Rohingya: What you need to know about the crisis*. https://www.bbc.com/news/world-asia-41566561

11 Bhatia, A., Mahmud, A., Fuller, A., Shin, R., Rahman, A., Shatil, T., ... Balsari, S. (2018). The Rohingya in Cox's Bazar: When the Stateless Seek Refuge. *Health and Human Rights Journal*, 20(2), 105–122.

12 Islam, M. M., & Yunus, M. D. Y. (2020). Rohingya refugees at high risk of COVID-19 in Bangladesh. *The Lancet Global Health*, 8(8), e993–e994. https://doi.org/10.1016/s2214-109x(20)30282-5

13 Steinberg, D. I. (2020). Myanmar | Facts, Geography, & History. Encyclope-dia Britannica. https://www.britannica.com/place/Myanmar

14 Khan, M. N., Islam, M. M., & Rahman, M. M. (2020). Risks of COVID19 outbreaks in Rohingya refugee camps in Bangladesh. *Public Health in Prac-tice*, 1, 100018. https://doi.org/10.1016/j.puhip.2020.100018

15 Cousins, S. (2020). Bangladesh's COVID-19 testing criticised. *The Lancet*, 396(10251), 591. https://doi.org/10.1016/s0140-6736(20)31819-5

16 *6 Months later: How has COVID-19 impacted the life of the first Rohingya patient?*. (2020, November 12). World Health Organization. https://www.who.int/bangladesh/news/detail/12-11-2020-6-months-later-how-has-covid-19-impacted-the-life-of-the-first-rohingya-patient

17 Khan, M. N., Islam, M. M., & Rahman, M. M. (2020). Risks of COVID19 outbreaks in Rohingya refugee camps in Bangladesh. *Public Health in Prac-tice*, 1, 100018. https://doi.org/10.1016/j.puhip.2020.100018

18 Cousins, S. (2020). Bangladesh's COVID-19 testing criticised. *The Lancet*, 396(10251), 591. https://doi.org/10.1016/s0140-6736(20)31819-5

19 Bhatia, A., Mahmud, A., Fuller, A., Shin, R., Rahman, A., Shatil, T., ... Balsari, S. (2018). The Rohingya in Cox's Bazar: When the Stateless Seek Refuge. *Health and Human Rights Journal*, 20(2), 105–122.

20 Islam, M. M., & Yunus, M. D. Y. (2020). Rohingya refugees at high risk of COVID-19 in Bangladesh. *The Lancet Global Health*, 8(8), e993–e994. https://doi.org/10.1016/s2214-109x(20)30282-5

21 Khan, M. N., Islam, M. M., & Rahman, M. M. (2020). Risks of COVID19 outbreaks in Rohingya refugee camps in Bangladesh. *Public Health in Prac-tice*, 1, 100018. https://doi.org/10.1016/j.puhip.2020.100018

22 Banik, R., Rahman, M., Hossain, M. M., Sikder, M. T., & Gozal, D. (2020). COVID-19 pandemic and Rohingya refugees in Bangladesh: What are the

major concerns? *Global Public Health*, *15*(10), 1578–1581. https://doi.org/1 0.1080/17441692.2020.1812103

23 Islam, M. M., & Nuzhath, T. (2018). Health risks of Rohingya refugee population in Bangladesh: a call for global attention. *Journal of Global Health*, *8*(2). https://doi.org/10.7189/jogh.08.020309

24 Islam, M. M., & Yunus, M. D. Y. (2020). Rohingya refugees at high risk of COVID-19 in Bangladesh. *The Lancet Global Health*, *8*(8), e993–e994. https://doi.org/10.1016/s2214-109x(20)30282-5

25 United Nations High Commissioner for Refugees. (2020). *Public Health during COVID-19.* UNHCR. https://www.unhcr.org/en-us/health-covid-19.html

26 Gregório, M.J., Irving, S., Teixeira, D., Ferro, G., Graça, P., & Freitas, G. (2021). The national food and nutrition strategy for the Portuguese COVID-19 response. *European Journal of Clinical Nutrition*. https://doi.org/10.1038/s41430-020-00818-w

27 Mahmood, H. N., Ibrahim, H., Goessmann, K., Ismail, A. A., & Neuner, F. (2019). Post-traumatic stress disorder and depression among Syrian refugees residing in the Kurdistan region of Iraq. *Conflict and Health*, *13*(1). https://doi.org/10.1186/s13031-019-0238-5

28 Reid, K. (2020, June 11). Syrian refugee crisis: Facts, FAQs, and how to help. https://www.worldvision.org/refugees-news-stories/syrian-refugee-crisis-facts#:~:text=The%20majority%20of%20Syria's%205.6,limited%20access%20to%20basic%20services

29 Janati, N., & Taylor, E., (2017, March 6). *New Study Documents Psychological Horrors of Six-Year War on Syrian Children.* https://www.savethechildren.org/us/about-us/media-and-news/2017-press-releases/new-study-documents-psychological-horrors-of-six-year-war-on-syr#:~:text=(March%206%2C%202017)%20%E2%80%94,today%20by%20Save%20the%20Children

30 Baker, A. (2014, March 14). *The Cost of War: Syria, Three Years On.* Time. http://time.com/24741/the-cost-of-war-syria-three-years-on/

31 Islam, M. M., & Nuzhath, T. (2018). Health risks of Rohingya refugee population in Bangladesh: a call for global attention. *Journal of Global Health*, *8*(2). https://doi.org/10.7189/jogh.08.020309

32 Mahmood, H. N., Ibrahim, H., Goessmann, K., Ismail, A. A., & Neuner, F. (2019). Post-traumatic stress disorder and depression among Syrian refugees residing in the Kurdistan region of Iraq. *Conflict and Health*, *13*(1). https://doi.org/10.1186/s13031-019-0238-5

33 Least Protected, Most Affected: Migrants and refugees facing extraordinary risks during the COVID-19 pandemic. (2020). International Federation of Red Cross and Red Crescent Societies.

34 Islam, M. M., & Nuzhath, T. (2018). Health risks of Rohingya refugee population in Bangladesh: a call for global attention. *Journal of Global Health*, *8*(2). https://doi.org/10.7189/jogh.08.020309

35 Bartovic, J., Datta, S. S., Severoni, S., & D'Anna, V. (2021). *Ensuring equitable access to vaccines for refugees and migrants during the COVID-19 pandemic.* World Health Organization. https://www.who.int/bulletin/volumes/99/1/20-267690/en/

36 Least Protected, Most Affected: Migrants and refugees facing extraordinary risks during the COVID-19 pandemic. (2020). International Federation of Red Cross and Red Crescent Societies.

37 Nezafat Maldonado, B. M., Collins, J., Blundell, H. J., & Singh, L. (2020). Engaging the vulnerable: A rapid review of public health communication

aimed at migrants during the COVID-19 pandemic in Europe. *Journal of Migration and Health*, 1–2, 100004. https://doi.org/10.1016/j.jmh.2020.100004

38 *Access and allocation: how will there be fair and equitable allocation of limited supplies?*. (2021, January 12). World Health Organization. https://www.who.int/news-room/feature-stories/detail/access-and-allocation-how-will-there-be-fair-and-equitable-allocation-of-limited-supplies

39 Nezafat Maldonado, B. M., Collins, J., Blundell, H. J., & Singh, L. (2020). Engaging the vulnerable: A rapid review of public health communication aimed at migrants during the COVID-19 pandemic in Europe. *Journal of Migration and Health*, 1–2, 100004. https://doi.org/10.1016/j.jmh.2020.100004

40 Least Protected, Most Affected: Migrants and refugees facing extraordinary risks during the COVID-19 pandemic. (2020). International Federation of Red Cross and Red Crescent Societies.

41 Least Protected, Most Affected: Migrants and refugees facing extraordinary risks during the COVID-19 pandemic. (2020). International Federation of Red Cross and Red Crescent Societies.

42 Cone, D. (2020, May 7). *Gender Matters: COVID-19's Outsized Impact on Displaced Women and Girls*. Refugees International. https://www.refugeesinternational.org/reports/2020/5/4/gender-matters-covid-19s-outsized-impact-on-displaced-women-and-girls

43 Ahmed, R. (2018). Challenges of migration and culture in a public health communication context. *Journal of Public Health Research*, all. https://doi.org/10.4081/jphr.2018.1508

44 *Access and allocation: how will there be fair and equitable allocation of limited supplies?*. (2021, January 12). World Health Organization. https://www.who.int/news-room/feature-stories/detail/access-and-allocation-how-will-there-be-fair-and-equitable-allocation-of-limited-supplies

45 Ahmed, R. (2018). Challenges of migration and culture in a public health communication context. *Journal of Public Health Research*, all. https://doi.org/10.4081/jphr.2018.1508

46 *COVID-19: Access to full mobile data and telecommunications in Myanmar and Bangladesh is essential to save lives, say 26 major aid groups - Bangladesh*. (2020, April 16). [Press release]. Relief Web. https://reliefweb.int/report/bangladesh/covid-19-access-full-mobile-data-and-telecommunications-myanmar-and-bangladesh

47 Sanchez-Paramo, C., & Legovini, A. (2021, January 12). Using social media to change norms and behaviors at scale. World Bank Blogs. https://blogs.worldbank.org/voices/using-social-media-change-norms-and-behaviors-scale

48 Least Protected, Most Affected: Migrants and refugees facing extraordinary risks during the COVID-19 pandemic. (2020). International Federation of Red Cross and Red Crescent Societies.

49 United Nations High Commissioner for Refugees. (2020). *Public Health during COVID-19*. UNHCR. https://www.unhcr.org/en-us/health-covid-19.html

50 Khan, M. N., Islam, M. M., & Rahman, M. M. (2020). Risks of COVID19 outbreaks in Rohingya refugee camps in Bangladesh. *Public Health in Practice*, 1, 100018. https://doi.org/10.1016/j.puhip.2020.100018

51 *COVID-19: Access to full mobile data and telecommunications in Myanmar and Bangladesh is essential to save lives, say 26 major aid groups - Bangladesh*. (2020, April 16). [Press release]. Relief Web. https://reliefweb.

int/report/bangladesh/covid-19-access-full-mobile-data-and-telecommuni-
cations-myanmar-and-bangladesh

52 Least Protected, Most Affected: Migrants and refugees facing extraordinary risks during the COVID-19 pandemic. (2020). International Federation of Red Cross and Red Crescent Societies.

53 Cone, D. (2020, May 7). *Gender Matters: COVID-19's Outsized Impact on Displaced Women and Girls.* Refugees International.https://www. refugeesinternational.org/reports/2020/5/4/gender-matters-covid-19s-outsized-impact-on-displaced-women-and-girls

54 Islam, M. M., & Yunus, M. D. Y. (2020). Rohingya refugees at high risk of COVID-19 in Bangladesh. *The Lancet Global Health, 8*(8), e993–e994. https://doi.org/10.1016/s2214-109x(20)30282-5

55 Least Protected, Most Affected: Migrants and refugees facing extraordinary risks during the COVID-19 pandemic. (2020). International Federation of Red Cross and Red Crescent Societies.

56 Bartovic, J., Datta, S. S., Severoni, S., & D'Anna, V. (2021). *Ensuring equitable access to vaccines for refugees and migrants during the COVID-19 pandemic.* World Health Organization. https://www.who.int/bulletin/ volumes/99/1/20-267690/en/

57 *Covid-19 Diagnostic Resources for Low- and Middle-Income Countries.* (2020, December 28). The Rockefeller Foundation. https://www. rockefellerfoundation.org/lmic-covid-19-diagnostic-resources/?utm_ source=MSH+Newsletter&utm_campaign=45dabacb6b-EMAIL_CAM-PAIGN_2017_04_GHSAC_COPY_01&utm_medium=email&utm_term= 0_869a96a773-45dabacb6b-120491829

58 Least Protected, Most Affected: Migrants and refugees facing extraordinary risks during the COVID-19 pandemic. (2020). International Federation of Red Cross and Red Crescent Societies.

59 Truelove, S., Abrahim, O., Altare, C., Lauer, S. A., Grantz, K. H., Azman, A. S., & Spiegel, P. (2020). The potential impact of COVID-19 in refugee camps in Bangladesh and beyond: A modeling study. *PLoS Medicine, 17*(6). https://doi.org/10.1371/journal.pmed.1003144

60 Sanchez-Paramo, C., & Legovini, A. (2021, January 12). Using social media to change norms and behaviors at scale. World Bank Blogs. https://blogs.world-bank.org/voices/using-social-media-change-norms-and-behaviors-scale

Recommended Readings

Ahmed, R. (2018). Challenges of migration and culture in a public health communication context. *Journal of Public Health Research.* https://doi.org/10.4081/ jphr.2018.1508

Centers for Disease Control and Prevention. (2021, January 14). *Refugee Health Profiles.* Centers for Disease Control and Prevention. https://www.cdc.gov/im-migrantrefugeehealth/profiles/index.html.

Islam, M. M., & Nuzhath, T. (2018). Health risks of Rohingya refugee population in Bangladesh: a call for global attention. *Journal of Global Health, 8*(2). https://doi.org/10.7189/jogh.08.020309

Least Protected, Most Affected: Migrants and refugees facing extraordinary risks during the COVID-19 pandemic. (2020). International Federation of Red Cross and Red Crescent Societies.

Spoerri, M., Ullah Y., & Nwangwu, C. (2020, July 27). *The Rohingya and COVID-19: Towards an inclusive and sustainable policy response.* Independent Diplomat. https://reliefweb.int/sites/reliefweb.int/files/resources/The%20 Rohingya%20and%20COVID-19%20-%20Towards%20an%20inclusive%20 and%20sustainable%20policy%20response.pdf

References

6 Months later: How has COVID-19 impacted the life of the first Rohingya patient?. (2020, November 12). World Health Organization. https://www.who. int/bangladesh/news/detail/12-11-2020-6-months-later-how-has-covid-19-impacted-the-life-of-the-first-rohingya-patient

Access and allocation: How will there be fair and equitable allocation of limited supplies?. (2021, January 12). World Health Organization. https:// www.who.int/news-room/feature-stories/detail/access-and-allocation-how-will-there-be-fair-and-equitable-allocation-of-limited-supplies

Ahmed, R. (2018). Challenges of migration and culture in a public health communication context. *Journal of Public Health Research.* https://doi. org/10.4081/jphr.2018.1508

Baker, A. (2014, March 14). *The cost of war: Syria, three years on.* Time. http:// time.com/24741/the-cost-of-war-syria-three-years-on/

Banik, R., Rahman, M., Hossain, M. M., Sikder, M. T., & Gozal, D. (2020). COVID-19 pandemic and Rohingya refugees in Bangladesh: What are the major concerns? *Global Public Health*, 15(10), 1578–1581. https://doi.org/ 10.1080/17441692.2020.1812103

Bartovic, J., Datta, S. S., Severoni, S., & D'Anna, V. (2021). *Ensuring equitable access to vaccines for refugees and migrants during the COVID-19 pandemic.* World Health Organization. https://www.who.int/bulletin/ volumes/99/1/20-267690/en/

BBC News. (2020, January 23). *Myanmar Rohingya: What you need to know about the crisis.* https://www.bbc.com/news/world-asia-41566561

Bhatia, A., Mahmud, A., Fuller, A., Shin, R., Rahman, A., Shatil, T., … Balsari, S. (2018). The Rohingya in Cox's Bazar: When the stateless seek refuge. *Health and Human Rights Journal*, 20(2), 105–122.

Cone, D. (2020, May 7). *Gender matters: COVID-19's outsized impact on displaced women and girls.* Refugees International. https:// www.refugeesinternational.org/reports/2020/5/4/gender-matters-covid-19s-outsized-impact-on-displaced-women-and-girls

Cousins, S. (2020). Bangladesh's COVID-19 testing criticised. *The Lancet*, 396(10251), 591. https://doi.org/10.1016/s0140-6736(20)31819-5

COVID-19: Access to full mobile data and telecommunications in Myanmar and Bangladesh is essential to save lives, say 26 major aid groups - Bangladesh. (2020, April 16). [Press release]. Relief Web. https://reliefweb.int/ report/bangladesh/covid-19-access-full-mobile-data-and-telecommunications-myanmar-and-bangladesh

Covid-19 Diagnostic Resources for Low- and Middle-Income Countries. (2020, December 28). The Rockefeller Foundation. https://www. rockefellerfoundation.org/lmic-covid-19-diagnostic-resources/?utm_ source=MSH+Newsletter&utm_campaign=45dabacb6b-EMAIL_CAM-

PAIGN_2017_04_GHSAC_COPY_01&utm_medium=email&utm_term=
0_869a96a773-45dabacb6b-120491829

Gregório, M. J., Irving, S., Teixeira, D., Ferro, G., Graça, P., & Freitas, G. (2021).
The national food and nutrition strategy for the Portuguese COVID-19 response. *European Journal of Clinical Nutrition.* https://doi.org/10.1038/
s41430-020-00818-w

Islam, M. M., & Nuzhath, T. (2018). Health risks of Rohingya refugee population in Bangladesh: a call for global attention. *Journal of Global Health, 8*(2).
https://doi.org/10.7189/jogh.08.020309

Islam, M. M., & Yunus, M. D. Y. (2020). Rohingya refugees at high risk of
COVID-19 in Bangladesh. *The Lancet Global Health, 8*(8), e993–e994.
https://doi.org/10.1016/s2214-109x(20)30282-5

Janati, N., & Taylor, E., (2017, March 6). *New study documents psychological
horrors of six-year war on Syrian children.* https://www.savethechildren.org/
us/about-us/media-and-news/2017-press-releases/new-study-documents-psy-
chological-horrors-of-six-year-war-onsyr#:~:text=(March%206%2C%20
2017)%20%E2%80%94,today%20by%20Save%20the%20Children

Khan, M. N., Islam, M. M., & Rahman, M. M. (2020). Risks of COVID19 outbreaks in Rohingya refugee camps in Bangladesh. *Public Health in Practice,
1,* 100018. https://doi.org/10.1016/j.puhip.2020.100018

*Least protected, most affected: Migrants and refugees facing extraordinary
risks during the COVID-19 pandemic.* (2020). International Federation of
Red Cross and Red Crescent Societies.

Lee, S., Wehrli, Z., & U.S. Global Leadership Coalition. (2020, December
14). COVID-19 Brief: Impact on refugees. USGLC. https://www.usglc.org/
coronavirus/refugees/

Mahmood, H. N., Ibrahim, H., Goessmann, K., Ismail, A. A., & Neuner, F.
(2019). Post-traumatic stress disorder and depression among Syrian refugees
residing in the Kurdistan region of Iraq. *Conflict and Health, 13*(1). https://
doi.org/10.1186/s13031-019-0238-5

Nezafat Maldonado, B. M., Collins, J., Blundell, H. J., & Singh, L. (2020). Engaging the vulnerable: A rapid review of public health communication aimed at
migrants during the COVID-19 pandemic in Europe. *Journal of Migration and
Health, 1–2,* 100004. https://doi.org/10.1016/j.jmh.2020.100004

Reid, K. (2020, June 11). Syrian refugee crisis: Facts, FAQs, and how to help.
https://www.worldvision.org/refugees-news-stories/syrian-refugee-cri-
sis-facts#:~:text=The%20majority%20of%20Syria's%205.6,limited%20
access%20to%20basic%20services

Sanchez- Paramo, C., & Legovini, A. (2021, January 12). Using social media to
change norms and behaviors at scale. World Bank Blogs. https://blogs.world-
bank.org/voices/using-social-media-change-norms-and-behaviors-scale

South Sudan Refugee Crisis: Aid, Statistics and News. (2020). UNHCR. https://
www.unrefugees.org/emergencies/south-sudan/

Steinberg, D. I. (2020). *Myanmar | Facts, Geography, & History.* Encyclopedia
Britannica. https://www.britannica.com/place/Myanmar

Truelove, S., Abrahim, O., Altare, C., Lauer, S. A., Grantz, K. H., Azman, A.
S., & Spiegel, P. (2020). The potential impact of COVID-19 in refugee
camps in Bangladesh and beyond: A modeling study. *PLoS Medicine, 17*(6).
https://doi.org/10.1371/journal.pmed.1003144

United Nations High Commissioner for Refugees. (2020). *Public Health during COVID-19*. UNHCR. https://www.unhcr.org/en-us/health-covid-19.html
United Nations High Commissioner for Refugees. (2020b). *South Sudan emergency*. UNHCR. https://www.unhcr.org/en-us/south-sudan-emergency.html
WHO Coronavirus Disease (COVID-19) Dashboard. (2020). WHO. https://covid19.who.int

13 Communicative Health Promotion for Refugee Children in Uganda

David Kaawa-Mafigiri, Francis Kato, Agnes Kyamulabi, Tamara Giles-Vernick, Ruth Kutalek, David Napier, and Eddie J. Walakira

Providing health care services to refugee children requires learning how to communicate to vulnerable populations and entails appreciating their expectations of the formal refugee support system and how they navigate it to access health care and maintain their health. We are guided by frameworks that advocate building trust among health care seekers and the relationship they have with the providers, in this case, the host community service providers. This chapter explores the ecosystem within which refugee children and their caretakers/parents gain access to health care in Uganda. This involves taking a holistic perspective of the person when examining lived experiences to understand the life circumstances they are facing and how these circumstances impact their health behavior. Some refugees are aware of where to get help regarding health care services. But many reports indicate a sense of being easily frustrated with the processes and related delays in service provision. To some, the health care seeking process feels like being 'tossed around' and reportedly contributes to them deciding against accessing care, as noted by two refugees:

> I am aware of the services I should be getting. Unfortunately, there is a lot of tossing especially at [Agency X]. [Agency X] is in charge of giving us documents that permit us to get services from public or formal organizations. They keep on telling us "come back tomorrow, come back next week, next month" eventually you get tired and stop following up support provision.
>
> (IDI_40-year-old male parent/caretaker Congolese Refugee)

> I live in a community that is highly dominated by refugees from different countries. But most of these refugees are in fear; they don't know the government's plans towards refugees. Personally I suspect they might poison us.
>
> (IDI_27-year-old female Congolese Refugee)

DOI: 10.4324/9781003230243-13

This outward frustration has an implication on the wellbeing of children who mostly depend on adult wisdom and decision for whatever is needed to address a health concern. At the same time, while some refugees may report awareness of the existence of points of health services support, a large number of refugees still do not know what services are within their immediate environment.

Additionally, unlike in refugee settlements, where attestation cards will easily facilitate health care especially during the clinical encounter, the experience for the urban (child) refugee can be different when navigating care-seeking. For instance, some refugees are very concerned about the behavior of some health service providers who reportedly may make solicitations for money on services known to be for 'free of charge'.

> There is a lot of corruption among these organisations that provide support to refugees e.g. if you want to see the chief for instance in charge of education, before seeing him/her, you're requested to pay something first or else you're tossed around. That's why you find refugees who are better off benefiting again from the service or support provision compared to those refugees who are poorer because the poorer ones have nothing to offer to the providers.
>
> (IDI_40-year-old male Congolese Refugee)

> [There is] selective provision of services e.g. providers target only those that are able to give kickbacks [unofficial payments]. The only trusted providers are the health workers at the [CITY] Health Center IV because they normally work on us with one heart.
>
> (IDI_22-year-old, female Somali Refugee)

It should be noted that what is regarded as corruption such as in the case above, is sometimes actually a known service user's cost-sharing strategy where service users pay out of pocket to bridge the gap in funding for public health services (Twimukye et al., 2017; Kavuma, Turyakira, Bills, & Kalanzi, 2020). Nonetheless, this may impact negatively on the health of the refugee as it prevents them from reaching out for services at a health facility (Gumisiriza, 2018; Nara, Banura, & Foster, 2020; Schoemaker, Baslan, Pon, & Dell, 2021). Such perceptions also influence the refugees' trust in the health care system and may negatively impact children's health care. Therefore, there should be a deliberate endeavor to work with other stakeholders to address the root causes of corruption. Any strategy to communicating health should be alive to the drivers of corrupt tendencies in any service provision. In cases where cost-sharing applies, it ought to be made clearly known to avoid misperceptions. It threatens the loss of trust in service delivery and may negatively impact any decision to reach out for services especially for the most vulnerable who have so little to facilitate access and use health or health-related services.

In this chapter, we begin by providing background literature on the refugee context and refugee health in Uganda. We discuss the influence of health communication on the health care-seeking patterns of parents and caretakers for their refugee children, and the means through which it happens. Additionally, we discuss what the current state of health communication implies for their vulnerability, exposure to health risk and consequences—a triple challenge in public health. We then discuss communicating health and the current and future implications for promoting the health of refugee children in a constrained environment. We conducted a vulnerability assessment study of urban refugees as part of the European Commission-funded project titled "A Global Social Sciences Network for Infectious Threats and Anti-Microbial Resistance (SONAR-Global)." One central activity of SONAR-Global is to adapt one vulnerability assessment (VA) tool[1] and appropriate community engagement (CE) models among multiple partners in preparation and response to epidemics.

As part of this activity, Makerere University with support from members from the SONAR-Global coordination team, and partners (UCL, MUW) conducted a Vulnerability Assessment (VA) in February-March 2020, just before the COVID-19 pandemic, in the five divisions of Kampala Capital City Authority (KCCA) namely: Central, Kawempe, Makindye, Nakawa, and Rubaga divisions. Ninety-nine in-depth interviews among residents originating from five different countries and living in urban and peri-urban zones within the city were conducted. Each of these divisions comprises low-income settlements (zones) with the highest population density in KCCA. More importantly, these zones are home to the largest population of urban migrant workers and international refugees who make their way to the city in Uganda (living outside government settlement camps). Similarly, these zones rank lowest in terms of poverty and SES indicators in the city.

Refugee Children in Uganda

Conflicts and wars in the Central and East African region have resulted in the widespread displacement of populations for years. Many governments and communities in the East African region have kept their borders and homes open, demonstrating remarkable generosity to their neighbors seeking safety from violence and persecution in line with long-standing traditions of hospitality and asylum. According to the UNHCR, by 1994 more than half of any refugee population were children, meaning that children likely face the biggest impact of conflict and the attendant displacement. These children are forced to flee, leaving behind their homes, communities, schools, friends, aspirations, sense of security and, often, their childhoods (UNHCR, 2014).

Interactions with displaced children reveal daily struggles faced in trying to live a normal life, particularly being deprived of their rights and violated. Their resilience and strength are an inspiration to those responding to their needs. Separation from family members, difficulty accessing basic services, and increased poverty make it more likely that children will get married early, work before the legal age or in dangerous and exploitative conditions, drop out of school or face violence in their schools. They also face risks of detention, trafficking, and other forms of exploitation during their displacement (UNHCR, 2014). The inadequate access to health services and the poor living conditions can lead to the deterioration of children's health. For these reasons, the United Nations High Commissioner for Refugees has adopted a policy on refugee children to improve their quality of life and enhance their protection and care (UNHCR, 1994).

Worldwide, Uganda is considered the third top refugee-hosting nation,[2] with more than a million refugees living in 11 camps.[3] The enormous influx of refugees is due to a combination of factors in Uganda and in neighboring countries: conflicts (war and violence), economic crisis, political instability, and most substantially, Uganda's 'friendly' policies, which provide rights to refugees: rights to education, work, private property, healthcare and other basic social services.[4] Most of the refugees in Uganda are from neighboring countries; 1,053,598 from South Sudan, 276,570 from DR Congo, 40,497 from Burundi, and a relatively minimum 37,193 from Somalia and 37,015 from other countries (Ethiopia, Eritrea, etc.).[5] The likelihood that Uganda will continue experiencing refugee influx remains pertinent, as the country continues to implement its open-door policy. By the end of 2018, the refugee population was expected to grow to over 1.8 million.[6] Like elsewhere in the region, most refugees in Uganda are hosted close to international borders (with a limited number recognized as urban refugees), in fragile communities facing poverty and unemployment, deficits in human capital development and social service delivery, and limited access to basic infrastructure. In some of these host communities, the refugee population outnumbers their hosts. Refugee-hosting districts are now recognized under the vulnerability criteria of Uganda's National Development Plan 2015/216–2019/2020 (NDP II), making them a priority for development intervention, targeting both refugees and host communities—including multi-sectoral and coordinated violence prevention, response and child protection services.

Refugees and Rights to Health

The Government of Uganda (GoU) is committed to the New York Declaration for Refugees and Migrants adopted by the United Nations General Assembly in 2016 and the Global Compact on Refugees that urges society to stand in solidarity with refugees and share responsibility and burden for hosting and supporting refugees. Translating these commitments into practice, Uganda implements the Comprehensive Refugee Response Framework (CRRF). As part of the CRRF, the Ministry of Health (MoH) in Uganda developed the Health Sector Integrated Refugee Response Plan (HSIRRP) to ensure equitable and well-coordinated access to health services for refugees and host communities (MoH, 2019). The CRRF like the other policy documents such as the Refugee Act 2006 and Refugee Regulations 2010 also provides space for refugees to access the same public services as nationals, including health services using a comprehensive approach where the whole society is involved in responding and finding solutions to refugee concerns (ibid). Whereas Uganda commits to hosting refugees, the country already faces constraints in delivering satisfactory health services to its own citizens. The additional need from the large numbers of refugees places a higher burden on capacities and resources of the state and host communities, most especially for health service delivery (HSIRRP 2019/2024).[7] Given these constraints, health communication should be sensitive to the dynamics of vulnerable populations like urban refugees. Tailoring health communication to the refugee context would add value to the strategies and efforts to promote the health of refugee children, as it increases effectiveness in terms of their health care and health care decisions (Johnson et al., 2004; Carroll et al., 2007; Juang et al., 2018; Bulled, 2016). This highlights the importance of health communication in refugee contexts.

Health communication is considered to be a practice of communicating promotional health information. Possible strategies to realize this include public health campaigns, health education, and interaction between health workers and patients. This kind of communication helps educate people about specific health issues and influences audiences to adopt healthier behaviors. They usually aim at impacting large audiences and require considerable resources and organizational partnerships.[8] Public health experts recognize health communication as vital to public health programs that address disease prevention, health promotion, and quality of life. It can make important contributions to promote and improve the health of individuals, communities, and society. The U.S. Department of Health and Human Services outlines critical ways health communication can enlighten people. In addition to increasing awareness about a health issue or solution, it can also shift social norms by influencing attitudes. For example, health communication campaigns have helped to reduce the stigma around HIV and AIDS, making it easier to convince people to get tested.

The HSIRRP aligns the refugee health response to the National Health Policy and Health Sector Development Plan and is rooted in values and principles of integration, equity, universal coverage, government leadership, mutual respect, and efficiency. It provides credibility to the use of the established decentralized health system and provides for a strengthened coordination mechanism at national, district or municipality, and sub-county levels. However, its role in supporting health communication both with parents/caretakers and among children in a refugee setting is not known. Health communication is ideally more critical in situations where the health services provision is constrained by resources because it will help promote good health and reduce the need for treatment.

Communicating to Refugees and Health of Refugee Children in Uganda: Reflections from the Vulnerability Assessment

Health communication as a way of impacting individuals, communities, and system health knowledge and practices follows different strategies and means in Uganda. The analysis of the VA data revealed that communication channels and forms really matter in the context of refugee experiences. For a long time, key health messages have been delivered through community sensitizations and dialogues. Educational institutions have also been leveraged upon as an avenue for improving health knowledge and health practices for both children and adult populations. Education in itself serves both the means to but also has direct health outcomes. For children whether refugee, migrant or otherwise, schools play a big role in promoting health behavior especially preventive but also knowledge on the relevance of seeking care. However, many refugee children especially in urban settings like Kampala, may be absent, abscond or drop out of school because their parents or host authorities are unable to meet the school requirements including tuition. These children are well aware of this danger.

> *In general, I do not think that there is enough help for people available where you live. Not really, in terms of basic needs like education because many of my fellow refugees without supporting families are lacking in this aspect. As for me, I get information about staying healthy from school. You know I go to XXXX – [School name left out due to confidentiality]. The Education itself that I get from school like science has all information on staying healthy e.g., sports, nutrition etc. Yes, the information is helpful because you get to know how to protect and prevent yourself from falling sick.*

(IDI_17-year-old male Eritrean refugee)

The children are therefore disadvantaged from benefiting from the health promotion work of the school setting. It means that other alternative strategies should be considered to reach the affected population if health is to be improved. Yet, this may also be hampered by other factors.

Language, Comprehension, and Adaptations

Many refugee households may have an interest in getting health information but remain challenged by the level of comprehension of the language used. It is not unusual that communication is insensitive to the language abilities of the refugee population (Chen, et al., 2018; Desai & Pandya, 2013; Mwenyango, 2020). Those who have managed to make adaptations to customs and traditions of the host communities including the language testify of a positive impact on their health.

> *By adapting to the customs and traditions of Ugandans e.g., many Somalis now speak Luganda (the most widely spoken local dialect) and eat their traditional food like matooke. To me, I think knowing how to speak Luganda is a bonus because it has helped us to survive in a foreign land.*
>
> (IDI_29-year-old male Somali Refugee)

However, several participants in the VA noted that they hear and see information about health from different media channels. Even then, for those who may hear or see other media channels, the language difference remains a constraint. One participant commenting about Ebola and the COVID-19 pandemic confessed that they have heard of the disease on television but could not comprehend the information due to language difficulties.

> *I heard about Ebola and COVID-19 from a Television though I couldn't understand the language. But I read from the internet that there is a disease called coronavirus which is very dangerous. They were saying we shouldn't touch infected people.*
>
> (IDI_22-year-old male Somali Refugee)

Others navigate the difficulties in language by resorting to communication channels back in their home countries, access through social media platforms, or just listening to information from their neighbors.

> *I hear about health events from my neighbors, news on Somali TV and YouTube. I heard and watched epidemics like Ebola that are so dangerous because they kill people instantly. So they were advising us to be very careful with our health.*
>
> (IDI_34-year-old female parent/caretaker, Somali refugee)

These various channels all carry implications regarding the content they carry and how easy it would be to determine the numerous interpretations that may emerge. In times of health emergencies, parents play a big role in ensuring the safety of their children. However, their role can only be effective if they are also equipped with the right information. Additionally, in urban settings where there are no de-marcated spaces for hosting refugees, many children live without any oversight or under the care of a formal organization. As such, it may be difficult to have targeted messaging for such refugees that reach their children. This is well represented by one participant who opined that:

> "[Health service] providers have to find means of working on lan-guage barrier because there could be some misinterpretation be-cause of not understanding each other".
> (IDI _19-year-old female, Somali refugee)

The effect of inadequate or lack of the (appropriate) information in health is well known. People are less likely to take the needed precau-tions (Orom, et al., 2018), and parents may not tend well to their own children and may not ensure that they seek attention from a health ser-vice provider (Amuge et al., 2004; Cook, Appleton, & Wiggs, 2020).

The vulnerability assessment also revealed that some refugee parents hold suspicions about the intent of health service provision reflected by perceptions of possible malpractices.

> "Somalis that are a bit rich go to Case Hospital because they believe that this facility does not provide fake drugs. They rarely give out drugs from India. So for that kind of Somalis, they have all their trust in Case Hospital than any other health facility. But of course this is a facility for wealthy people".
> (IDI_19-year-old Female Somali refugee)

In one interview, one participant was concerned about possible poison-ing if they visited a health facility. This reflects poor trust in the existing care system, and the refugee community is aware of the downside of such a message.

> "They [health care providers] must find a way of relating with us [refugees) so that we gain trust in them. They should be on the same level with us, understand us than judging us. [...] learn how to treat refugees and to ensure that we get access to all services that we may need. Without that, would-be receivers of support are likely to miss out on support because of being suspicious of the providers.

Such mistrust in the health system can complicate health care access for refugee children, largely because they rely heavily on, and trust in health information that is provided to them by their parents (Al-subhi, Goldthorpe, Epton, Khanom, & Peters, 2020; Mwenyango &

Palattiyil, 2019). Without the parents getting to understand (well) the information, there is likely to be a persistent unawareness or possible misinformation about the prevailing condition, and may result delays to take appropriate steps and, in some cases, inappropriate steps may be taken. Ultimately, misinformation and the associated mistrust in the health system negatively impact the health of refugee children. Such concerns need to be reflected upon when communicating health with the refugee populations.

   Lack of knowledge about who has the responsibility to intervene also remains at large. In one conversation, when asked if he was aware of any organization with the responsibility to intervene in conditions of health emergencies, a participant bluntly noted that:

"I have no idea because I don't understand how Ugandan systems operates".

In such situations, awareness of communities of support for health among the refugee communities is important. The VA revealed that through mobilizing their (refugee) social networks, refugees were more successful in addressing the health concerns of their children:

"Yes, I participate e.g. I contribute towards a given cause for example my neighbor had a sick child and didn't have money to take the child for medication. So we mobilized ourselves to support our neighbor. I participate because helping is at my heart.
(IDI_40-year old, Male refugee from DRC)

This reflects the value of social networks and the positive effect on the health of any population (Hanley et al., 2018; Sierau, Schneider, Nesterko, & Glaesmer, 2019; Sengoelge, Solberg, Nissen, & Saboonchi, 2020). Through their networks, refugee children also learn about the existence of health services and are supported to access and use them. With support from friends, they are in a position to navigate the language barrier or cover communication gaps during health services delivery, such as where there may not be interpreters.

"One of my friends had told me about the free health services they [Kisenyi Health Center IV] provide. I contacted them. I actually went with an interpreter to help me out. I received antenatal, postnatal and malaria treatment services. I was helped to deliver all my four children without paying any single coin; went back for postnatal services and I have always gone there in case I have malaria. In fact, even now when my children fall sick, it is the same health center I go to".
(IDI_34-year-old female, Somali refugee)

The question should be how such thin networks can be harnessed to communicate and promote health in a larger group of refugees who may be scattered in an urban setting not and, therefore, not well organized.

Dual Health Practices Necessary to Satisfy Patient Expectation

Utilizing multiple treatment resorts when seeking health care for children featured prominently among refugees as revealed by the VA data. Duality in health practices is one other concern that health communication ought to reconcile with. It was revealed that refugees, like any other population, are able to evaluate their own health conditions and then determine which health practice to follow for an *appropriate* response. There will be conditions linked to spirituality or faith and/or may not be conceived as having solutions in modern medicine. For instance, a condition perceived to be demonic would call for spiritual intervention including seeking attention from the religious front (like church, mosque) or from traditional/local spiritualists such as known among the Kuku refugees from South Sudan as 'Buni.' The latter are reportedly contacted for anything related to poison, but could also be engaged in situations believed to be arising from demons or evil spirits. Accordingly, there are known conditions such as malaria that are considered a preserve for modern medicine and thus lie in the purview of modern health care providers. Such perceptions were particularly common among a number of refugee groups including the Democratic Republic of Congo and the Somalis.

> "Yes, for fever and strong headache they go to hospitals. But things like stress, they normally go to neighbors, friends, pastors or an elder in church. Sometimes people can go to local healers. When someone has malaria or [high blood] pressure, he/she will go to hospital but if someone is bewitched, she will definitely go to a local healer. A local healer handles issues of poison and "ettalo" [Local Luganda word for a situation where someone claims to be bewitched evidenced by a swelling on the leg]. She/he normally uses a mixture of herbs".
> (IDI_40-year-old, Congolese refugee)

> Yes, for example for a pregnant woman who is about to deliver a baby, I hire a uber car to take her to a hospital but for someone with malaria, I can just move with him/her to the hospital. Being pregnant is a serious condition in the sense that when you do not hurry, a woman can give birth along the way unlike malaria.
> (IDI_33-year old male, Congolese refugee).

You are considered seriously ill when you are bedridden. When you are bedridden, people panic and look for health care from specialists and invite even your relatives. For those not considered seriously ill, they can support in terms of providing food and funds for use.

(IDI_29-year-old male, Somali refugee)

For instance, if it is devil attacks, some people will read the Quran, others will lock the patient in the room. If it is HIV/AIDS, some will enroll on ARVs and others will take herbs.

(IDI _19-year-old male, Somali refugee)

Yes, for devil attacks, we take the patients to mosques and we read the Quran to calm down the situation. For malaria, we take them to hospital.

(IDI_34-year-old female, Somali refugee)

Duality in health care seeking presents a delicate situation and misdiagnosis or tensions regarding disease etiology or recommendation of inappropriate response. On the other hand, a feeling that a particular practice is an imposition may threaten the health of the refugee child. For instance, it was revealed that decisions to take one to a hospital would depend on the severity, in many cases defined as involving vomiting, diarrhea or being bedridden. By implication, a child who may not present with such symptoms may not be given immediate attention on the assumption that he or she has demonic or spiritual issues leading to the delayed clinical encounter. In turn, such delays in seeking appropriate biomedical treatment may result in negative outcomes, which usually become severe by the time the child accesses appropriate health intervention. Moreover, the experience described above when a child develops a severe condition may also play a role in where one decides to take their child for health services. A perceived failure on the part of a particular practice may mean seeking alternatives elsewhere for the current ailment or when the condition reoccurs. One participant cited a scenario when a relative first sought care from the hospital. When they perceived that no diagnosis was given regarding the presenting illness/sickness, a decision was made to consider visiting a traditional healer or sorcerer.

Like last year [2019] for example; my cousin sister fell seriously sick. Her father took her to that witch doctor and the witch doctor told him that she [the cousin sister] had been bewitched. Because this condition at first, they took her hospital and the doctors said that there was no sickness, then they brought her to Mulago hospital here in Kampala and still they doctor said no disease. So, the father decided to take her to the witch doctor. The witch doctor gave them medicine which was suggested to be used while bathing. She used that medicine and up to now, she is okay.

(IDI_20-year-old female, South Sudan refugee)

In cases where the conditions culminate in the worst possible scenario - death, the cultural practices around burials/funerals also stood out among some refugee groups as being worth paying attention to especially where epidemics are involved. Whereas these practices of revering the dead may be well-meaning, they carry the risk of becoming superspreading events (Moran, 2017; Park, 2020). For instance, among the Kuku, it was noted that certain rituals are undertaken as a form of social pathology and postmortem to prevent a life-threatening disease such as Ebola or COVID-19 from affecting any other person especially the young ones.

When someone dies, the community need to understand what caused that death. And then how to organize the burial, they need the uncle of the dead person to be around and if this uncle is not around then the burial does not take place. Then after the burial, the community members (the relatives) will gather and try to understand if there is any problem with this family if someone died of like Ebola or Corona virus. Diseases like those ones, I heard that after the burial, they slaughter a goat so that that disease stops with that person and does not affect the young ones.

(IDI_20-year-female, South Sudan refugee)

When engaging refugee communities, the focus should be put on understanding how refugees determine child health care choices. For this to happen, it is critical to identify and work with leaders of the refugee populations. They bring to bear important resources such as the collective need to help but also helps in building trust (Park, 2020; Feinberg et al., 2021) and can prevent the consequences of mistrust such as boycotting services due to suspicion (Browne et al., 2016; Earnshaw, Bogart, Klompas, & Katz, 2019; Karim, Boyle, Lohan, & Kerr, 2020) as illustrated by these Somali refugees:

"To promote health there is need collaborate with the refugees themselves. To be specific LC1 leaders should work hand in hand with the support providers instead of the middlemen who do not know what is happening here. Support providers should contact local leaders to understand who is eligible for services/support provided and who is not. Remember we trust our local leaders so if the providers of support go through our leaders, it becomes easier for us to trust them".

(IDI_22-year-old, Somali refugee)

"I normally trust doctors because they are in a position to tell me what is happening with my life. For example, it is only them with the mandate to tell whether I have malaria or not. I also gave birth to four children; if I didn't have trust in them, how was I going to deliver these children by myself? [However), support providers should focus on moving with interpreters that we trust most. Remember language is still a challenge to many of us. So moving with interpreters can greatly improve on the trust we have for them because we shall be sure of what they are saying."

(IDI_34-year-old Female, Somali refugee)

Recommendations for Communicative Health Promotion among Refugee Children

Child abuse, sexual and domestic violence are among the most destructive experiences afflicting children. The wide prevalence of such violence takes an enormous toll on the lives of individual survivors as well as the larger society, through innumerable behavioral, health, psychological, and economic consequences. All these consequences affect the health of refugee children. We note that child protection, prevention, and response services in refugee-hosting communities in Uganda show the reach of health communication and justify the need to understand and improve existing health communication practices to better align them to the wellbeing of the refugee children. Therefore, it is important to understand how these children navigate and whether there is any health communication that is directly related to prevention or mitigation of the effects of these within the refugee setting.

Like many children, the preference to accept information from a trusted source is not new. Mwenyango and Palattiyil (2019) show that refugee children, especially adolescents, prefer their parents as the source of information on sexual and reproductive health (SRH). The challenge that emerges is parents may also find it difficult to freely communicate about SRH comprehensively with their children because of cultural norms and beliefs that inhibit such discussion between parents and their children. Such an inhibiting cultural context has a bearing on health-seeking practices and thus the behavior of the children as well as their caregivers. The very young children who do not make any key health decisions rely heavily on their parents or caregivers' health knowledge for their own health and wellbeing. There was no evidence particularly in urban settings that indicate deliberate effort to target the refugee parents with health promotion messages particularly outside of a clinical setting. When refugee parents have a clinical encounter, it often provided the most obvious opportunity to hear from the attending health worker regarding any health concern for sick children. Given the provision for interpreters within the refugee settlements (Mwenyango & Palattiyil, 2019), communicating health between the health care providers and child patients (with the caregivers) can be smooth including in VAC related concerns. On the other hand, urban settings may present difficulties as there may not be any special consideration for interpreters. As a result, the kind of health messages that a parent receives during the clinical encounter and how they translate it to address a health challenge affecting their child can also yield a lot of misinformation and infidelity in practices including poor adherence to prescription. This is notwithstanding the influence of poverty levels as parents may not afford the prescription even with the right information.

Generally, participants in the VA conducted within suburban areas of Kampala City indicated that they did not know of organizations that would offer help even though there exists a number of organizations involved in health promotion work around the city. There appear to be no deliberate targeting of refugee children and their families in the urban setting with health communication. Yet, whereas urban refugees might be clustered with the general population, health promotion through communication appears to unfold without necessarily considering the unique position and communication needs of the refugee children and their respective families.

Communication, Continuity of Care, and Confidence

Knowledge on health alone may not mean better health outcomes. Health communication should be coupled with other efforts that address the broader social determinants of health. After all, parents' decision-making processes regarding the health of their children occur within a broader social context (Renner & McGill, 2016; WHO 2016). For example, efforts to address livelihood concern including income-generating activities can yield dividends when they integrate health messages since they have the potential to strengthen the economic wellbeing (WHO 2016), which is crucial to the urban refugee's care-seeking decisions. Data from the VA highlighted instances where some refugee parents resorted to faith or prayer waiting for God's intervention for their sick child when they could not afford the cost of biomedical intervention or any other alternative medicine. All these limitations have implications for the health of the refugee children. It may also mean that, if communicating health is effective, it must be considered in a broad sense to address the factors that impact the decision-making regarding health choices and practices for refugee children and their families.

Notes

1 David Napier, *The Barefoot Manual* (University College London).
2 www.newvision.co.ug/new_vision/news/1456081uganda-3rd-refugee-hosting-nation-world
3 http://ugandarefugees.org/
4 http://www.amnesty.org/en/latest/campaigns/2017/06/8-things-you-need-to-know-about-refugees-in-uaganda/
5 http://ugandarefugees.org/
6 UNHCR/OPM March 2018
7 file:///C:/Users/user/Downloads/Final-HSIRRP-31-Jan-2019-MASTER.pdf
8 https://publichealth.tulane.edu/blog/health-communication-effective-strategies/

Recommended Readings

Karim, N., Boyle, B., Lohan, M., & Kerr, C. (2020). Immigrant parents' experiences of accessing child healthcare services in a host country: A qualitative thematic synthesis. *Journal of Advanced Nursing, 76*(7), 1509–1519.

Mwenyango, H. (2020). The place of social work in improving access to health services among refugees: A case study of Nakivale settlement, Uganda. *International Social Work*. https://doi.org/10.1177/0020872820962195

Napier, A. D., Depledge, M., Knipper, M., Lovell, R., & Ponarin, E., Sanabria, E., & Thomas, F. (2017). *Culture matters: Using a cultural contexts of health approach to enhance policy-making.* 10.13140/RG.2.2.17532.74881.

Renner, L. A., & McGill, D. (2016). Exploring factors influencing health-seeking decisions and retention in childhood cancer treatment programmes: perspectives of parents in Ghana. *Ghana Medical Journal, 50*(3), 149–156.

References

Alsubhi, M., Goldthorpe, J., Epton, T., Khanom, S., & Peters, S. (2020). What factors are associated with obesity-related health behaviours among child refugees following resettlement in developed countries? A systematic review and synthesis of qualitative and quantitative evidence. *Obesity Reviews, 21*(11), e13058.

Amuge, B., Wabwire-Mangen, F., Puta, C., Pariyo, G. W., Bakyaita, N., Staedke, S., et al. (2004). Health-seeking behavior for malaria among child and adult headed households in Rakai district, Uganda. *African Health Sciences, 4*(2), 119–124.

Browne, A. J., Varcoe, C., Lavoie, J., Smye, V., Wong, S. T., Krause, M., et al. (2016). Enhancing health care equity with Indigenous populations: evidence-based strategies from an ethnographic study. *BMC Health Service Research, 16*(1), 544.

Bulled, N. (2016). *Prescribing HIV Prevention: Bringing Culture into Global Health Communication.* Page 273. New York: Routledge. doi: https://doi.org/10.4324/9781315421971

Carroll, J., Epstein, R., Fiscella, K., Gipson, T., Volpe, E., & Jean-Pierre, P. (2007). Caring for Somali women: Implications for clinician–patient communication. *Patient Education and Counseling, 66*(3), 337–345.

Chen, X., Hay, J. L., Waters, E. A., Kiviniemi, M. T., Biddle, C., Schofield, E., et al. (2018). Health literacy and use and trust in health information. *Journal of Health Communication, 23*(8), 724–734.

Cook, G., Appleton, J. V., & Wiggs, L. (2020). Parentally reported barriers to seeking help and advice for child sleep from healthcare professionals. *Child: Care, Health and Development, 46*(4), 513–521.

Desai, P. P., & Pandya, S. V. (2013). Communicating with children in healthcare settings. *Indian Journal of Pediatrics, 80*(12), 1028–1033.

Earnshaw, V. A., Bogart, L. M., Klompas, M., & Katz, I. T. (2019). Medical mistrust in the context of Ebola: Implications for intended care-seeking and quarantine policy support in the United States. *Journal of Health Psychology, 24*(2), 219–228.

Feinberg, I. Z., Owen-Smith, A., O'Connor, M. H., Ogrodnick, M. M., Rothenberg, R., & Eriksen, M. P. (2021). Strengthening culturally competent health communication. *Health Security, 19*(S1), 41–49.

Gumisiriza, P. (2018). Challenges and emerging issues affecting the management of Refugees in Uganda. *The Ugandan Journal of Management and Public Policy Studies*, 4, 40–54. https://www.researchgate.net/publication/348432460_Challenges_and_Emerging_Issues_Affecting_the_Management_of_Refugees_in_Uganda

Hanley, J., Al Mhamied, A., Cleveland, J., Hajjar, O., Hassan, G., Ives, N., et al. (2018). The social networks, social support and social capital of Syrian refugees privately sponsored to settle in Montreal: Indications for employment and housing during their early experiences of integration, 50(2), 123–148. *Canadian Ethnic Studies, 50*(2), 123–148.

Johnson, J. L., Bottorff, J. L., Browne, A. J., Grewal, S., Hilton, B. A., & Clarke, H. (2004). Othering and being othered in the context of health care services. *Health communication, 16*(2), 255–271.

Juang, L. P., Simpson, J. A., Lee, R. M., Rothman, A. J., Titzmann, P. F., Schachner, M. K., ... & Betsch, C. (2018). Using attachment and relational perspectives to understand adaptation and resilience among immigrant and refugee youth. *American Psychologist, 73*(6), 797.

Karim, N., Boyle, B., Lohan, M., & Kerr, C. (2020). Immigrant parents' experiences of accessing child healthcare services in a host country: A qualitative thematic synthesis. *Journal of Advanced Nursing, 76*(7), 1509–1519.

Kavuma, P., Turyakira, P., Bills, C., & Kalanzi, J. (2020). Analysis of financial management in public emergency medical services sector: Case study of the department of emergency medical services, Uganda. *African Journal of Emergency Medicine, 10*, S85–S89.

MoH. (2019). Health Sector Integrated Refugee Response Plan 2019–2024. *The Republic of Uganda, Ministry of Health*. Available at: https://www.health.go.ug/cause/health-sector-integrated-refugee-response-plan/

Moran, M. H. (2017). Missing bodies and secret funerals: The production of "safe and dignified burials" in the Liberian Ebola crisis. *Anthropological Quarterly, 90*(2), 399–421.

Mwenyango, H., & Palattiyil G. (2019). Health needs and challenges of women and children in Uganda's refugee settlements: Conceptualising a role for social work. *International Social Work*, 62(6), 1535–1547.

Mwenyango, H. (2020). The place of social work in improving access to health services among refugees: A case study of Nakivale settlement, Uganda. *International Social Work,* https://doi.org/10.1177/0020872820962195

Nara, R., Banura, A., & Foster, A. M. (2020). Exploring Congolese refugees' experiences with abortion care in Uganda: a multi-methods qualitative study. *Sexual and Reproductive Health Matters, 27*(1), 262–271.

Orom, H., Schofield, E., Kiviniemi, M. T., Waters, E. A., Biddle, C., Chen, X., ... Hay, J. L. (2018). Low health literacy and health information avoidance but not satisficing help explain "Don't Know" responses to questions assessing perceived risk. *Medical Decision Making, 38*(8), 1006–1017.

Park, C. (2020). Traditional funeral and burial rituals and Ebola outbreaks in West Africa: A narrative review of causes and strategy interventions. *Journal of Health and Social Sciences, 5*(1), 073–090.

Renner, L. A., & McGill, D. (2016). Exploring factors influencing health-seeking decisions and retention in childhood cancer treatment programmes: Perspectives of parents in Ghana. *Ghana Medical Journal, 50*(3), 149–156.

Schoemaker, E., Baslan, D., Pon, B., & Dell, N. (2021). Identity at the margins: data justice and refugee experiences with digital identity systems in Lebanon, Jordan, and Uganda. *Information Technology for Development, 27*(1), 13–36.

Sengoelge, M., Solberg, Ø., Nissen, A., & Saboonchi, F. (2020). Exploring Social and Financial Hardship, Mental Health Problems and the Role of Social Support in Asylum Seekers Using Structural Equation Modelling. *International Journal of Environmental Research and Public Health, 17*(19), 6948.

Sierau, S., Schneider, E., Nesterko, Y., & Glaesmer, H. (2019). Alone, but protected? Effects of social support on mental health of unaccompanied refugee minors. *European Child & Adolescent Psychiatry, 28*(6), 769–780.

Twimukye, A., King, R., Schlech, W., Zawedde, F. M., Kakaire, T., & Parkes-Ratanshi, R. (2017). Exploring attitudes and perceptions of patients and staff towards an after-hours co-pay clinic supplementing free HIV services in Kampala, Uganda. *BMC Health Services Research, 17*(1), 580.

UNHCR. (1994). *Refugee Children: Guidelines on protection and care.* Available at: https://www.unhcr.org/protect/PROTECTION/3b84c6c67.pdf

UNHCR. (2014). *Protection of refugee children in the Middle East and North Africa.* Available at: https://www.refworld.org/pdfid/54589a6a4.pdf

WHO. (2015). *Toolkit on mapping legal, health and social services responses to child maltreatment.* Available at: http://apps.who.int/iris/bitstream/handle/10665/155237/9789241549073_eng.pdf;jsessionid=640D5B1B44D999FF64A339E5769A9BEC?sequence=1

WHO. (2016). *INSPIRE: Seven strategies for ending violence against children.* Available at: http://apps.who.int/iris/bitstream/handle/10665/207717/9789241565356-eng.pdf;jsessionid=768770D74C1FEC2A71312F-CEA58391DC?sequence=1

14 South-South Migration and the Health Communication Concerns Confronting Venezuelan Refugees in Peru

Hilda Patricia Garcia Cosavalente and Gary L. Kreps

Introduction

There has been a growing health crisis with Venezuelan refugees in Peru (Mendoza, 2019). Venezuelan refugees, who have escaped the many dangers from the expanding political, economic, cultural, and safety crises they faced living in Venezuela by migrating to live in Peru, have encountered many different difficult and continuing physical and mental health problems in their new home country (Peru), especially while being forced to navigate the serious and evolving social and health repercussions from the COVID-19 pandemic (Vázquez-Rowe & Gandolfi, 2020). Many of these health problems have been exacerbated by poor health communication practices, where refugees' health concerns have not been heard and attended to, relevant health information and support have not been provided very well to these refugees, and there has been a dire need for working collaboratively with members of the refugee community to introduce important health risk prevention, detection, and treatment programs to promote wellbeing. This chapter examines these complex health communication issues and recommends strategies for health communication intervention to improve health outcomes.

Refugee Health Threats

Becoming a refugee often involves facing serious challenges to maintaining optimal health and wellbeing (Efird & Bith-Melander, 2018; Bender, 2021). Even though refugees are typically very relieved to be able to relocate from tremendously difficult destabilized (and often deadly) conditions in their former home countries to safer national homes, their health and wellbeing often suffers tremendously from the migration process (Guo, Al Ariss, & Brewster, 2020). It is even often difficult for refugees to just leave their home countries that are reeling from terrible problems, such as economic meltdowns, environmental crises, government takeovers, food deprivation, violence, and active warfare, as we recently witnessed with the many impediments that faced the thousands

DOI: 10.4324/9781003230243-14

of frightened citizens of Afghanistan who tried in vain to leave their dangerously destabilized country. Some refugees are forced to find nefarious illegal and dangerous paths to escape from their countries, often feeling forced to embark on difficult, exhausting, and perilous trips to new lands (Olwig, 2021). Many refugees perish during these dangerous journeys, and the ones who arrive in the countries of asylum are often ill, injured, weak, and exhausted both physically and mentally (Lori & Boyle, 2015; Olwig, 2021).

Once arriving in their new host country, refugees often encounter tremendous problems with bureaucracy, resistance, hostility, and stigma from officials and from many local residents, creating very cold welcomes to their new countries, even when they have been offered official asylum (Baranik, Hurst, & Eby, 2018; Bemak & Chung, 2021). Due to fears about immigrants, residents of many countries have not been eager to accept poor, troubled, and needy refugees (Esses, Hamilton, & Gaucher, 2017). Sadly, refugees often experience severe anti-immigrant public sentiment, prejudice, and resentment from xenophobic residents in their adopted countries (Cowling, Anderson, & Ferguson, 2019).

It is well documented that perceived discrimination can affect mental and physical health in many different contexts. For example, the work by Agudelo-Suarez and colleagues (2011) found that immigrants in Spain who experienced higher discrimination were more likely to experience health problems such as poor mental health. Comparing to their health status in their home country to their health status in their new country, the respondents affirmed their health declined in Spain. This shows the vulnerabilities in health that many immigrants face when moving to a different country. The association between reported discrimination and poor health is consisted with other findings on immigrants' health (Gonzalez-Castro & Ubillos, 2011; Williams, Neighbors & Jackson, 2003). Likewise, the systematic review by Paradies (2006) illustrates how self-reported racism and poor health are often linked.

Immigration management policies, regulations, and practices too often treat refugees roughly, focusing more on policing, herding, and controlling refugees than on helping to resettle them safely into their new countries (Ambrosini, 2021). Even in the rare, but happy, situations when refugees are warmly welcomed to their new country, the refugees often arrive in very poor health, both physically and mentally, due to often severe conditions of deprivation, violence, and trauma they experienced in their home country that led them to seek asylum from a new country (Matlin, Depoux, Schütte, Flahault, & Saso, 2018). In addition, the refugee travel and relocation processes that enable them to physically get to their new country can often be grueling and brutally dangerous (Olwig, 2021). Too often, refugees do not have comfortable and hygienic places to live upon entry to their new country, with many refugees forced to live in crowded resettlement camps or even on the streets, sometimes hiding from local police and immigration officials (Blitz, d'Angelo, Kofman, & Montagna, 2017). These refugees also often do not have access to healthy foods and high-quality needed health care services (Blitz, d'Angelo, Kofman, & Montagna, 2017; Feinberg, O'Connor, Owen-Smith, & Dube, 2021).

To further complicate matters for refugee health and wellbeing today, we are living though an especially difficult time due to current health and environmental threats to the public that add additional health risks for refugees. For example, the current COVID-19 pandemic has complicated refugee health issues by adding serious health risks from contagion for these already vulnerable groups of people who are often living in high-risk crowded and unhygienic circumstances (Freier & Brauckmeyer, 2020; Lupieri, 2021; Saifee, Franco-Paredes, & Lowenstein, 2021). Public lockdowns, business shutdowns, and social distancing regulations established in host countries to combat the pandemic have also made it increasingly difficult for refugees to integrate into their new home countries. In addition, the growing negative influences from climate change on severe weather and environmental conditions (hurricanes, earthquakes, floods, tsunamis, etc.) have also complicated the health of refugee populations (Bhowmik, 2020; Brickhill-Atkinson & Hauck, 2020). Refugees are often highly vulnerable to serious health risks and need strong prevention, detection, and treatment services and support to promote their wellbeing.

The Health Issues Confronting Venezuelan Refugees in Peru

In recent years, Venezuela has been facing serious socioeconomic, political, cultural, and public safety crises that have caused significant pain and suffering for the Venezuelan people (Ellis, 2017). These evolving problems in Venezuela have led to an outpouring of Venezuelan refugees and migrants, many of whom have moved to nearby Peru to seek relief and a better life, especially since Peru was one of the only countries in South America that welcomed Venezuelan citizens with open immigration policies for them to escape the crises in their home country (Bahar, Piccone, & Trinkunas, 2018, Mendoza, 2019, Sanchez Cardenas, 2019). According to a report from the World Bank (2021a) there are more than 1.2 million Venezuelan refugees/immigrants now living in Peru. This is also an especially challenging time for Venezuelan refugees living in Peru due to dangers and public restrictions related to the current coronavirus pandemic leading to widespread infections, hospitalizations, and deaths for many residents, but especially for refugees (Mendoza, 2019). Due to their often crowded and dangerous living conditions, there have been high rates of COVID-19 infections among Venezuelan refugees in Peru (Vázquez-Rowe & Gandolfi, 2020).

There are many other serious health and safety problems the Venezuelan refugees have confronted, including discrimination, xenophobia, as well as food and job insecurity that negatively affect Venezuelan's health in Peru (Mendoza, 2019). For example, food security has been a major health problem for refugees. According to a recent report of the World Food Program, two-thirds of the 2.8 million refugees and immigrants living in Colombia, Ecuador, and Peru are facing serious health and food safety problems related to the COVID-19-19 pandemic (Programa Mundial de Alimentos, 2020). Schmitt (2021) documents the dire problems with food insecurity that Venezuelan migrants and refugee are facing in Peru leading to hunger, stress, and malnutrition for these vulnerable refugees.

Venezuelan immigrants in Peru also have severely limited access to high quality health care services (Zambrano-Barragán et al. 2021). If Venezuelans get sick, only 33% of them seek medical care in contrast with 48% of native Peruvians (World Bank, 2021b). A study by Larenas-Rosa and Cabieses Valdés (2019) found that undocumented immigrants usually use health care less frequent than citizens. In turn, this makes immigrants socioeconomically vulnerable and has negative influences on their health and wellbeing. Cabieses, Bernales, and van der Laat (2016) saw immigration as an important determinant of health. They affirmed that Latin America is a region that has inconsistent policies regarding human rights and health for immigrants. This makes it a challenge for governments in the American Region to assure immigrants and local populations have equal access to needed health care services.

Venezuelan immigrants in Peru have also faced problems with discrimination. One study by Mougenot, Amaya, Mezones-Holguin, Rodriguez-Morales, and Cabieses (2021) showed that there was an association between perceived discrimination and presenting mental health problems among the Venezuelan immigrant population in Peru. Having health problems is not uncommon for Venezuelan immigrants. The "Survey of the Venezuelan Population Residing in Peru" 2018 by Hernández-Vásquez and colleagues (2019) found that 50% of Venezuelans immigrants in Peru affirmed having health problems such as chronic diseases and mental health issues. In the same sense, Mougenot and colleagues (2021) found that Venezuelan immigrants living in Peru who perceived that they were being discriminated against also experienced mental health issues. Their study found that especially Venezuelan females reported higher rates of mental health problems. It is very important to pay attention to the discrimination that Venezuelans are experiencing in Peru. According to the report by QR Consulting (2020) Venezuelan refugees in Peru perceive high levels of discrimination, nearly 48% of female Venezuelans and 41% of male Venezuelans living in Peru have experienced discrimination. Moreover, according to Delgado-Flores, Cutire, Cvetkovic-Vega, and Nieto-Gutierrez (2021) Venezuelans who perceive discrimination in Peru are less likely to seek and follow adequate treatment for their chronic illness which can have adverse effects on their overall health and wellbeing. In a recent qualitative study by Freier and Pérez (2021) the researchers found that Venezuelans immigrants in Peru who experience xenophobic discrimination also experienced criminalization because of their nationality. Participants in this study affirmed they experienced verbal abuse when taking public transportation, and when accessing public services in healthcare and public education. This shows that Venezuelans might not access healthcare because of concerns about the potential discrimination they could face when receiving these services. Moreover, a survey developed by the World Food Program (2020) found that Venezuelan immigrants in Peru face many resettlement challenges, such as lack of employment, discrimination, and exploitation. All these factors can combine to harm the physical and mental health of Venezuelan refugees in Peru.

The ethnographic work by Zambrano-Barragán and colleagues (2021) shows that COVID-19 has worsened Venezuelans' health in Peru and Colombia. Venezuelans perceived they had better health in their home country than they do in Peru. In their study, discrimination also played an important role in whether Venezuelan refugees access health care in Peru. Moreover, one of the major barriers to accessing healthcare for Venezuelan immigrants is their undocumented status in the country.

Besides limited access to healthcare, Venezuelans also face job insecurity. The Think Tank Equilibrium Centro para el Desarrollo Económico (2020) performed an Opinion Survey with Venezuelan immigrants in Peru and found that 37% of the respondents affirmed that they worked as street vendors (out of 406 Venezuelan respondents in urban Peru). Concerning job security, 86.7% affirmed they didn't have a formal work contract. This shows that Venezuelans immigrants in Peru have limited access to formal employment and thus they cannot access health care and health insurance. Discrimination was also mentioned by the respondents in this survey, with 40.6% affirming that discrimination was limiting their access to formal work and 87.4% of the respondents affirming that the did not have access to health insurance. These striking numbers show that there is low access to health and job security among Venezuelan immigrants in Peru.

COVID-19 and Other Health Problems

In March 2020, the Peruvian Government (Gobierno del Perú, 2021) declared a state of emergency and public lockdown for 90 days. This was later extended due to the high levels of COVID-19 transmission in the country. With the highest death rates from COVID-19 in the world (New York Times, 2021), Peru has suffered an economic downturn. Peru's GDP sank 40% in April 2020 (Instituto Peruano de Economia, 2020) due to COVID-19 restrictions. According to the World Bank, the strict quarantine implemented in Peru decreased the country's GDP by 11.1% in 2020. Unemployment increased and the restrictions pushed almost 2 million people into poverty, raising the poverty rate in the country to 27%. One of the reasons the state of emergency and lockdown affected Peru is because the economy is highly informal, with those doing work having little or no job security, not having a contract, and no guarantee that they will have the same employer for more than a few weeks or months. In fact, 72% of the Peruvian economy is informal (Manky, 2020) and in some provinces such as Huancavelica, the rate of informal employment is even higher, up to 91.2%. Individuals lack social protection because the informal jobs they have lack social benefits. The Government launched social and economic support to citizens to lessen the burdens caused by the informal economy. However, these programs did not apply to Venezuelan immigrants since national identification was needed to access these programs (Freier & Espinoza, 2021). Venezuelan immigrants have been more harmed by the COVID-19 pandemic than other segments of the Peruvian population because of their lack of social protection and legal status (Freier, Jara, & Luzes (2020).

Immigrant women face larger challenges when accessing health care services. For example, unplanned pregnancy is a health problem that can affect immigrant women more often than local women since immigrants are vulnerable to economic insecurity (Irons, 2021). In her qualitative study on reproductive health services in Peru, Irons (2021) affirmed that there is a deficit of relevant health information for Venezuelan women when they arrived in Peru. Most of the respondents affirmed they seek contraceptives in pharmacies and only a small number of the total respondents went to the MINSA (Ministry of Health). There is also lack of information about the free access of contraceptives by MINSA in Peru. For example, almost half of the interviewees didn't know about the free access of reproductive services (Irons, 2021). It is not uncommon for women to get health information and reproductive health information at the pharmacies. For example, according to the Instituto Nacional de Estadistica (2019) more than half of Venezuelan women (55.1%) seek health information at the pharmacies and only 17.7% seek health information at MINSA centers.

Moreover, Moquillaza-Alcántara and Soria-Gonzales (2019) affirmed that pregnant Venezuelan women in Peru don't access prenatal health care because of a lack of health information, high costs of healthcare, and their fears about facing discrimination when seeking health care. As revealed by these studies, Venezuelan immigrants don't have adequate access to health care in Peru. Most of them perceived high levels of xenophobia and discrimination in Peru. They also usually don't have health insurance and access to relevant health information that helps them make informed decisions about their health.

Media and Health Information Seeking

It is not uncommon for the news media in Peru to show negative portrayals of Venezuelan refugees in Peru such as in an articles published in main newspapers in Peru El Comercio (2021) and "La Republica" (2021b). Because of this kind of negative portrayal, many Venezuelan immigrants prefer not to obtain information through the local media or Peruvian newspapers. Capsula Migrante (Migrant Capsule), an account in Twitter funded by Venezuelan journalists in Peru (La Republica, 2021a), was formed as an alternative communication channel for Venezuelans in Peru after analyzing the situation where these immigrants don't have positive perceptions about other local media channels.

In an attitudinal study designed and conducted by the Instituto de Opinión Pública (IOP) and Instituto de Democracia y Derechos Humanos PUCP (2020), researchers found that 89% of respondents in Peru thought that "many Venezuelans are engaged in criminal activities in Peru." Furthermore, 77% affirmed that they believed that "Venezuelans are taking away job opportunities from Peruvians." These numbers show that there are widespread discriminatory negative attitudes that Peruvians hold regarding Venezuelan immigrants that are often supported by mainstream media channels in Peru.

There is a need to create more democratic mass media and local media that fulfill immigrants' health information needs. As explained previously, Venezuelans in Peru perceive that mass media contribute to xenophobia because of how they are portrayed in the media (Salazar, 2018). It is also recommended to offer more specific health messages to immigrants considering their unique health information needs. As an example, we can cite the 'HealthyMe' smartphone health application developed at the University of Maryland as an example of a program that could be started in Peru (University of Maryland, 2021). This project aims to provide personalized health information to immigrants and underserved population in the DC area, Maryland and Virginia, and similar programs could be used in Peru too.

Communication Strategies for Reducing Venezuelan Refugee Health Risks

Relevant information is needed to guide health communication efforts to address the health risks facing Venezuelan refugees in Peru. Formative health communication research should be conducted as an important first-step towards addressing the serious health problems facing Venezuelan refugees in Peru (Kreps, 2014; Kreps & Neuhauser, 2015). For example, it is important to carefully examine the nature of the health problems that Venezuelan refugees confront by conducting in-depth needs analysis research. Needs analysis should be used to collect data from members of the refugee community, local public health officials, and through examination of health and epidemiological records to determine the specific kinds of health problems that are harming members of this population, to find out what is known about how these health problems spread within the refugee population, and what the best strategies available are for preventing and treating these specific health problems.

In addition to conducting needs analysis studies, audience analysis research is needed to connect with and learn more about members of the refugee community. Audience analysis research can collect information about the unique perceived health needs, concerns, beliefs, values, attitudes, and health promotion strategies that are likely to work well with members of this population. Audience analysis can also be used to collect relevant information about audience communication skills and preferences to inform use of the best communication strategies for providing refugees with relevant health information and support. For example, audience analysis research can identify trusted information sources, preferred channels of communication, and messaging strategies that will resonate with different segments of the refugee population (Kreps, 2014, 2021). In addition, audience analysis research can help identify allies within the refugee community for providing culturally sensitive information, advice, and support in developing, implementing, evaluating, and sustaining health promotion programs for this vulnerable population (Neuhauser, Kreps, & Syme, 2013; Kreps & Sparks, 2008).).

Working in close collaborations with members of the refugee community is an essential strategy for not only learning more about their unique needs and preferences, but also is an important strategy for empowering members of this community to design and implement needed changes to improve refugee health and wellbeing. It is important to work as partners with members of cultural groups to design the best health promotion interventions for this group, as well as to encourage a sense of ownership and commitment to these programs among the population (Neuhauser, Kreps, & Syme, 2013). Members of the refugee group population often have high credibility within the refugee community and are likely to possess cultural sensitivity needed to communicate effectively to disseminate relevant health information to and influence other members of the community. They are more likely to be trusted than government officials or other experts who are not members of the cultural group. Community partners can gather relevant information, share information, and help to implement and sustain important culturally sensitive health promotion programs with other refugees.

These collaborative research efforts can help guide the development of culturally appropriate and effective new policies for communication, health care, education, employment, nutrition, and other social processes that are relevant to improving the health and wellbeing of refugee communities. Moreover, these partnerships are a good way to initiate the development of meaningful and cooperative relationships between members of the refugee community and members of the broader Peruvian population, promoting acculturation and providing new opportunities for refugee participation in their new countries. Eventually, they should lead to increased participation in the Peruvian workforce, education system, and even the health care and political systems, enabling these social systems to better serve the needs of the Venezuelan refugees, as well as to enhance refugee health and wellbeing.

Recommended Readings

Bemak, F., & Chung, R. C. Y. (2021). Contemporary refugees: Issues, challenges, and a culturally responsive intervention model for effective practice. *The Counseling Psychologist*, *49*(2), 305–324.

Camino, P., & Montreuil, U. L. (2020). Asylum under pressure in Peru: the impact of the Venezuelan crisis and COVID-19. *Forced Migration Review*, *65*, 53–56.

Feinberg, I. Z., Owen-Smith, A., O'Connor, M. H., Ogrodnick, M. M., Rothenberg, R., & Eriksen, M. P. (2021). Strengthening culturally competent health communication. *Health Security*, *19*(S1). DOI: 10.1089/hs.2021.0048

Kreps, G. L., & Neuhauser, L. (2015). Designing health information programs to promote the health and well-being of vulnerable populations: The benefits of evidence-based strategic health communication. In C. A. Smith & A. Keselman (Eds.), *Meeting health information needs outside of healthcare: Opportunities and challenges* (pp. 3–17). Waltham, MA: Chandos Publishing.

Kreps, G. L., & Sparks, L. (2008). Meeting the health literacy needs of vulnerable populations. *Patient Education and Counseling*, *71*(3), 328–332.

Mendoza, W. (2019). Venezuelan immigration in Peru from a health perspective. *Revista peruana de medicina experimental y salud pública*, *36*, 3. DOI: 10.17843/rpmesp.2019.363.4812

Vázquez-Rowe, I., & Gandolfi, A. (2020). Peruvian efforts to contain COVID-19 fail to protect vulnerable population groups. *Public Health in Practice*, *1*, 100020.

References

Agudelo-Suárez, A. A., Ronda-Pérez, E., Gil-González, D. *et al.* (2011). The effect of perceived discrimination on the health of immigrant workers in Spain. *BMC Public Health*, *11*, 652. DOI: 10.1186/1471-2458-11-652

Ambrosini, M. (2021). The battleground of asylum and immigration policies: A conceptual inquiry. *Ethnic and Racial Studies*, *44*(3), 374–395.

Bahar, D., Piccone, T., & Trinkunas, H. (2018). Venezuela: a path out of misery. *Brookings Policy Brief*. https://www.brookings.edu/research/venezuela-a-path-out-of-misery/

Baranik, L. E., Hurst, C. S., & Eby, L. T. (2018). The stigma of being a refugee: A mixed- method study of refugees' experiences of vocational stress. *Journal of Vocational Behavior, 105,* 116–130.

Bemak, F., & Chung, R. C. Y. (2021). Contemporary refugees: Issues, challenges, and a culturally responsive intervention model for effective practice. *The Counseling Psychologist, 49*(2), 305–324.

Bender, F. (2021). Should refugees govern refugee camps? *Critical Review of International Social and Political Philosophy,* 1–24. DOI: 10.1080/13698230.2021.1941702

Bhowmik, D. (2020). Problems of refugee and the climate change. In *Refugee crises and third-world economies* (pp. 45–72). Emerald Publishing Limited. DOI: 10.1108/978-1-83982-190-520201008

Blitz, B. K., d'Angelo, A., Kofman, E., & Montagna, N. (2017). Health challenges in refugee reception: Dateline Europe 2016. *International Journal of Environmental Research and Public Health, 14*(12), 1484.

Brickhill-Atkinson, M., & Hauck, F. R. (2021). Impact of COVID-19 on resettled refugees. *Primary Care, 48*(1), 57.

Cabieses, B., Bernales, M., & van der Laat, C. (2016). Health for all migrants in Latin America and the Caribbean. *Lancet Psychiatry, 3,* 5. DOI: 10.1016/S2215-0366

Camino, P., & Montreuil, U. L. (2020). Asylum under pressure in Peru: the impact of the Venezuelan crisis and COVID-19. *Forced Migration Review, 65,* 53–56.

Cowling, M. M., Anderson, J. R., & Ferguson, R. (2019). Prejudice-relevant correlates of attitudes towards refugees: A meta-analysis. *Journal of Refugee Studies, 32*(3), 502–524.

Delgado-Flores, C., Cutire, O. S., Cvetkovic-Vega, A., & Nieto-Gutierrez, W. (2021). Perceived discrimination as a barrier for the adequate treatment of chronic diseases in Venezuelan migrants from Peru. *Revista Brasileira de Epidemiologia, 24,* e210029–e210029. DOI: 10.1590/1980-549720210029

Efird, J. T., & Bith-Melander, P. (2018). Refugee health: an ongoing commitment and challenge. *International Journal of Environmental Research and Public Health, 15*(1), 131. DOI: 10.3390/ijerph15010131

El Comercio (2021, July 23). Capturan a delincuentes. https://elcomercio.pe/videos/pais/sjm-capturan-a-banda-delincuencial-que-practicaba-rituales-antes-de-realizar-asaltos-nnav-latv-venezolanos-en-peru-delincuentes-ritual-de-santeria-noticia/

Ellis, R. E. (2017). The collapse of Venezuela and its impact on the region. *Military Review, 97*(4), 22.

Equilibrium CenDe. (2020). Encuesta de Opinión a Población Migrante Venezolana en Perú - Junio, 2020. https://equilibriumcende.com/resultados-de-la-encuesta-de-opinion-a-poblacion-migrante-venezolana-en-peru-junio-2020/. Accessed 25 November 2020.

Esses, V. M., Hamilton, L. K., & Gaucher, D. (2017). The global refugee crisis: Empirical evidence and policy implications for improving public attitudes and facilitating refugee resettlement. *Social Issues and Policy Review, 11*(1), 78–123.

Feinberg, I., O'Connor, M. H., Owen-Smith, A., & Dube, S. R. (2021). Public health crisis in the refugee community: little change in social determinants of health preserve health disparities. *Health Education Research, 36*(2), 170–177.

Feinberg, I. Z., Owen-Smith, A., O'Connor, M. H., Ogrodnick, M. M., Rothenberg, R., & Eriksen, M. P. (2021). Strengthening culturally competent health communication. *Health Security*, 19(S1). DOI: 10.1089/hs.2021.0048

Freier, L. F., & Brauckmeyer, G. (2020). Migrantes venezolanos y COVID-19: impacto de la cuarentena y propuestas para la apertura in *Por una nueva convivencia. La sociedad peruana en tiempos de COVID-19: escenarios, propuestas de política y acción pública*. Editors M. Burga, F. Portocarrero, & A. Panfichi. Lima: Fondo Editorial PUCP.

Freier, L. F., & Espinoza, M. V. (2021). COVID-19 and immigrants' increased exclusion: The politics of immigrant integration in Chile and Peru. *Frontiers in Human Dynamics*, *3*. DOI: 10.3389/fhumd.2021.606871

Freier, L. F., Jara, S. C., & Luzes, M. (2020). The plight of migrants and refugees in the pandemic. *Current History*, *119*(820), 297–302.

Freier, L. F., & Pérez, L. M. (2021). Nationality-based criminalization of south-south migration: The experience of Venezuelan forced migrants in Peru. *European Journal on Criminal Policy and Research*, *27*, 1. DOI: 10.1007/s10610-020-09475-y

Gobierno del Perú. (2021, July 20). Archivo. Declaratoria de Emergencia Sanitaria Nacional. https://www.gob.pe/institucion/mtc/informes-publicaciones/1074671-declaratoria-de-emergencia-sanitaria-nacional.

Gonzalez-Castro, J. L., & Ubillos, S. (2011). Determinants of psychological distress among migrants from Ecuador and Romania in a Spanish city. *International Journal of Social Psychiatry*, *57*, 1. DOI: 10.1177/0020764010347336

Guo, G. C., Al Ariss, A., & Brewster, C. (2020). Understanding the global refugee crisis: Managerial consequences and policy implications. *Academy of Management Perspectives*, *34*(4), 531–545.

Hernández-Vásquez, A., Vargas-Fernández, R., Rojas-Roque, C., & Bendezu-Quispe, G. (2019). Factores asociados a la no utilización de servicios de salud en inmigrantes venezolanos en Perú. *Revista Peruana de Medicina Experimental y Salud Publica*, *36*(4), 583–591. DOI: 10.17843/rpmesp.2019.360.4654

Instituto de Opinión Pública (IOP) and Instituto de Democracia y Derechos Humanos PUCP. (2020). Cambios en las actitudes hacia los inmigrantes venezolanos en Lima-Callao 2018–2019. http://repositorio.pucp.edu.pe/index/bitstream/handle/123456789/169459/IOP_1119_01_R2.pdf?sequence=1&isAllowed=y (Accessed July 20, 2021).

Instituto Nacional de Estadística e Informática. (2019). Condiciones de vida de la población Venezolana que reside en Perú. Lima; 2019. https://www.inei.gob.pe/media/MenuRecursivo/publicaciones_digitales/Est/Lib1666/. Retrieved July 21, 2021.

Instituto Peruano de Economía. (2020). Boletín IPE. Impacto del COVID en Perú y Latinoamérica. https://www.ipe.org.pe/portal/boletin-ipe-impacto-del-covid-19-la-economia-peruana-y-latinoamerica/ Retrieved July 20, 2021.

Irons, R. (2021). Venezuelan Women's Perception of sexual and reproductive health services in Lima, Peru. *Revista Peruana de Medicina Experimental y Salud Publica*, *38*, 2.

Kreps, G. L. (2014*).* Evaluating health communication programs to enhance health care and health promotion. *Journal of Health Communication*, *19*(12), 1449–1459.

Kreps, G. L. (2021). The role of strategic communication to respond effectively to pandemics. *Journal of Multicultural Discourses, 16*(1), 12–19. DOI: 10.1080/17447143.2021.1885417

Kreps, G. L., & Neuhauser, L. (2015). Designing health information programs to promote the health and well-being of vulnerable populations: The benefits of evidence-based strategic health communication. In C. A. Smith & A. Keselman (Eds.), *Meeting health information needs outside of healthcare: Opportunities and challenges* (pp. 3–17). Waltham, MA: Chandos Publishing.

Larenas-Rosa, D., & Cabieses Valdés, B. (2019). Salud de migrantes internacionales en situación irregular: una revisión narrativa de iniciativas. *Revista Peruana de Medicina Experimental y Salud Publica, 36*, 3. DOI: 10.17843/rpmesp.2019.363.4469

La Republica. (2021a, June 24). Cápsula Migrante, un proyecto al servicio de la comunidad venezolana en Perú. https://larepublica.pe/mundo/2021/06/24/capsula-migrante-un-proyecto-al-servicio-de-la-comunidad-venezolana-en-peru/

La Republica. (2021b, January 18). Han llegado delincuentes que desprestigian la comunidad venezolana. https://larepublica.pe/sociedad/2020/01/21/venezolanos-en-el-peru-carlos-moran-han-llegado-delincuentes-que-desprestigian-la-comunidad-venezolana-delincuencia/

Lori, J. R., & Boyle, J. S. (2015). Forced migration: Health and human rights issues among refugee populations. *Nursing Outlook, 63*(1), 68–76.

Lupieri, S. (2021). Refugee health during the Covid-19 pandemic: A review of global policy responses. *Risk Management and Healthcare Policy, 14*, 1373.

Matlin, S. A., Depoux, A., Schütte, S., Flahault, A., & Saso, L. (2018). Migrants' and refugees' health: towards an agenda of solutions. *Public Health Reviews, 39*(1), 1–55.

Manky, O. (2020). Los trabajadores informales in *Por una nueva convivencia. La sociedad peruana en tiempos de COVID-19: escenarios, propuestas de política y acción pública.* Editors M. Burga, F. Portocarrero, & A. Panfichi. Lima: Fondo Editorial PUCP.

Mendoza, W. (2019). Venezuelan immigration in Peru from a health perspective. *Revista peruana de medicina experimental y salud pública, 36*, 3. DOI: 10.17843/rpmesp.2019.363.4812

Moquillaza-Alcántara, V. H., & Soria-Gonzales, L. A. (2019). Características asociadas a la presencia de atención prenatal en gestantes venezolanas residentes en el Perú, 2018. *Anales de la Facultad de Medicina, 80*, 4. DOI: 10.15381/anales.v80i4.16940

Mougenot, B., Amaya, E., Mezones-Holguin, E., Rodriguez-Morales, A. J., & Cabieses, B. (2021). Immigration, perceived discrimination and mental health: Evidence from Venezuelan population living in Peru. *Globalization and Health, 17*, 1. DOI: 10.1186/s12992-020-00655-3

Neuhauser, L., Kreps, G. L., & Syme, S. L. (2013). Community participatory design of health communication interventions. In D. K. Kim, A. Singhal, & G. L. Kreps (Eds.), *Health communication: Strategies for developing global health programs* (pp. 227–243). New York: Peter Lang Publishers.

New York Times. (2021, July 8). Coronavirus Briefing, what happened today. What we know about the Lambda variant, first discovered in Peru. https://www.nytimes.com/2021/07/08/us/coronavirus-briefing-what-happened-today.html

Olwig, K. F. (2021). The end and ends of flight. Temporariness, uncertainty and meaning in refugee life. *Ethnos*, 1–17. DOI: 10.1080/00141844.2020. 1867606

Paradies, Y. (2006). A systematic review of empirical research on self-reported racism and health. *International Journal of Epidemiology*. DOI: 10.1093/ije/dyl056

Programa Mundial de Alimentos. (2020). Crisis sin precedentes por la COVID-19 afecta gravemente la seguridad alimentario de migrantes en América del Sur. https://es.wfp.org/noticias/crisis-sin-precendentes-covid-19-golpea-alimenta-cion-migrantes-America-del-Sur

QR Consulting. (2020). *Estudio de Georreferenciación y Caracterización de la Población Venezolana en Situación de Movilidad Humana y Población Receptora*. Lima y Quito: Plan International.

Saifee, J., Franco-Paredes, C., & Lowenstein, S. R. (2021). Refugee Health During COVID-19 and Future Pandemics. *Current Tropical Medicine Reports*, 1–4. DOI: 10.1007/s40475-021-00245-2

Salazar, D. (2018, April 12). La xenofobia nuestra de cada día o cómo los medios han renunciado a sus responsabilidades editoriales. *Radio Ambulante*. https://radioambulante.org/extras/laxenofobianuestra

Sanchez Cardenas, M. (2019). Case Study: Migration from Venezuela to Peru "profound economic instability, shortages and human rights viola-tions as the main pushing factors for migration from Venezuela to Peru. ResearchGate/341537652.

Schmitt, A. (2021). The Peruvian Government's exacerbation of food insecurity among Venezuelan migrants and refugees during COVID-19. *Anthropology Department Honors Papers 19*. Retrieved January 18, 2022 from https://dig-italcommons.conncoll.edu/anthrohp/19

University of Maryland. (2021, July 23). A smartphone health information application for African Americans and Hispanics. https://sph.umd.edu/research-impact/research-centers/horowitz-center-health-literacy/projects-center-health-literacy/welcome-healthymemisalud-center-health-literacy

Vázquez-Rowe, I., & Gandolfi, A. (2020). Peruvian efforts to contain COVID-19 fail to protect vulnerable population groups. *Public Health in Practice*, 1, 100020.

Williams, D. R., Neighbors, H. W., & Jackson, J. S. (2003). Racial/ethnic dis-crimination and health: Findings from community studies. *American Journal of Public Health*, 93, 2. DOI: 10.2105/ajph.93.2.200

World Bank. (2021a). *Migrantes y refugiados venezolanos en el Perú: el impacto de la crisis del COVID-19*. Retrieved July 20, 2021 https://documents1.worldbank.org/curated/en/647431591197541136/pdf/Migrantes-y-Refugia-dos-Venezolanos-en-El-Peru-El-Impacto-de-la-Crisis-del-Covid-19.pdf.

World Bank. (2021b). *The World Bank in Peru*. https://www.worldbank.org/en/country/peru/overview. Retrieved July 20, 2021.

Zambrano-Barragán, P., Ramírez Hernández, S., Freier, L. F., Luzes, M., Sobczyk, R., Rodríguez, A., & Beach, C. (2021). The impact of COVID-19 on migrants' access to health: A qualitative study in Colombian and Peru-vian cities. *Journal of Migration and Health*, 3, 100029. DOI: 10.1016/j.jmh.2020.10w0029

15 Ecological Message Design Strategies Based on Narrative Evidence from Immigrants and Refugees in Diverse Socio-Cultural Contexts

Soo Jung Hong

Julia is a 37-year-old foreign domestic worker in Singapore. She is from the Philippines and has been working in Singapore for about eight years. She has a close friend from Indonesia but found it difficult to discuss health with her friend because they speak different native languages. She explained, "Sometimes [my friend] cannot understand what I feel and what kind of sickness I have now. I just leave it alone and go to my boss. I don't want to argue…" When foreign domestic workers search for health information online, they experience language barriers and often have difficulty deciphering medical information and complex terms. Julia also noted, "Some of the [medical terms are] so hard to understand. Some medical terms, [I] need to check Google [to find out] what is the meaning…"

Julia's story illustrates the hardship an immigrant experiences when trying to communicate about health in a new environment, and how the communication is affected by unfamiliar social contexts. This may have an effect on the immigrant's beliefs, behaviors, and even health outcomes. Globalization has deeply influenced not only financial capital and social organization, but also the mobility of people, products, occupations, and information (Castells, 2000). In many countries, immigrants and refugees – who seek diverse opportunities in a new environment – work and live together with host communities. In addition, as part of economic migration, a large number of the global poor cross borders to find employment opportunities; this is essential to globalization (Dutta, 2016). For example, as of 2020, the total foreign workforce in Singapore was 1,351,800, making up nearly 24% of the country's population (Department of Statistics Singapore, 2020). Although Singapore is known to be a country with a *melting pot of cultures and nationalities* (Hirschmann, 2020), these immigrants and refugees still have difficulties adapting to their new environment for various reasons such as differences in social system, language, religion, and cultural norms.

DOI: 10.4324/9781003230243-15

An ecological perspective can explain individuals' health and well-being based on multiple levels – individual, institutional, community, and policy – within the larger social environment (Bronfenbrenner, 1979; McLeroy et al., 1988; Street, 2003). Although scholars and researchers have emphasized the importance of an ecological approach to health communication and have considered diverse social and cultural influences on individuals' health and well-being, previous literature on the effects of health messages has made little or partial efforts to reflect this integrative view on health message design. Therefore, this chapter argues that an ecological approach should be adopted to create effective health messages for immigrants and refugees in diverse socio-cultural contexts.

This chapter discusses and illustrates my experience as a resident and researcher in three countries: South Korea, the United States, and Singapore. Throughout the experience, I learned that health communication interventions, including messaging strategies, should consider and reflect the lived experiences of these refugees and immigrants. This chapter discusses how we can apply an ecological model to health message design based on narrative evidence, and concluded with pertinent suggestions for integrative messaging strategies based on both an ecological approach and theoretical robustness for future research and debate.

Applying an Ecological Perspective to Message Design for Immigrants and Refugees

Health communication interventions require a multidisciplinary approach that considers both the individual (i.e., prior experience, efficacy beliefs, knowledge, etc.) and the macro-social (i.e., interpersonal relationships, cultural patterns, social norms) levels (Rimal & Lapinski, 2009). Nevertheless, the initial studies of health communication reflected the basic premises and questions of psychological studies just as the field of human communication partly developed as a branch of psychology (Obregon & Waisbord, 2012). Although social marketing has emphasized audience research and the segmentation of target publics (Kotler & Zaltman, 1971), existing theories and models of changes to health behavior based on this approach still support individualism as well as individual psychology (Airhihenbuwa et al., 2000). As an alternative model, an ecological perspective (Bronfenbrenner, 1979; McLeroy et al., 1988; Street, 2003) provides a framework not only to focus on individual health behavior, but also to identify the multiple contextual and macro-social factors that influence that behavior. However, the ecological approach has rarely been applied to designing health messages in combination with rigorous theoretical approaches. This chapter suggests that adopting an ecological model based on narrative evidence can complement the existing health-messaging strategies that largely embrace individual psychology and social marketing.

Although health communication was originated from the apparent influence of social psychology (Obregon & Waisbord, 2012), the *social* aspect of health communication has been less emphasized, particularly in the studies of message effect and behavioral changes. In the existing health communication research that mostly focuses on behaviorist theories and goals, researchers often assume the universal effectiveness of cognitive and affective strategies in designing health messages. However, these strategies may bring about limited effects on desired outcomes given the potential diversity in the target audience's cultures and contexts. In addition, while there have been some efforts to design effective messages by emphasizing similarities between the target audience and speakers or characters in the messages, these attempts are often limited in that the similarities stay at the level of demographic correspondence, such as gender, age, and ethnicity. Therefore, this chapter suggests a way to broaden the scope of the audience's sympathy as well as further develop existing theories of message design by employing an ecological approach and narrative evidence.

An ecological perspective posits that an individual's health and well-being are influenced by not just individual factors but support through social networks, environmental factors, and policies. Therefore, an ecological approach allows researchers to examine the various social contexts that influence health and health-related communication. This chapter discusses how the embeddedness of the ecological approach can be applied to message design strategies.

Ecological Message Design for Immigrants and Refugees and Applicable Narrative Evidence

According to Bandura's (1977a) social learning theory, individuals learn others' behavior by observing role models. Soap opera stories, which are often used for entertainment, and education programs that expect imitations and influences, are all well-aligned with the major standard of social learning theory. These stories take advantage of role models who vicariously experience benefits and risks of recommended behaviors, address potential structural problems that hinder the characters' change, and help improve self-efficacy to complete recommended actions (Bandura, 1977b; Maibach & Murphy, 1995).

While entertainment programs have used their forum to educate in a way that has been developed for the public at large (e.g., SARS transmission on *Law & Order*, and breast cancer in *The Young & the Restless*), others have targeted specific groups, including youth, gay men, and ethnic minorities (Unger et al., 2013). Nevertheless, the creative process of entertainment education (e.g., multiple formative studies and tests on narratives) is often time-consuming, costly, and difficult (Green, 2021). Given the difficulty, targeting specific and/or small minority groups such as immigrants and refugees may not always be a viable option for media-based entertainment education. Therefore, this chapter recommends that health communication researchers use narrative evidence as a format to design effective messages for immigrants and refugees.

Unlike most research studies that explain narratives based on plot structures, a few researchers viewed narratives as a form of evidence that describes a speaker's inner portrayal, views and perspectives, and goals in their studies (e.g., Fludernik, 1996; Schank, 1990). Schank and Berman (2002) defined a story as "a structured, coherent retelling of an experience or a fictional account of an experience" (p. 288), which reflects some characteristics of narrative evidence. In narrative evidence, the claims of a speaker are supported by the narrator's views, perspectives, and experiences (see Schank, 1990). Schank (1990) identified five types of stories (i.e., official, invented, firsthand experiential, secondhand, and culturally common) that can be used as narrative evidence. In particular, culturally common stories are pervasive in particular cultural environments, and thus are generalized due to its exceptional salience in the specific culture (e.g., Jewish people who use Yiddish phrases) (Schank, 1990).

Narrative evidence that aids in persuasion may vary across cultures. By focusing on Schank's (1990) culturally common story and Gordon and Paci's (1997) cultural narrative described below, this chapter discusses using a narrative as a form of evidence for effective health message design. *Master narrative* is a term coined by a French philosopher, Lyotard (1979). This type of narrative functions as legitimated knowledge, and in our society, the myths in the narrative help legitimize the existing power relations/structure and social practices (Lyotard, 1979). The role of the master narrative can be understood in relation to the function of Gordon and Paci's (1997) *cultural narrative*. Gordon and Paci (1997) investigated cultural narratives regarding open and closed medical disclosure in Tuscany, Italy, and classified cultural narratives as "usually taken for granted and invisible, operating in the background of attention" (p. 1434). More specifically, their study revealed the significant role of master narratives in society along with cultural narratives in Tuscany regarding traditional silence around a cancer diagnosis.

My previous studies (Hong, 2018, 2020) adopted *cultural narrative* as a form of culturally common story as well as narrative evidence to design culturally tailored messages to promote family health history communication among Asians living in the US. The next sections detail how different types of cultural narratives can be used for message design for immigrants and refugees by illustrating my previous studies, while suggesting health-messaging strategies based on both the ecological approach and narrative evidence. The strategies include the following three dimensions: (1) intrapersonal factors, (2) interpersonal and community factors, and (3) structural limitations. The first dimension covers existing studies based on my previous research that employed cultural narrative evidence and social psychological factors (i.e., Hong, 2018, 2020). This chapter provides a detailed thought process that theorizes and rationalizes cultural narrative evidence in these previous studies. With regard to the second and third dimensions, this chapter suggests a few ecological message design strategies based on my previous research regarding Asian and African immigrants in the US, migrant workers in Singapore, and North Korean refugees in South Korea.

Social Cognition and Culture: Intrapersonal Factors

From an ecological perspective, intrapersonal factors encompass an individual's knowledge, attitudes, behaviors, and skills. This means, although researchers emphasize a socio-cultural approach to health messaging, it is impossible to exclude these intrapersonal factors from potential influences on individuals' health and well-being or vice versa. Social psychology played a substantial role in the creation and progress of health communication (Obregon & Waisbord, 2012). Social cognitive theory (Bandura, 1986) is one of the most foundational approaches to health communication. Although social cognitive theory addresses structuration and/or interactive processes between individuals and social environments, behaviorist theories have played a pivotal role in health communication research, using their basic premises and questions as a vital foundation (Obregon & Waisbord, 2012). As social cognitive theory suggests, intrapersonal factors, including individuals' knowledge, attitudes, behaviors, and skills, cannot be understood separately from social and environmental influences. There is a need for reinterpretation, as well as reapplication, of social cognitive theory to the field of health communication in order to address an ecological paradigm in health messaging strategies. To link social cognitive theory and an ecological model, this chapter focuses on the concept of agency (Bandura, 2000).

Manipulating Agency in Cultural Narrative Evidence

Bandura (2000) defines human agency as an individual's capacity to influence and shape their lives and environments. The concept of agency links an intrapersonal factor to environmental influences because the individual's capacity to influence the environment is shaped by the environment as well. According to social cognitive theory, individuals' functions reflecting attitudes and behavioral characteristics are socially situated and not free from their environment (Bandura, 2006). Then, how can we design messages by considering the environmental and/or socio-cultural influences that may affect individuals' attitudinal and behavioral outcomes? We may be able to find the answer from the concept of *agency*. More specifically, this chapter introduces health-messaging strategies to promote agency of audiences who live in an unfamiliar culture or a new living environment, like immigrants and refugees. Consistent with the concept of contextual embeddedness, individuals' agency – which is viewed as an intrapersonal psychological factor – is situated within the socio-cultural contexts as well as individuals' minds. To manipulate the agency in a cultural narrative message, this chapter focuses on cultural archetypes and linguistic agencies used for health messages.

Cultural Exemplars Promoting Agency

The most essential characteristic of agency is an individual's metacognitive capability to evaluate the adequacy of his or her thoughts and actions (Bandura, 2006). Although individuals learn others' behavior by observing role models (Bandura, 1986), the influences and cases of modeling are situated within social contexts, and thus social cognitions are socially embedded (Bandura, 2006). Therefore, immigrants and refugees often experience difficulties in finding appropriate role models as well as health information in their new living environment, and often try to solve health issues by themselves. For example, our recent collected data in Singapore is consistent with previous findings that foreign domestic workers often undergo self-treatment (e.g., Bernadas & Jiang, 2016). Many migrant workers prefer home remedies and traditional methods, as they perceive them to be cheaper and more effective in soothing body pain (Dutta et al., 2018). North Korean refugees are also significantly influenced by their previous medical and cultural experiences, which makes them self-diagnose and resort to self-treatments (Hong, 2015, 2017). These can be considered the results of immigrants' and refugees' relegating agency to shape their lives by interacting with their new social and cultural environment.

Socio-cultural approaches to health messaging strategies provide relevant information in the context of the socio-cultural characteristics of the intended audience (Kreuter & McClure, 2004). Similarly, existing approaches, such as the cultural sensitivity approach (Dutta, 2007; Resnicow et al., 1999), have emphasized the importance of cultural tailoring based on cultural values and beliefs and message processing via identification and engagement. If health communication interventions try to promote agency via cultural tailoring, they can benefit from discursive messaging strategies that acknowledge complex societal factors affecting behavior beyond personal willpower (Guttman & Ressler, 2001).

According to Resnicow and colleagues (1999), cultural values and norms are comprised of the *deep structure* of cultural sensitivity that can be incorporated into health communication interventions to convey salience to the target population. While conducting my doctoral research, I found that family health history communication for people of Korean or Chinese descent may vary from that of an American family (Hong, 2016). To address this in the health messages targeting Korean, Chinese, and European Americans in the US and to promote the audience's agency, my dissertation research utilized the two types of cultural narratives described and investigated in Gordon and Paci's (1997) study. These two types of narratives (i.e., autonomy control narrative and social-embeddedness narrative) are good examples of culturally common narratives that can be used as narrative evidence. According to Gordon and Paci (1997), cultural narratives are contested with other multiple co-existing narratives from organizations and experiences of self and others causing conflicting perspectives. Gordon and Paci (1997) also clarify the two main constructs of cultural narrative as follows: "we use *narrative* in order to capture the types of stories people live in or are trying to construct (Mattingly, 1994), not necessarily a *reality* that exists; the *cultural* refers to societal, meta-narratives of broad or deep cultural influence" (p. 1433).

To describe the *social-embeddedness narrative*, Gordon and Paci (1997) focus on the traditional practice in Tuscany of non-disclosure of a cancer diagnosis. The silence around cancer can be interpreted as a method of group protection, which reflects reality, truth, morality, and emotions that are socially created and defined. Then, they contrast the social-embeddedness narrative to the *autonomy-control narrative*, which challenges the traditional group protection and promotes open disclosure and medical/social practices that support patients' self-determination. To develop the agency-based cultural narratives reflecting conflicting values within the context of family history communication, several formative interviews were conducted with Korean and Chinese participants, and a few cultural archetypes relevant to the agency that can be used as cultural exemplars were identified (Hong, 2016). As described, Gordon and Paci's (1997) cultural narratives and Schank's (1990) culturally common stories are referents that were captured as influences and values embedded within Korean and Chinese cultures that contribute to the collective decision-making of family history communication. For example, both Korean and Chinese participants said that talking about family history is not easy because health is not an appropriate issue for open discussion in their culture, and their patriarchic/hierarchic family culture makes it difficult for male family members to disclose their diseases. To be contrasted with the Korean and Chinese social-embeddedness narratives, an autonomy-control narrative – which emphasizes individual power, control, and decision-making – was also developed by employing values identified from an existing US family history campaign targeting the general public.

Agency and Linguistic Strategies

In addition to the cultural referents, my dissertation research focused on language styles that may affect the agency of participants to theorize agency-based cultural narrative evidence further. Linguistic strategies for message design should focus on immigrants' and refugees' culture, knowledge, literacy, and native language. Immigrants often have difficulties obtaining and comprehending health information in multicultural societies like the US and Singapore due to language barriers as well as having to familiarize themselves with a complicated new healthcare system (Ang et al., 2020; Kim et al., 2015). For those with these difficulties, it would be helpful for health communication researchers and practitioners to use plain language strategies or mother-tongue- based approaches (Costa, 2010; Stableford & Mettger, 2007). At the same time, linguistic strategies can address various aspects of the ecological approach and social cognitive theory by highlighting individuals' cultures and values as well as social and environmental influences.

Although Resnicow and colleagues (1999) categorized linguistic features as the surface structure of cultural sensitivity, these features have a powerful influence on individuals' agency. Linguistically, the concept of agency indicates who is framed as capable of and responsible for a change and its occurrence and processes (Ahearn, 2001; Al Zidjaly, 2009). According to Al Zidjaly (2009), agency is a basic concept that explains every type of social interaction and is mediated by language that determines social actors linguistically as well as socio-culturally. In the same vein, Bandura's (2000) concept of personal and collective efficacy helps link the linguistic concept of agency to the personal and collective capacity to act, or the agency from the sociocultural perspective. With this in mind, I developed different types of cultural narrative evidence that include an agency component as a linguistic index explaining the socio-cultural capacity to act.

Complex societal factors beyond personal willpower can promote agency as well as influence collective behavior (Guttman & Ressler, 2001). Collective agency, the locus of which dwells in group members' minds as the agentic form of *we*, involves people's shared beliefs in their ability to produce the desired results collectively, while agency includes agent and the capability of *I* to influence (Bandura, 2000). Based on this insight, I manipulated the agentic forms (*I* vs. *we* or *I* vs. *my family*) embedded in varying cultural exemplars to design and test the autonomy-control narrative and social-embeddedness narrative. As expected, these cultural narrative messages showed meaningful results in persuading those for whom the cultural referents used in the message have cultural meanings through identification and engagement under the influence of socio-psychological factors (Hong, 2018, 2020).

Social Relationships and Message Sources: Interpersonal and Community Factors

From the ecological view, an individual's health is influenced by several social contexts, including social networks and communities. Adapting to a new host culture, however, simultaneously separates an individual from one's traditional social networks and fosters a sense of isolation (Berry, 2005). Previous studies have found that social disengagement leads to higher risks of cognitive decline, morbidity, and mortality (Shor & Roelfs, 2015; Tomaka et al., 2006). Therefore, foreign workers often call their families living in their homeland and seek support from them (Dutta et al., 2018; Iyer et al., 2004). This suggests the difficulty of building relationships and communities in their new living environment. It would be helpful for health communication researchers and practitioners to recognize migrants' and refugees' difficulty in building relationships and take advantage of the technological ecology for messaging strategies.

Trust is another issue to consider in terms of social networks and communities. Minorities, including immigrants and refugees, often mistrust healthcare systems in their host country. A lack of trust in existing healthcare systems can be a barrier to their medical care. For example, North Korean refugees were not satisfied with their South Korean providers who depend on computerized medical technology, and therefore relied on their own self-diagnoses instead of listening to their doctors' recommendations (Hong, 2015, 2017). In the US, racial discrimination toward African American patients has been historically pervasive and has contributed to minority patients' mistrust (Stepanikova et al., 2006). Therefore, racial minority groups are often unwilling to participate in medical treatments or research because of privacy concerns, and feel they need more transparency and control over their data (Lemke et al., 2010). According to my previous study that investigated diverse patients' preferences over the different types of consent forms, African Americans needed more control over their donated sample when compared to European Americans (Hong et al., 2020).

Unlike in the informed consent situation, however, it is not easy to use and manipulate perceived controllability in health messages covering diverse health- and risk-related issues. Although control is an individual characteristic that can hardly be manipulated for message appeals, we can instead focus on the reason why African Americans needed more control over their sample and preferred an informed consent model in order to obtain this control. For example, according to the study mentioned above, mistrust was an important predictor of participants' needs for control over their samples (Hong et al., 2020).

In a similar vein, one way to include interpersonal and/or community factors in health-messaging strategies would be considering who would be the speaker in a message and what would be the target audience's perceptions of the source. The elaboration likelihood model and the heuristic-systematic model suggest that source credibility is one of the most important message-related characteristics that affect the persuasion process (Chaiken, 1980; Petty & Cacioppo, 1986). Health communication researchers and practitioners need to establish ways to work with various communities and find the most trusted sources of information among immigrants and refugees. In addition, trustworthiness – defined as a perception inspiring trust – should be considered as well (Levine et al., 2018). The three dimensions of trustworthiness include ability, benevolence, and integrity (Gefen, 2002; Mayer et al., 1995). These qualities can translate into the sources' expertise, goodwill, and honesty that are reflected in narrative evidence based on a speaker's experiences, testimonies, perspectives, views, etc.

A *role model story* may incorporate these qualities within a format of narrative evidence. To increase source credibility, role model stories, which are based on social learning theory (Bandura, 1986), combine a model individual's experiences with recommended behaviors in a narrative form by incorporating local relevancy and culturally appropriate language and values for targeted communities (Corby et al., 1996; Kreuter & McClure, 2004). As discussed earlier, the characteristics of these stories are well-aligned with those of cultural narrative evidence. According to previous literature, role model stories effectively increase an audience's knowledge about health issues, identification with speakers, engagement in storylines, and information retention (Berkley-Patton et al., 2009; Hoe et al., 2021). Although role model stories have been mostly applied to health interventions targeting ethnic minorities (e.g., Berkley-Patton et al., 2009; Hoe et al., 2021), it would be an effective approach for immigrants and refugees that are usually ethnic and cultural minorities in many societies. Moreover, in addition to finding trusted sources, working with various communities such as non-profit and/or governmental organizations and religious institutions in addition to understanding their technological ecology will be helpful in the distribution of role model stories to further increase the receptivity of health messages by finding effective channels of communication in various settings.

Overcoming Structural Limitations

From the ecological standpoint, an individual's health is influenced by social structures, processes, and policies. Although policy and structural changes would be the top priority to solve relevant problems, this chapter shares a few strategies that may help overcome these structural limitations. One important way to overcome these barriers would be *empowerment*. As shown in the beginning of this chapter, migrant workers, immigrants, and refugees in many countries face longstanding issues of restricted legal and human rights, a poor understanding of the local language, barriers to access to health care and information, different cultural beliefs, and economic problems (Ang et al., 2017; Laverack, 2018). This provides important insights for practical and theoretical messaging strategies.

To be empowered, however, people should first understand the sources of their own power, feel valued, and have the necessary knowledge (Laverack, 2019). To meet this goal, this chapter suggests a participatory message design/production. As discussed in terms of agency and linguistic features, using multi-lingual messages based on these groups' mother-tongues will help. At the same time, if these individuals are able to express their thoughts, perspectives, and experiences with their own voices, the empowerment effect of narrative messages will be heightened. A few previous health promotion efforts adopted a technology-based participatory approach (e.g., photography and video production) in different steps of the production process and provided meaningful results for strengthening targeting groups' capacity and identity and engaging communities (Chiu, 2009; Duffy, 2010). Moreover, social media such as YouTube has expanded the participatory opportunities and possibilities of refugee and migrant communities from culturally and linguistically diverse backgrounds (Burgess & Green, 2009).

Although these previous studies have highlighted the importance of the participatory process and analyzing the produced data to empower target audiences and engage communities, the stories, footages, or photos – including narrators' experiences, views, and perspectives – have hardly been developed or used as narrative evidence in health interventions. The produced data, which reflect immigrants' and refugees' experiences, thoughts, and views as the socially weak and alienated, have the power to persuade other community members in the same situation. The data can support an argument for the goal of health interventions (see Toulmin, 1958). As discussed earlier, narrative evidence (Schank, 1990) will be an effective bowl where immigrant and refugee groups' views, perspectives, and experiences can be stored for an ecological message design. Migrants' and refugees' stories are their own cultural narratives and culturally common stories (Gordon & Paci, 1997; Schank, 1990).

In conclusion, this chapter makes a few suggestions on integrative messaging strategies based on both the ecological approach and theoretical robustness for future research. As discussed above, the first suggestion is adopting social cognitive theory to identify and manipulate message factors (e.g., agency, controllability, etc.) that combine and connect individual characteristics to social and contextual influences. The process of combining social cognitive factors into message contents will need health communication researchers' thorough investigation of these groups as well as community members' active participation in the messaging and production process. In addition, it is necessary to think about how to theoretically analyze and evaluate the narrative messages based on cultural narrative evidence. For example, the strategies suggested in this chapter utilize a combined message processing based on both central and peripheral routes. More specifically, message contents within cultural narrative evidence can be systematically evaluated for its quality, while perceptions about source characteristics are affected by surface cues. Although an ecological approach, social cognitive theory, and message effects based on heuristic/systematic processing have been understood and investigated separately in previous literature, these can be combined with the use of cultural narrative evidence, both theoretically and practically. The potential effect of this integrative approach includes message-related outcomes derived from existing theories (e.g., ELM) as well as the complementary impact expected from the empowerment effect of the combined strategies.

Acknowledgement

I would like to recognize Jean Chia Yee Hwa, my former student at the National University of Singapore, who collected the interview data referred in this chapter.

Recommended Readings

Bandura, A. (1986). *Social foundations of thought & action: A social cognitive theory*. Prentice Hall.

Bandura, A. (2006). Toward a psychology of human agency. *Perspectives on Psychological Science, 1*, 164–180.

Gordon, E. R., & Paci, E. (1997). Disclosure practices and cultural narratives: Understanding concealment and silence around cancer in Tuscany, Italy. *Social Science & Medicine, 44*, 1433–1452.

Hong, S. J. (2020). Developing a mediation model for narrative evidence processing based on social cognitive variables and agency-based cultural exemplars. *International Journal of Communication, 14*, 3819–3842.

McLeroy, K. R., Bibeau, D., Steckler, A., & Glanz, K. (1988). An ecological perspective on health promotion programs. *Health Education Quarterly, 15*, 351–377.

References

Ahearn, L. M. (2001). Language and agency. *Annual Review of Anthropology, 30*, 109–37.

Airhihenbuwa, C. O., Makinwa, B. and Obregon, R. (2000). Toward a new communications framework for HIV/AIDS. *Journal of Health Communication, 5*(1), 101–111.

Al Zidjaly, N. (2009). Agency as an interactive achievement. *Language in Society, 38*, 177–200.

Ang, J., Chia, C., Koh, C. J., Chua, B. W., Narayanaswamy, S., Wijaya, L., ..., Vasoo, S. (2017). Healthcare-seeking behaviour, barriers and mental health of non-domestic migrant workers in Singapore. *BMJ Global Health*, 2, e000213.

Ang, J., Koh, C., Chua, B., Narayanaswamy, S., Wijaya, L., Chan, L., ..., Vasoo, S. (2020). Are migrant workers in Singapore receiving adequate healthcare? A survey of doctors working in public tertiary healthcare institutions. *Singapore Medical Journal*, 61(10), 540–547.

Bandura, A. (1977a). *Social learning theory*. Prentice-Hall.

Bandura, A. (1977b). Self-efficacy: toward a unifying theory of behavioural change. *Psychological Review*, 84(2), 191–215.

Bandura, A. (1986). *Social foundations of thought & action: A social cognitive theory*. Prentice Hall.

Bandura, A. (2000). Exercise of human agency through collective efficacy. *Current Directions in Psychological Science*, 9, 75–78.

Bandura, A. (2006). Toward a psychology of human agency. *Perspectives on Psychological Science*, 1, 164–180.

Berkley-Patton, J., Goggin, K., Liston, R., Bradley-Ewing, A., & Neville, S. (2009). Adapting effective narrative-based HIV-prevention interventions to increase minorities' engagement in HIV/AIDS services. *Health Communication*, 24(3), 199–209.

Bernadas, J. M., & Jiang, L. C. (2016). "Of and beyond medical consequences": Exploring health information scanning and seeking behaviors of Filipino domestic service workers in Hong Kong. *Health Care for Women International*, 37(8), 855–871.

Berry, J. W. (2005). Acculturation: Living successfully in two cultures. *International Journal of Intercultural Relations*, 29(6), 697–712.

Bronfenbrenner, U. (1979). *The ecology of human development: Experiments by nature and design*. Harvard University Press.

Burgess, J., & Green, J. (2009). *YouTube: Online video and participatory culture*. Polity.

Castells, M. (2000). Information technology and global capitalism. In W. Hutton & A. Giddens (Eds.), *On the edge: Living with global capitalism* (pp. 52–75). The New Press.

Chaiken, S. (1980). Heuristic versus systematic information processing and the use of source versus message cues in persuasion. *Journal of Personality & Social Psychology*, 39(5), 752–766.

Chiu, L. (2009). Culturally competent health promotion: The potential of participatory video for empowering migrant and minority ethnic communities. *International Journal of Migration, Health and Social Care*, 5(1), 5–14.

Corby, N. H., Enguídanos, S. M., & Kay, L. S. (1996). Development and use of role model stories in a community level HIV risk reduction intervention. *Public Health Reports*, 111(Suppl 1), 54–58.

Costa, B. (2010). Mother tongue or non-native language? Learning from conversations with bilingual/multilingual therapists about working with clients who do not share their native language. *Journal of Ethnicity and Inequalities in Health and Social Care*, 3(1), 15–24.

234 *Soo Jung Hong*

Department of Statistics Singapore. (2020). *Population and population struc-ture*. Retrieved from https://www.singstat.gov.sg/find-data/search-by-theme/population/population-and-population-structure/latest-data

Duffy, L. (2010). Hidden heroines: lone mothers assessing community health using photovoice. *Journal of Health Promotion Practice, 11,* 788–797.

Dutta, M. J. (2007). Communicating about culture and health: Theorizing culture-centered and cultural sensitivity approaches. *Communication Theory, 17,* 304–328.

Dutta, M. J. (2016). *Neoliberal health organizing: Communication, meaning, and politics*. Routledge.

Dutta, M. J., Comer, S., Teo, D., Luk, P., Lee, M., Zapata, D., … Kaur, S. (2018). Health meanings among foreign domestic workers in Singapore: A culture-centered approach. *Health Communication, 33*(5), 643–652.

Fludernik, M. (1996). *Towards a "natural" narratology*. Routledge.

Gefen, D. (2002). Nurturing clients' trust to encourage engagement success during the customization of ERP systems. *Omega: The International Journal of Management Science, 30*(4), 287–299.

Gordon, E. R., & Paci, E. (1997). Disclosure practices and cultural narratives: Understanding concealment and silence around cancer in Tuscany, Italy. *Social Science & Medicine, 44,* 1433–1452.

Green, D. P. (2021). In search of entertainment-education's effects on attitudes and behaviors. In L. B. Frank & P. Falzone (Eds.), *Entertainment-education behind the scenes: Case studies for theory and practice*. Palgrave Macmillan.

Guttman, N., & Ressler, W. H. (2001). On being responsible: Ethical issues in appeals to personal responsibility in health campaigns. *Journal of Health Communication, 6,* 117–136.

Hoe, D. F., Johari, K., Rahman, A., & Enguidanos, S. (2021). Theory-driven role model stories improve palliative care knowledge among a diverse older population. *Palliative & Supportive Care, 19*(1), 34–40.

Hong, S. J. (2015). Not at all effective: Differences in views on the causes of prescription non-adherence between North Korean defectors and medical providers in South Korea. *Journal of Immigrant & Minority Health, 17*(3), 867–884.

Hong, S. J. (2016). *Developing and testing cultural narrative messages within the context of family health history communication* [Doctoral dissertation, Pennsylvania State University].

Hong, S. J. (2017). I want an omnipotent doctor: North Korean defectors' unmet expectations of South Korean medical providers. *The Qualitative Report, 22*(10), 2612–2628.

Hong, S. J. (2018). Culturally tailored narrative evidence about family health history: A moderated mediation analysis. *Asian Journal of Communication, 28*(4), 377–396.

Hong, S. J. (2020). Developing a mediation model for narrative evidence processing based on social cognitive variables and agency-based cultural exemplars. *International Journal of Communication, 14,* 3819–3842.

Hong, S. J., Drake, B., Goodman, M., & Kaphingst, K. (2020). Race, trust in doctors, privacy concerns, and consent preferences for biobanks. *Health Communication, 35*(10), 1219–1228.

Iyer, A., Devasahayam, T. W., & Yeoh, B. S. (2004). A clean bill of health: Filipinas as domestic workers in Singapore. *Asian and Pacific Migration Journal, 13*(1), 11–38.

Kim, W., Kreps, G. L., & Shin, C. (2015). The role of social support and social networks in Health Information–seeking behavior among Korean AMERICANS: A qualitative study. *International Journal for Equity in Health, 14*(1), 1–10.

Kotler, P., & Zaltman, G. (1971). Social marketing: An approach to planned social change. *Journal of Marketing, 35*(3), 3–12.

Kreuter, M. W., & McClure, S. M. (2004). The role of culture in health communication. *Annual Review of Public Health, 25*, 439–455.

Laverack, G. (2018). The challenge of promoting the health of refugees and migrants in Europe: A review of the literature and urgent policy options. *Challenges, 9*(2), 32.

Laverack, G. (2019). *Public health: Power, empowerment and professional practice*. Macmillan International Higher Education.

Lemke, A. A., Wolf, W. A., Hebert-Beirne, J., & Smith, M. E. (2010). Public and biobank participant attitudes toward genetic research participation and data sharing. *Public Health Genomics, 13*, 368–377.

Levine, E. E., Bitterly, T. B., Cohen, T. R., & Schweitzer, M. E. (2018). Who is trustworthy? predicting trustworthy intentions and behavior. *Journal of Personality and Social Psychology, 115*(3), 468–494.

Lyotard, J. F. (1984). *The postmodern condition: A report on knowledge* (Vol. 10). University of Minnesota Press.

Maibach, E., & Murphy, D. A. (1995). Self-efficacy in health promotion research and practice: conceptualization and measurement. *Health Education Research, 10*(1), 37–50.

Mattingly, C. (1994). The concept of therapeutic 'emplotment.' *Social Science & Medicine, 38*, 811–822.

Mayer, R. C., Davis, J. H., & Schoorman, F. D. (1995). An integrative model of organizational trust. *Academy of Management Review, 20*(3), 709–734.

McLeroy, K. R., Bibeau, D., Steckler, A., & Glanz, K. (1988). An ecological perspective on health promotion programs. *Health Education Quarterly, 15*(4), 351–377.

Obregon, R., & Waisbord, S. R. (2012). *Theoretical divides and convergence in global health communication*. In R. Obregon & S. R. Waisbord (Eds.), *The handbook of global health communication* (Vol. 29). Wiley-Blackwell.

Petty, R. E., & Cacioppo, J. T. (1986). *Communication and persuasion: Central and peripheral routes to attitude change*. Springer-Verlag.

Resnicow, K., Baranowski, T., Ahluwalia, J. S., & Braithwaite, R. L. (1999). Cultural sensitivity in public health: Defined and demystified. *Ethnicity & Disease, 9*, 10–21.

Rimal, R., & Lapinski, M. (2009). *Why health communication is important in public health*. WHO; World Health Organization. https://www.who.int/bulletin/volumes/87/4/08-056713/en/

Schank, R. C. (1990). *Tell me a story: A new look at real and artificial memory*. Scribner.

Schank, R. C., & Berman, T. R. (2002). The pervasive role of stories in knowledge and action. In M. C. Green, J. J Strange, & T. C. Brock (Eds.), *Narrative impact: Social and cognitive foundations* (pp. 287–314). Lawrence Erlbaum Associates.

Shor, E., & Roefls, D. J. (2015). Social contact frequency and all-cause mortality: A meta-analysis and meta-regression. *Social Science & Medicine, 128,* 76–86.

Stableford, S., & Mettger, W. (2007). Plain language: a strategic response to the health literacy challenge. *Journal of Public Health Policy*, 28(1), 71–93.

Stepanikova, I., Mollborn, S., Cook, K. S., Thom, D. H., & Kramer, R. M. (2006). Patients' race, ethnicity, language, and trust in a physician. *Journal of Health and Social Behavior, 47,* 390–405.

Street, R. L. (2003). Communication in medical encounters: An ecological perspective. In T. L. Thompson, R. Parrott & J. F. Nussbaum (Eds.), *Handbook of health communication* (2nd ed., pp. 63–89). Routledge.

Tomaka, J., Thompson, S., & Palacios, R. (2006). The relation of social isolation, loneliness, and social support to disease outcomes among the elderly. *Journal of Aging and Health, 18*(3), 359–384.

Toulmin, S. (1958). *The uses of argument.* Cambridge University Press.

Unger, J. B., Cabassa, L. J., Molina, G. B., Contreras, S., & Baron, M. (2013). Evaluation of a fotonovela to increase depression knowledge and reduce stigma among Hispanic adults. *Journal of Immigrant and Minority Health, 15*(2), 398–406.

16 Health Campaigns and Message Design for Immigrant Populations

Xiaomei Cai, Xiaoquan Zhao, Kyeung Mi Oh, and Emily B. Peterson

Health Campaigns and Message Design for Immigrant Populations

Health disparities experienced by immigrants pose pressing public health and social equity challenges in the United States (U.S.). Compared to their U.S.-born counterparts, immigrants are more likely to be uninsured, are less likely to have a regular healthcare provider, use less health care services, receive poorer quality health care, and take part in less preventive care services (Batalova et al., 2021; Hall & Cuellar, 2016). Moreover, immigrants encompass a constellation of social and cultural backgrounds. Differences in language, religion, income, education, country of origin, English proficiency, and other factors contribute to the complexity of immigrant health. Efforts to promote immigrant health, consequently, cannot adopt a one-size-fits-all strategy and need to attend to the unique characteristics of the target population (Institute of Medicine, 2002; Kreps & Neuhauser, 2015)

This chapter focuses on message and program design issues in health communication campaigns targeting immigrant populations in the U.S. It first presents a case study of a culturally tailored smoking cessation program for first-generation, male immigrant smokers from China and Korea, which illustrates several broad principles for campaign and message design targeting immigrant populations. It then describes the general approach to health campaigns and discusses the role of theory in campaign and message development for immigrant populations. Finally, the chapter concludes by making recommendations to inform future intervention efforts seeking to improve immigrant health in the U.S.

Case Study: An East Asian Immigrant Smoking Cessation Intervention

Background

Asian Americans are the fastest growing immigrant group in the U.S. since 2010, with China ranking second and Korea ninth on the list of

DOI: 10.4324/9781003230243-16

top source countries in 2015 (López & Bialik, 2017). China and Korea both have strikingly high smoking rates among their male populations. In 2017, the age-standardized prevalence estimates for current tobacco smoking among persons aged 15 and above were 48.0% for men and 1.8% for women in China and 39.3% for men and 5.9% for women in Korea (WHO, 2019). By comparison, in the U.S., cigarette smoking rates among adults 18 years or older were 15.3% for men and 12.7% for women in 2019 (Cornelius et al., 2020). Pro-tobacco cultural norms, the stress of immigration, and continuing behavioral habits lead to prevalent tobacco use among first-generation Chinese and Korean male immigrants. Promoting smoking cessation among these groups can make important contributions to community health, cancer control, and the reduction of health disparities in the U.S.

Approach and Rationale

We developed and pilot tested a program that used graphic, native-language, mobile messaging to promote smoking cessation among first-generation Chinese and Korean male immigrant smokers. There is evidence that text messaging is an effective method for promoting smoking cessation (DHHS, 2014; Whittaker et al., 2012). Prior to our work, no smoking cessation interventions had used text or mobile messaging as a primary intervention tool to target Asian immigrants in the U.S. However, a large trial in China that modeled an existing general-population text-messaging program in the U.S. has produced encouraging results (Augustson et al., 2017). The favorable outcome of this intervention lends confidence that a similar approach may also work with Asian immigrants in the U.S.

The use of graphics was included in the intervention, as health education efforts targeting immigrant groups are often hampered by low literacy levels among the target population (Kreps & Sparks, 2008). Although Asian Americans are generally known for high educational attainment, many new immigrants, particularly undocumented immigrants from China, have low levels of education and poor literacy in both English and their native language. These low education and low literacy groups are also at high risk for cigarette smoking (Zhang & Wang, 2008). Our program used native languages primarily to address linguistic and literacy barriers. But the use of graphics could further enhance intervention effectiveness by improving message attention, comprehension, and recall among the target population in general and those facing literacy challenges in particular.

The design of our mobile messaging intervention was guided by the extended parallel process model (EPPM), a theory about threat appeals in health communication (Witte, 1992, 1994). According to EPPM, threat message design should aim to elicit not only a sufficient level of perceived threat, but also an adequate level of perceived efficacy. Lacking either may result in ineffective intervention messages. Existing evidence has largely supported the importance of both threat and efficacy in health message design and effectiveness (Peters et al., 2013; Witte & Allen, 2000), including in the context of smoking cessation messaging (e.g., Gharlipour et al., 2015).

In addition to presenting threatening graphic images and efficacy information, our program displayed cultural sensitivity. Tobacco use among immigrants is influenced by a complex web of social, economic, and cultural factors (NCI, 2017). As a result, it is imperative for tobacco control efforts targeting these populations to adopt culturally appropriate intervention strategies that are responsive to the norms, values, and life experiences of the target groups (Institute of Medicine, 2002; NCI, 2017). We made cultural sensitivity and appropriateness a central consideration in our intervention design and implementation.

Message Development

Guided by EPPM, we developed 16 graphic threat messages and eight efficacy messages. The graphic threat messages included both existing health warnings from around the world and newly designed, culturally tailored messages focusing on themes salient to Asian smokers as identified in previous literature, such as the health effects on family, financial costs of smoking, and the stigmatization of smoking in the U.S. (Ferketich et al., 2004; Kim et al., 2007). The efficacy messages were text-only and included six specific quitting tips adapted from existing text messaging programs (Augustson et al., 2017) and two messages introducing an Asian-language quitline (Zhu et al., 2012). All texts in the messages were in Chinese or Korean. A total of eight focus groups (five Chinese and three Korean; N = 45) were conducted with members of the Chinese and Korean immigrant communities in the Washington DC metropolitan area to pretest these messages (Peterson et al., 2018). Based on feedback from the focus groups, we dropped low-performing messages, revised others, and created a message library for field testing.

Pilot Testing

The pilot test featured a 2 (threat: graphic + text vs. text-only) X 2 (efficacy: quitline vs. tips) factorial design. Participants (N = 71; 39 Chinese and 32 Korean first-generation male immigrant smokers) were recruited from the Washington DC metropolitan area and randomized to condition. The pilot intervention delivered a total of 30 messages over four weeks. Self-reported quitting behaviors, attitudes, and beliefs as well as expired air CO were measured at both baseline and one-month follow-up.

While all participants were currently smoking at baseline, 10 (14.1%) reported abstinence from smoking in the past seven days at follow-up. Nine of the ten participants returned CO readings at 7 ppm or below, lower than the cutoff range (8–10 ppm) for current smoking based on established standards in the literature (SRNT Subcommittee on Biochemical Verification, 2002). Full sample analysis showed that, from baseline to follow-up, participants' average expired air CO levels decreased ($p = .001$), and their attitudes toward quitting became more positive ($p = .028$).

Analysis focusing on condition differences showed no significant difference in quitting outcomes. However, differences in seven-day point prevalence abstinence (20% vs. 8.3%, $p = .23$) and currently trying to quit (55.9% vs. 44.4%, $p = .18$) trended in favor of the graphic messaging condition as compared to the text-only condition. Furthermore, the graphic messaging condition produced greater positive change in quitting attitudes ($p = .039$) and fear ($p = .005$). It also led to greater regret among the participants ($p = .076$) and higher ratings of message persuasiveness ($p = .077$), although these differences did not reach statistical significance. Additional results from this pilot study are available elsewhere (Zhao et al., 2019).

Findings from this study were overall supportive of the efficacy of our intervention approach. First, it is encouraging to see that a brief, one-month pilot intervention was able to produce biochemically verifiable quitting behavior among the target population. Second, the data showed consistent trends that graphic risk messaging was able to induce more favorable cognitive and emotional responses. However, these responses did not translate into clear, statistically discernible impact on quitting behavior, likely due to sample size constraints. Third, receptivity data showed that the intervention was overall well received and participants were comfortable with the mobile messaging method and the frequency with which the messages were delivered. Overall, the findings of the pilot testing demonstrated strong potential for this culturally tailored, graphic mobile messaging intervention to promote smoking cessation among first-generation Chinese and Korean male immigrant smokers.

Health Communication Campaigns for Immigrant Populations

Health communication campaigns typically include four related tasks: (1) identifying campaign objectives; (2) developing message strategies; (3) disseminating campaign messages through appropriate channels; and (4) conducting systematic research to inform and evaluate campaign activities (Hornik, 2002b; Institute of Medicine, 2002; Rice & Atkin,

2013; Zhao, 2020). Whether targeting the general population or specific immigrant groups, health communication campaigns will need to make informed decisions on all four fronts.

Identifying Campaign Objectives

Campaign objectives are measurable outcomes that a campaign seeks to achieve given available time and resources. The identification of campaign objectives often begins with identifying a target population and a health condition that requires remedy and/or improvement within that population. Immigrant populations are often defined and labeled based on the source country and/or region in public discourse. But for campaign purposes, this crude classification is often inadequate because substantial heterogeneity might exist on other dimensions within such populations, such as race/ethnicity, gender, religion, and social economic status (Institute of Medicine, 2002). One or more of these additional characteristics might significantly contribute to the relevant health issue, thus requiring careful attention in audience segmentation and analysis. For example, the smoking cessation program described earlier targeted only a small segment of the Asian immigrant population, jointly defined by two neighboring source countries (China and Korea), one biological sex (men), and a common health behavior (cigarette smoking). As narrowly defined as the population was, one might still argue that Chinese and Korean male immigrants should be further divided into two distinct target populations. While the intervention separated the two groups by the languages used in the messages, we found sufficient homogeneity between the two groups for them to be considered a unified target population and to be addressed with the same set of messages (Zhao et al., 2019).

Almost all campaign decisions depend on a deep understanding of the factors that influence the health condition in question within the target population. National surveillance data can provide important information for general population campaigns, but comprehensive data are rarely available for immigrant populations to inform campaign decisions. Indeed, even large national surveillance systems may lack adequate and accurate representation of diverse immigrant groups due to small sample sizes for these groups and important biases in the sampling process (e.g., failure to include non-English-speaking members of these communities) (Chae et al., 2006; Lew & Tanjasiri, 2003). For this reason, it is critically important for campaign designers to conduct primary research with the target population to inform campaign objectives and strategies.

Developing Message Strategies

Campaigns for immigrant populations should build message strategies based on a careful assessment of the behavioral norms, belief systems, cultural influences, and the general social-ecological environment surrounding the target population. Message strategies represent decisions on two fronts: content focus and executional styles. The content focus of campaign messages pinpoints the specific kinds of health information that the messages should convey. In the campaign literature, the content focus is often represented by a relatively small and well-defined set of target beliefs. Hornik and Woolf (1999) proposed three criteria for the selection of promising target beliefs for campaigns. First, a promising belief should be strongly correlated with the focal behavior or behavioral intention that the campaign seeks to influence. Second, a promising belief should have sufficient room for change. In other words, a reasonably large portion of the target population should currently hold less than ideal positions on the belief, thus making it movable by campaign messaging. Third, a promising belief must lend itself to the construction of persuasive messages. Some beliefs, such as those deeply rooted in the culture of the immigrant population, are unlikely to be changed by persuasive messaging. This approach has been adopted by a number of large-scale campaigns with demonstrated success (Brennan et al., 2017; Parvanta et al., 2013; Vallone et al., 2018).

Campaign messages can be executed in many different styles. The same core information may be conveyed through statistics, infographics, testimonials, or even fictional storylines in entertainment media. Creativity is often at the core of executional and stylistic decisions, but research in communication and persuasion provides ample evidence-based guidance for message execution (Dillard & Shen, 2013; Maibach & Parrott, 1995; O'Keefe, 2016). Given that many immigrant populations suffer from cultural barriers and literacy challenges, we would like to draw particular attention to the power of narratives and visual messaging.

Narratives derive their power of persuasion from the fact that humans are hard-wired to be influenced by story-telling. Compared to other forms of persuasion, narratives have distinct advantages in gaining and maintaining interest, facilitating information processing, overcoming resistance and counterarguing, and providing opportunities for emotional connections (Kreuter et al., 2007; Slater & Rouner, 2002). These advantages are particularly important for campaigns targeting immigrant populations because these target groups often find traditional forms of health communication messages difficult to understand and lacking personal relevance. Engaging narratives featuring personalities and voices from within the community can help overcome these barriers. As described in the smoking cessation case study, visual representation of health messages affords some of these same advantages and is particularly helpful when communicating with immigrant groups that face literacy challenges. More comprehensive treatment of visual persuasion can be found in Messaris's work (1997).

Disseminating Campaign Messages

Health intervention efforts targeting immigrant populations can occur in many contexts, from healthcare settings, to group counseling at community centers, to local or national campaigns. At the core of any campaign dissemination is the concept of exposure (Hornik, 2002c; Slater, 2004). What communication channels to use and how to use them for message dissemination are fundamentally governed by concerns over the quantity and quality of exposure generated through campaign activities.

While the idea of quantity in exposure is straightforward, it can be difficult to achieve. Indeed, evidence shows that many campaigns, even those with ample resources, have had difficulty generating sufficient exposure among their target audiences (Hornik, 2002a). Achieving high exposure in immigrant populations is particularly challenging because of limited campaign resources, lack of centralized media systems, income barriers and literacy challenges among the audiences, and limited reach of available communication channels. However, the rapid advancement of the Internet and digital technologies have provided new opportunities to reach immigrant populations. Recent statistics show that minority groups in the U.S. now have similar levels of access to the Internet, often through the use of mobile phones (Perrin & Turner, 2019). This trend holds great promise for health campaigns targeting immigrant populations to generate substantial exposure using internet- and mobile-based media platforms.

Quality in exposure refers to the extent to which exposure to campaign messages would lead to additional engagement, such as attention and message comprehension. For campaigns to work, mere exposure is not enough; the message has to go through a series of additional processes to generate expected campaign outcomes (McGuire, 2013). For immigrant populations, quality exposure often depends on the placement of campaign messages in informational environments that foster attention and interest and facilitate understanding, such as ethnic media or community events. But other channel characteristics may also come into play. For example, focus group participants in our intervention said they would be more likely to pay attention to incoming text messages than new messages received on social media (i.e., WeChat for Chinese and KakaoTalk for Korean immigrants), precisely because text messaging is used less often and thus is more likely to signal something important to them (Peterson et al., 2018). Based on this finding, we made a decision to use text messaging to deliver intervention messages so that the exposure would be of higher quality.

Conducting Systematic Research

While we discuss research last, it is essential for the entire campaign process. For campaigns targeting immigrant populations, research is particularly important because existing knowledge on these populations is often limited and many of the lessons learned from general population campaigns may not apply. Campaign research generally falls into three categories: formative research, process evaluation, and outcome evaluation (National Cancer Institute, 2002). Formative research includes research activities that inform and support campaign development, including audience analysis and message pretesting. Careful audience analysis, as discussed earlier, will assist in the proper setting of campaign objectives and inform message design. Message pretesting allows campaign planners to systematically evaluate candidate messages and decide whether they need to be further revised or even discarded.

Process evaluation includes research activities that monitor campaign progress, with particular attention to campaign performance on exposure. Outcome evaluation assesses the extent to which the campaign has successfully achieved its objectives. For campaigns targeting immigrant populations, evaluation may be particularly challenging because of difficulties in sample recruitment and retention. Indeed, the smoking cessation study showed that, even for a modest sample size, recruitment could take a substantial amount of time. While many strategies were tried in that study, in the end, it was personal contact and assistance from a local community center that provided the strongest recruitment results (Zhao et al., 2019). Evaluation efforts for immigrant population campaigns should conscientiously leverage the power of social networks and partner with local organizations to increase community participation.

Finally, some have argued that long-running real-world campaigns, because of their complexity and constant interactions with environmental influences, may not lend well to highly controlled evaluation designs, such as randomized controlled trials (Hornik, 2002a). This may be particularly the case for immigrant populations because many immigrant communities are close-knit, thus extremely vulnerable to cross-contamination across intervention arms. Campaign evaluators should be cognizant of the relative strengths and weaknesses of different research designs and consider utilizing less-controlled designs if needed.

Theory in Health Campaigns for Immigrant Populations

Theories informing health communication campaigns generally fall in two categories: behavioral theories that identify the most important drivers of health behaviors, and communication theories that illuminate the processes and effects of campaign activities. Examples of influential behavioral theories in the campaign literature include the reasoned action approach to behavior prediction (Fishbein & Ajzen, 2010), health belief model (Champion & Skinner, 2008), social cognitive theory (Bandura, 1998), and stages of changes model (DiClemente & Prochaska, 1998). Together, these theories seek to provide a systematic account of the motivational basis for health behaviors and point to potential pathways for health behavior change.

While the focus of behavioral theories is largely unified, the role of communication theories in the development and implementation of health campaigns is more diversified. The elaboration likelihood model (Petty & Cacioppo, 2011), for example, is often used to guide message decisions that may impact how the audiences process and respond to campaign messages. The extended parallel process model (EPPM) (Witte, 1992), which was used in the case study, offers important guidance on the construction and effects of threat appeals. Diffusion of innovations (Rogers, 2003) provides useful perspectives on both the desirable features of the health product or service that is being promoted and the value of social networks in the dissemination and amplification of important campaign messages. Agenda-setting theory (McCombs & Shaw, 1972) and media advocacy (Wallack & Dorfman, 1996) shed light on the media processes thorough which campaign activities can influence public opinion and policy initiatives. The possibility and benefits of engaging communication theories in campaign research and practice are vast.

Applying Behavioral Theory in Immigrant Campaigns

Behavioral theories are generally focused on identifying the most powerful sources of motivation behind health behaviors and behavior change. The influence of these theories is often reflected in the kinds of beliefs that are considered in campaign development. These beliefs are typically organized around key constructs that are believed to exist on a higher level and represent more proximal predictors of behavior. In the reasoned action framework, for example, these beliefs typically cluster around the constructs of attitude, norms, and self-efficacy, which in turn predict behavioral intention. The relevance of any given belief, thus, resides on two different levels: whether the belief contributes to a higher-level construct that matters for behavioral prediction and whether the belief is important to the higher-level construct among other beliefs within the same domain.

When designing campaigns for immigrant populations, interventionists should consider the dynamics on both levels. First, the relative importance of higher-level constructs might differ from the mainstream population. For example, for immigrant communities with a strong collectivist culture, social norms might carry greater weight in behavioral decision making. Second, within each construct, which beliefs are influential need to be carefully assessed through primary research, as many of the existing belief assessment instruments are developed using mainstream population samples. While carefully validated, these tools may not be appropriate to use when conducting audience analyses with immigrant populations. In the smoking cessation case study, focus group participants generally found health effects on their offspring to be a highly motivating message concept. Although second-hand smoke is a broad concern, this particular belief is not included in many of the existing assessment tools for smoking consequences (e.g., Brandon & Baker, 1991; Myers et al., 2003). Without careful formative research, this important belief and its messaging potential could have been easily overlooked in the intervention.

Applying Communication Theory in Immigrant Campaigns

The application of communication theories needs to be adaptive to and respectful of the cultural norms and lived experience of the target communities. We will discuss two illustrative issues here, one on message content, the other message execution. EPPM is a widely used theory to guide the design of threat-based health messages, as was the case in the smoking cessation program described earlier. While most applications of EPPM emphasize the importance of balancing efficacy-building and threat induction, constructing threat messages for the immigrant populations demands extra focus on efficacy. Immigrant communities are often disenfranchised on multiple dimensions and face complex vulnerabilities originating from cultural, linguistic, and economic barriers (Kreps & Sparks, 2008; Liu et al., 2013; Pitkin Derose et al., 2009). For this reason, many immigrant communities may trend toward low baseline efficacy on many health issues. To serve these communities, extraordinary care should be taken to ensure that the efficacy information in threat messages is sufficiently strong and culturally appropriate to channel audience response in a productive direction. Absent adequate efficacy-building capacity, threat messaging could easily lead to maladaptive reactions from immigrant audiences such as risk minimization, defensive avoidance, and psychological reactance (Witte, 1992; Witte & Allen, 2000).

Health campaigns targeting immigrant populations also require careful attention to the structural features of their messages. Culture is a meaning system, and sources of meaning in a particular culture often transcend the semantic content of the message. The meaning carried by the structural features of campaign messages are often patently clear to those living in that culture but completely invisible to those living outside it. According to the elaboration likelihood model (Petty & Cacioppo, 2011), motivation (such as personal relevance) and ability (such as prior knowledge) are critical determinants of the mode in which a message may be processed. Message characteristics that may influence appraisals of motivation and ability, thus impact depth of processing, however, are likely to be culturally defined within immigrant populations. For example, calligraphy is a rich art form in many Asian cultures. To the Chinese communities, the font type chosen for health messages carries nontrivial supra-linguistic meaning because different fonts are associated with messaging conventions from different sources. Government documents in China, for example, are often printed in an "official" font type that implies seriousness and authority. Community engagement materials, on the other hand, may be printed in more lively fonts that signal warmth or even humor. In the smoking cessation case study, the font type used in the Chinese graphic text messages was carefully chosen to be clear, sincere but non-edgy, and consistent in tone with the content of the messages. Although no data were gathered on this particular front, we believe that the font type chosen contributed to favorable audience reception to the messages in the study.

Recommendations for Practice

In this chapter, we used a case study to share our experience in designing and pilot testing a culturally tailored, graphic text-messaging-based, smoking cessation intervention for first-generation Chinese and Korean male immigrant smokers. We then presented a framework for health communication campaigns and discussed important areas of adaptation for immigrant populations. Next, we examined the role of behavioral and communication theories in the development, implementation, and evaluation of health communication campaigns, with attention to tailored application of these theories for campaigns targeting immigrant populations. We conclude this chapter by offering several recommendations for practice. Instead of attempting to provide comprehensive recommendations for the entire campaign process, we focus on a few key decision points where interventionists may benefit particularly strongly from insights and evidence from the communication science.

1   Use empirical data to inform message content strategy. The Hornik and Woolf (1999) approach described earlier has proven useful in identifying promising target beliefs for message development (Brennan et al., 2017; Parvanta et al., 2013; Vallone et al., 2018). This and/or other systematic empirical approaches should be adopted to help ascertain the content focus of campaign messages targeting immigrant populations.

2   Consider using narratives and visual messages in campaign materials. As discussed earlier, these two types of message execution have important advantages in communication interventions targeting populations facing cultural barriers and literacy challenges. There is

good evidence for their general effectiveness as means of persuasive messaging in important health contexts (Noar et al., 2016; Shen et al., 2015).

3   Make sure that exposure to campaign messages is of sufficient quantity and quality. Many health communication programs are ineffective because they have failed to generate enough exposure (Hornik, 2002a, 2002c). Finding innovative ways to reach and engage immigrant populations is critically important to campaign success. Mobile technologies and ethnic social media appear to be promising vehicles for message dissemination among immigrant populations (Perrin & Turner, 2019).

4   Plan for process and outcome evaluation from the very beginning. It is often difficult to implement highly controlled research designs in campaign evaluation when working with immigrant populations (Hornik, 2002b). Evaluators should be open to alternative designs and tolerant of imprecise but useful findings.

Recommended Readings

Hornik, R. C. (Ed.). (2002a). *Public health communication: Evidence for behavior change.* Lawrence Erlbaum Associates.

Kreps, G. L., & Neuhauser, L. (2015). Designing health information programs to promote the health and well-being of vulnerable populations. In *Meeting health information needs outside of healthcare* (pp. 3–17). Elsevier. https://doi.org/10.1016/B978-0-08-100248-3.00001-9

Institute of Medicine. (2002). *Speaking of health: Assessing health communication strategies for diverse populations.* National Academies Press. http://site.ebrary.com/id/10032363

NCI. (2017). *A Socioecological approach to addressing tobacco-related health disparities* (No. 22; Tobacco Control Monographs). National Cancer Institute. https://cancercontrol.cancer.gov/brp/tcrb/monographs/22/docs/m22_complete.pdf

Zhao, X., Peterson, E. B., Oh, K. M., & Cai, X. (2019). Using graphic text-messaging to promote smoking cessation among first-generation Chinese and Korean male immigrants. *Health Education Research, 34*(3), 332–344. https://doi.org/10.1093/her/cyz006

References

Augustson, E., Engelgau, M. M., Zhang, S., Cai, Y., Cher, W., Li, R., Jiang, Y., Lynch, K., & Bromberg, J. E. (2017). Text to Quit China: An mHealth Smoking Cessation Trial. *American Journal of Health Promotion, 31*(3), 217–225. https://doi.org/10.4278/ajhp.140812-QUAN-399

Bandura, A. (1998). Health promotion from the perspective of social cognitive theory. *Psychology & Health, 13*(4), 623–649. https://doi.org/10.1080/08870449808407422

Batalova, J., Hanna, M., & Levesque, C. (2021, February 9). *Frequently Requested Statistics on Immigrants and Immigration in the United States.* Migrationpolicy.Org. https://www.migrationpolicy.org/article/frequently-requested-statistics-immigrants-and-immigration-united-states-2020

Brandon, T. H., & Baker, T. B. (1991). The smoking consequences questionnaire: The subjective expected utility of smoking in college students. *Psychological Assessment: A Journal of Consulting and Clinical Psychology, 3*(3), 484–491.

Brennan, E., Gibson, L. A., Kybert-Momjian, A., Liu, J., & Hornik, R. C. (2017). Promising Themes for Antismoking Campaigns Targeting Youth and Young Adults. *Tobacco Regulatory Science, 3*(1), 29–46. https://doi.org/10.18001/TRS.3.1.4

Chae, D. H., Gavin, A. R., & Takeuchi, D. T. (2006). Smoking Prevalence Among Asian Americans: Findings from the National Latino and Asian American Study (NLAAS). *Public Health Reports, 121*(6), 755–763.

Champion, V. L., & Skinner, C. S. (2008). The health belief model. In K. Glanz, B. K. Rimer, & K. Viswanath (Eds.), *Health behavior and health education: Theory, research, and practice* (4th ed., pp. 45–65). Jossey-Bass.

Cornelius, M. E., Wang, T. W., Jamal, A., Loretan, C. G., & Neff, L. J. (2020). Tobacco Product Use Among Adults—United States, 2019. *MMWR. Morbidity and Mortality Weekly Report, 69.* https://doi.org/10.15585/mmwr.mm6946a4

DHHS. (2014). *Using health text messages to improve consumer health knowledge, behaviors, and outcomes: An environmental scan.* U.S. Department of Health and Human Services. Health Resources and Services Administration. http://www.hrsa.gov/healthit/txt4tots/environmentalscan.pdf

DiClemente, C. C., & Prochaska, J. O. (1998). Toward a comprehensive, transtheoretical model of change: Stages of change and addictive behaviors. In W. R. Miller & N. Heather (Eds.), *Treating addictive behaviors (2nd ed.)* (pp. 3–24). Plenum Press.

Dillard, J. P., & Shen, L. (2013). *The SAGE handbook of persuasion: Developments in theory and practice* (2nd ed.). SAGE Publications, Inc.

Ferketich, A. K., Wewers, M. E., Kwong, K., Louie, E., Moeschberger, M. L., Tso, A., & Chen, M. S. (2004). Smoking cessation interventions among Chinese Americans: The role of families, physicians, and the media. *Nicotine & Tobacco Research, 6*(2), 241–248. https://doi.org/10.1080/1462220040010 01676350

Fishbein, M., & Ajzen, I. (2010). *Predicting and changing behavior: The reasoned action approach* (1st ed.). Psychology Press.

Gharlipour, Z., Hazavehei, S. M. M., Moeini, B., Nazari, M., Beigi, A. M., Tavassoli, E., Heydarabadi, A. B., Reisi, M., & Barkati, H. (2015). The effect of preventive educational program in cigarette smoking: Extended Parallel Process Model. *Journal of Education and Health Promotion, 4.* https://doi.org/10.4103/2277-9531.151875

Hall, E., & Cuellar, N. G. (2016). Immigrant Health in the United States: A Trajectory Toward Change. *Journal of Transcultural Nursing, 27*(6), 611–626. https://doi.org/10.1177/1043659616672534

Hornik, R. C. (Ed.). (2002a). *Public health communication: Evidence for behavior change.* Lawrence Erlbaum Associates.

Hornik, R. C. (2002b). Public health communication: Making sense of contradictory evidence. In R. C. Hornik (Ed.), *Public health communication: Evidence for behavior change* (pp. 1–22). Lawrence Erlbaum Associates.

Hornik, R. C. (2002c). Exposure: Theory and evidence about all the ways it matters. *Social Marketing Quarterly, 8*(3), 31–37. https://doi.org/10.1080/15245000214135

Hornik, R. C., & Woolf, K. D. (1999). Using cross-sectional surveys to plan message strategies. *Social Marketing Quarterly, 5*(2), 34–41. https://doi.org/10.1080/15245004.1999.9961044

Institute of Medicine. (2002). *Speaking of Health: Assessing Health Communication Strategies for Diverse Populations.* National Academies Press. http://site.ebrary.com/id/10032363

Kim, S., Ziedonis, D., & Chen, K. (2007). Tobacco use and dependence in Asian Americans: A review of the literature. *Nicotine & Tobacco Research, 9*(2), 169–184. https://doi.org/10.1080/14622200601080323

Kreps, G. L., & Neuhauser, L. (2015). Designing health information programs to promote the health and well-being of vulnerable populations. In *Meeting Health Information Needs Outside Of Healthcare* (pp. 3–17). Elsevier. https://doi.org/10.1016/B978-0-08-100248-3.00001-9

Kreps, G. L., & Sparks, L. (2008). Meeting the health literacy needs of immigrant populations. *Patient Education and Counseling, 71*(3), 328–332. https://doi.org/10.1016/j.pec.2008.03.001

Kreuter, M., Green, M., Cappella, J., Slater, M., Wise, M., Storey, D., Clark, E., O'Keefe, D., Erwin, D., Holmes, K., Hinyard, L., Houston, T., & Woolley, S. (2007). Narrative communication in cancer prevention and control: A framework to guide research and application. *Annals of Behavioral Medicine, 33*(3), 221–235. https://doi.org/10.1007/BF02879904

Lew, R., & Tanjasiri, S. P. (2003). Slowing the Epidemic of Tobacco Use Among Asian Americans and Pacific Islanders. *American Journal of Public Health, 93*(5), 764–768. https://doi.org/10.2105/AJPH.93.5.764

Liu, J. J., Wabnitz, C., Davidson, E., Bhopal, R. S., White, M., Johnson, M. R. D., Netto, G., & Sheikh, A. (2013). Smoking cessation interventions for ethnic minority groups—A systematic review of adapted interventions. *Preventive Medicine, 57*(6), 765–775. https://doi.org/10.1016/j.ypmed.2013.09.014

López, G., & Bialik, K. (2017, May 3). Key findings about U.S. immigrants. *Pew Research Center.* http://www.pewresearch.org/fact-tank/2017/05/03/key-findings-about-u-s-immigrants/

Maibach, E., & Parrott, R. (Eds.). (1995). *Designing health messages: Approaches from communication theory and public health practice.* Sage Publications.

McCombs, M. E., & Shaw, D. L. (1972). The agenda-setting function of mass media. *Public Opinion Quarterly, 36*(2), 176–187. https://doi.org/10.1086/267990

McGuire, W. J. (2013). McGuire's classic input-output framework for constructing persuasive messages. In R. E. Rice & C. K. Atkin (Eds.), *Public Communication Campaigns* (Fourth Edition, pp. 133–145). Sage Publications, Inc.

Messaris, P. (1997). *Visual persuasion: The role of images in advertising.* Sage Publications.

Myers, M. G., MacPherson, L., McCarthy, D. M., & Brown, S. A. (2003). Constructing a short form of the Smoking Consequences Questionnaire with adolescents and young adults. *Psychological Assessment*, 15(2), 163–172. https://doi.org/10.1037/1040-3590.15.2.163

National Cancer Institute. (2002). *Making health communication programs work: A planner's guide* (Rev. December 2001). U.S. Department of Health & Human Services.

NCI. (2017). *A Socioecological Approach to Addressing Tobacco-Related Health Disparities* (No. 22; Tobacco Control Monographs). National Cancer Institute. https://cancercontrol.cancer.gov/brp/tcrb/monographs/22/docs/m22_complete.pdf

Noar, S. M., Hall, M. G., Francis, D. B., Ribisl, K. M., Pepper, J. K., & Brewer, N. T. (2016). Pictorial cigarette pack warnings: A meta-analysis of experimental studies. *Tobacco Control*, 25(3), 341–354. https://doi.org/10.1136/tobaccocontrol-2014-051978

O'Keefe, D. J. (2016). *Persuasion: Theory and research* (3rd ed.). SAGE Publications, Inc.

Parvanta, S., Gibson, L., Forquer, H., Shapiro-Luft, D., Dean, L., Freres, D., Lerman, C., Mallya, G., Moldovan-Johnson, M., Tan, A., Cappella, J., & Hornik, R. (2013). Applying Quantitative Approaches to the Formative Evaluation of Antismoking Campaign Messages. *Social Marketing Quarterly*, 19(4), 242–264. https://doi.org/10.1177/1524500413506004

Perrin, A., & Turner, E. (2019). Smartphones help blacks, Hispanics bridge some – but not all – digital gaps with whites. *Pew Research Center*. https://www.pewresearch.org/fact-tank/2019/08/20/smartphones-help-blacks-hispanics-bridge-some-but-not-all-digital-gaps-with-whites/

Peters, G.-J. Y., Ruiter, R. A. C., & Kok, G. (2013). Threatening communication: A critical re-analysis and a revised meta-analytic test of fear appeal theory. *Health Psychology Review*, 7(sup1), S8–S31. https://doi.org/10.1080/17437199.2012.703527

Peterson, E. B., Zhao, X., Cai, X., & Oh, K. M. (2018). Developing a graphic text messaging intervention for smoking cessation targeting first-generation chinese immigrant men: Insights from focus group interviews. *Studies in Media and Communications*, 15, 241–264. https://doi.org/10.1108/S2050-206020180000015005

Petty, R. E., & Cacioppo, J. T. (2011). *Communication and persuasion: Central and peripheral routes to attitude change* (Softcover reprint of the original 1st ed. 1986). Springer.

Pitkin Derose, K., Bahney, B. W., Lurie, N., & Escarce, J. J. (2009). Review: Immigrants and health care access, quality, and cost. *Medical Care Research and Review*, 66(4), 355–408. https://doi.org/10.1177/1077558708330425

Rice, R. E., & Atkin, C. K. (Eds.). (2013). *Public communication campaigns* (4th ed.). SAGE Publications, Inc.

Rogers, E. M. (2003). *Diffusion of Innovations* (5th ed.). Free Press.

Shen, F., Sheer, V. C., & Li, R. (2015). Impact of narratives on persuasion in health communication: A meta-analysis. *Journal of Advertising*, 44(2), 105–113. https://doi.org/10.1080/00913367.2015.1018467

Slater, M. D. (2004). Operationalizing and analyzing exposure: The foundation of media effects research. *Journalism and Mass Communication Quarterly; Thousand Oaks, 81*(1), 168–183.

Slater, M. D., & Rouner, D. (2002). Entertainment—Education and elaboration likelihood: Understanding the processing of narrative persuasion. *Communication Theory, 12*(2), 173–191. https://doi.org/10.1111/j.1468-2885.2002.tb00265.x

SRNT Subcommittee on Biochemical Verification. (2002). Biochemical verification of tobacco use and cessation. *Nicotine & Tobacco Research, 4*(2), 149–159. https://doi.org/10.1080/14622200210123581

Vallone, D., Cantrell, J., Bennett, M., Smith, A., Rath, J. M., Xiao, H., Greenberg, M., & Hair, E. C. (2018). Evidence of the impact of the truth FinishIt campaign. *Nicotine & Tobacco Research, 20*(5), 543–551. https://doi.org/10.1093/ntr/ntx119

Wallack, L., & Dorfman, L. (1996). Media advocacy: A strategy for advancing policy and promoting health. *Health Education & Behavior, 23*(3), 293–317.

Whittaker, R., McRobbie, H., Bullen, C., Borland, R., Rodgers, A., & Gu, Y. (2012). Mobile phone-based interventions for smoking cessation. *Cochrane Database of Systematic Reviews, 2012*(11). http://onlinelibrary.wiley.com/doi/10.1002/14651858.CD006611.pub3/abstract

WHO. (2019). *WHO report on the global tobacco epidemic, 2019: Offer help to quit tobacco use.* World Health Organization. https://www.who.int/tobacco/global_report/en/

Witte, K. (1992). Putting the fear back into fear appeals: The extended parallel process model. *Communications Monographs, 59*(4), 329–349.

Witte, K. (1994). Fear control and danger control: A test of the extended parallel process model (EPPM). *Communications Monographs, 61*(2), 113–134.

Witte, K., & Allen, M. (2000). A meta-analysis of fear appeals: Implications for effective public health campaigns. *Health Education & Behavior, 27*(5), 591–615.

Zhang, J., & Wang, Z. (2008). Factors associated with smoking in Asian American adults: A systematic review. *Nicotine & Tobacco Research, 10*(5), 791–801. https://doi.org/10.1080/14622200802027230

Zhao, X. (2020). Health communication campaigns: A brief introduction and call for dialogue. *International Journal of Nursing Sciences, 7*, S11–S15. https://doi.org/10.1016/j.ijnss.2020.04.009

Zhao, X., Peterson, E. B., Oh, K. M., & Cai, X. (2019). Using graphic text-messaging to promote smoking cessation among first-generation Chinese and Korean male immigrants. *Health Education Research, 34*(3), 332–344. https://doi.org/10.1093/her/cyz006

Zhu, S.-H., Cummins, S. E., Wong, S., Gamst, A. C., Tedeschi, G. J., & Reyes-Nocon, J. (2012). The effects of a multilingual telephone Quitline for Asian smokers: A randomized controlled trial. *JNCI: Journal of the National Cancer Institute, 104*(4), 299–310. https://doi.org/10.1093/jnci/djr530

Index

For Product Safety Concerns and Information please contact our EU
representative GPSR@taylorandfrancis.com
Taylor & Francis Verlag GmbH, Kaufingerstraße 24, 80331 München, Germany

www.ingramcontent.com/pod-product-compliance
Ingram Content Group UK Ltd.
Pitfield, Milton Keynes, MK11 3LW, UK
UKHW021450080625
459435UK00012B/434